Cattle Behaviour and Welfare

Cattle Behaviour and Welfare

Second Edition

CLIVE PHILLIPS BSc, MA, PhD
Department of Clinical Veterinary Medicine,
University of Cambridge, United Kingdom

Blackwell
Science

First Edition published as *Cattle Behaviour* by
the Farming Press 1993
Second Edition published 2002 by Blackwell
Science Ltd

Library of Congress
Cataloging-in-Publication is available

ISBN 0-632-05645-2

A catalogue record for this title is available
from the British Library

Set in Times and produced by
Gray Publishing, Tunbridge Wells, Kent
Printed and bound in Great Britain
by MPG Books Ltd, Bodmin, Cornwall

For further information on
Blackwell Science, visit our website:
www.blackwell-science.com

Contents

Preface

This book evolved from an initial publication on cattle behaviour (Phillips, 1993), which was written primarily for farmers and students of farming systems. The intimate relationship between the behaviour of cattle and their welfare encouraged me to develop the original text into one dealing with the welfare of cattle and its relation to their behaviour. The welfare of cattle has been much studied in the last decade, as farm animal welfare has been a prominent topic for debate and research, and this book attempts to review the recent research. Welfare can mean different things to different people and this is discussed as the topic is placed in context. It would be impossible to describe all the possible adverse conditions that could affect the welfare of cattle, so the principal influences are summarised for the different types of production – dairy, beef, calves and draft oxen. Two particularly important influences – humans and transport systems – are given chapters of their own.

In the increasing pressure to intensify cattle production, people often ignore the fact that the unit in the factory production system is a higher mammal, with complex mental and physical needs. An attempt to evaluate the welfare of cattle in a system of production must start with their perception of the system, progress to their choice of components of the system and end with a description of their behavioural reaction to the system. Their physiological response can also be measured and may be related to their metabolism and even production rate, but it usually bears little relationship to behaviour and to the adequacy of the environment. The latter is best indicated by the ability to display normal behaviour patterns and the absence of abnormal, deleterious behaviour. For humans, the behaviour of cattle is a signal about their well-being; for cattle, it is the reaction to the environment as they perceive it, modified by the innate motivation to perform the behaviours.

Studying the behaviour of cattle is probably one of the youngest and also one of the oldest sciences. The first students of cattle behaviour were undoubtedly our primeval ancestors. Many of the physical attributes of cattle rendered them unsuitable for domestication, in particular their large size and the low proportion of muscle tissues in the areas giving desirable meat cuts, such as the loin. However, aspects of cattle behaviour and their ability to thrive on grasses of little value to man led early man to choose cattle as the major domesticated animal. Their limited agility, gregarious social structure, the promiscuity of the male and extravert receptivity display by the female, as well as the precocial development of the young, are probably responsible for the relative ease with which they must have entered into a symbiotic relationship with man. The passion for salt, which they shared with man, provided an easy means of controlling them which is still in use with the relatives of cattle nowadays. Domestication therefore led to significant benefits to both cattle and man and a mutual respect evolved.

Nowadays the study of cattle behaviour is no less important. Cattle are still our major domesticated animal, contributing worldwide almost 18% of man's protein intake and 9% of our energy intake, as well as draft power, hides and dung for fuel. Veterinarians utilise cattle behavioural signals for disease diagnosis, and livestock handlers and farmers can derive useful information on the health of the stock in their charge from their behaviour. As well as discussing the major influences on welfare, this book describes the major behaviour patterns in cattle, their ontogeny and their purpose. It is intended for all involved in the study of animal welfare and ethology, as well as students of animal science, agriculture and veterinary medicine. It is also hoped that it will be of interest to advisers in cattle husbandry and leading farmers.

I acknowledge CAB International for permission to reproduce part of an article already published (Phillips, 1997).

Clive Phillips
Cambridge, UK

Chapter 1
Introduction to Cattle Welfare

Definition and measurement

The welfare of an animal relates primarily to its ability to cope, both with its external environment, including housing, weather and the presence of other animals, and with its internal environment, such as specific pains, fever and nutritional status. An instantaneous assessment of the welfare of cattle would ideally concentrate on their feelings at the time, which would be influenced by their genetic predisposition, by recent experiences, by their environment at the time of assessment and by any anticipation of future events, such as feeding. However, feelings are difficult to measure and the assessment is more likely to concentrate on more easily quantified parameters, such as the strength of their preference for different environments.

A long-term assessment of welfare, for example over the lifetime of an animal, should evaluate the degree to which the animal has been in harmony with its environment, and will include such aspects as whether it could perform behaviours to which it is genetically predisposed, e.g. suckling in infancy, whether the prevalence of disease was unacceptably high, and the extent to which it achieved nutritional and thermal comfort and homeostasis, and adequate rest and exercise (Fig. 1.1).

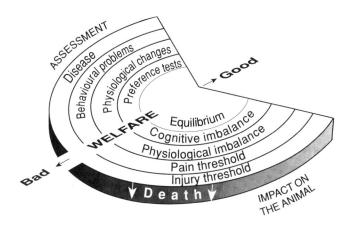

Fig. 1.1   The different degrees of welfare, assessment and the impact on the animal.

As the animal passes from a good to a worse environment it moves from a state of harmony, or equilibrium, to one where it recognises an environmental deterioration. This can be detected experimentally by preference tests, indicating which environment the animal prefers. These must be treated with caution for several reasons: animals may give an exaggerated or diminished response according to previous experience, they may not be sufficiently experienced to choose the best environment for themselves in the long term and their immediate reaction may differ substantially from their long-term one if they are attracted by the novelty of one or more of the environments. A cognitive imbalance may turn into a physiological imbalance if the environment progressively deteriorates. Later pain may be felt and injuries sustained, both of which will tend to cause abnormal behaviour. Disease may follow and may result ultimately in death of the animal.

We may also evaluate the extent to which an animal is able to perpetuate the bovine species through reproduction. This is related to welfare, because courtship and copulation are natural behaviours that cattle have a strong drive to perform. However, it cannot be claimed that the welfare of a semen-donating bull is necessarily any greater than a bull slaughtered for meat. It is likely to be worse if he becomes lame. It is therefore not a simple relationship between reproductive behaviour and welfare, but man often assumes the management of reproduction as part of their 'domestic contract' with animals. In this contract, we provide basic requirements – food, water, a suitable environment, medical care and companionship – but we take away freedoms that the animal would have in the wild – choice of mate, companion, food, freedom of movement, etc. We also reduce the longevity of cattle kept for the production of beef, because as they get older their growth rate declines and they have increasingly more fat in the carcase. Most dairy cows have a short life, because of the stress of many lactations and the poor conditions that they are often kept in. In intensive dairy systems they only last on average for about three lactations in the milk-producing herd. This will be considered by many to be evidence of inadequate welfare.

The management of the domestic contract, and the issue of whether cattle should be allowed to reproduce naturally, are principally moral issues. In the case of reproduction, the opportunities for highly selective breeding by artificial means not only prevent cows from performing natural copulation, but also may compromise the future of the species by limiting the genotype diversity. Presently cattle are selectively bred to be either high milk producers or fast growing meat animals. In future, their ability to survive on by-products, straw, human food residues, etc., may be of greater importance if increased population pressure dictates that land can no longer be used solely to grow feed for cattle. Also, the efficient use of nutrients such as nitrogen may be of special importance to increase production efficiency and reduce nitrogen pollution in excreta.

The future welfare of the species should be considered in relation to breeding policies, but this is unlikely to be done by individual farmers who cannot be expected to predict or respond to the economic situation in the distant future. A prudent approach would be to maintain sufficient cattle breed diversity for all future eventualities. Maintaining diversity in the cattle genotypes is an important aspect of long-term breeding policy in which central government intervention could be beneficial to the species in the long term.

Modern breeding techniques may also create dilemmas for the welfare of individual animals. For example, if a cow were selected to donate embryos for genetic manipulation, there could be an increase in the welfare of the donor cow, since she would have to be well managed to produce the best embryos. However, there might be a decrease in the welfare of the offspring as a result of the genetic manipulation, if it led, for example, to a large increase in milk production potential. This moral dilemma must be addressed on an individual case basis.

Humans manage both the genotype and phenotype of cattle, and they have perhaps modified the genotype more than in any other species for their own benefit. It should not be forgotten that in modifying cattle to the farm environment, we have improved their welfare. Selection for a suitable temperament, and in particular docility, has enabled cattle to co-exist with humans in an environment where ancient *Bos aurochs* cattle would have found the conditions very difficult to cope with. The ease with which cattle can be managed in dairy and beef farms is in marked contrast to other species that have not been extensively domesticated, such as deer, ostriches, mink and foxes. These species are all difficult to farm and individuals show high levels of aggression to each other and their keepers.

Our modification of the cattle genotype has enabled us to keep them in a large variety of conditions and environments. In environments where many people would consider that cattle are not well adapted, they still produce economic quantities of milk or grow at an economically acceptable rate. Production is largely a function of nutrient supply, and although cattle kept in adverse conditions can have low levels of immunity, and a high incidence of diseases, such as lameness, there is little evidence that any productive function is affected. This does not mean that such systems are morally justified, just because the cattle do not overtly manifest their difficulties in coping with the system. That cattle suffer in silence is partly due to the influence of domestication, and partly due to the evolutionary forces pre-domestication – prey animals grazing in open grassland would not wish to attract attention to themselves by excessive vocalisation or other display if they are having trouble coping with the environment. A survey of cattle vocalisations at abattoirs found that very few cattle (10%) vocalise there, despite the stressful conditions (Grandin, 1998). However, they do emit fear pheromones in their urine that can indicate danger to conspecifics, but not potential predators (Boissy *et al.*, 1998).

Determining the optimum welfare for cattle – moral issues

There is no universal guide to the minimum level of conditions that is acceptable for the adequate welfare of cattle. This is a moral decision that people have to take, and it will vary with nationality, gender, previous experiences, age, etc. Usually the moral viewpoint prevailing in any one situation is the majority view. The type of system that is used is largely free for the farmer to choose, but in some regions societal values are taken into account, and legal restrictions are imposed, e.g. on calf accommodation and diet in the European Union. Above any legal limit it would be ideal if animal products were available to a range of international welfare standards, so that consumers could choose according to their moral persuasion and means. However, this is not practical as we do not have international welfare standards yet and consumers want simple choices. Probably the most successful method so far by which consumers can buy products from animals with guaranteed high welfare is when the welfare standards are incorporated into more general environmental control, as in organic produce.

When considering the optimum level of welfare for cattle, there are both altruistic and moral considerations:

(1) Cattle kept in poor conditions are more susceptible to disease, which may reduce the quality of the product. They are more susceptible to zoonoses, such as tuberculosis and paratuberculosis, which may be transmitted in milk to people. Although much progress in controlling zoonoses has been made over the last 50 years, in particular by milk pasteurisation, new pathogens are emerging, e.g. *Escherichia coli* 0157, largely present in faecal contamination of pelts and carcases.

(2) Societal values will be improved if we care for others, animals and humans, in at least as good a manner as we wish to be cared for ourselves. Contact with animals is an important part of a child's emotional development and it positively shapes their future personality. It can also act as a releaser for individual frustrations, and in children violence towards animals is closely linked with violence to people (Miller, 2001). Cattle are an essential part of human society, helping us by providing food, clothing, fuel, traction and companionship, often using resources that would be of little or no value to ourselves. They also act as genetic insurance for the future. Focusing the world's genetic resources into a small number of genotypes dominated by man is dangerous, since future events may favour different genotypes.

Some farmers may justify low welfare standards for cattle within their care because they are acting for their individual benefit, or that of their families, rather than society as a whole. Because they run businesses, profit is the ultimate objective, not animal welfare, but the approach is not acceptable to societies which have respect for animal welfare. For most of our evolution, humans lived in less complex societies, where self-preservation was more important genetically than acting for the benefit of society. In many cases the two were compatible, as they often are today. However, in an age when society demands conformity to a common purpose, there may be conflict between the inherent desire for self-preservation and the need to support the society. Societal values are portrayed through religious organisations, government, non-government organisations and perhaps most important of all, the media, but they can easily be ignored by individuals in large, loosely configured social groups.

Individuals, and their dependants, may benefit physically if they spend as little as possible on food from animals, which might be best obtained from farming systems that had scant regard for the animals' welfare. However, societal values would also benefit from keeping animals in good conditions. Thus the individual consumer is presented with a moral dilemma, the outcome of which may be determined by the extent of their commitment to society and their disposable income.

(3)   Many believe that humans have a God-given duty to care for animals, as prescribed in most of the major religions. However, the Judaeo-Christian religion emphasises man's dominion over nature that is not apparent in older religions, which emphasise careful stewardship of resources. Some argue that the Genesis reference in the King James' version of the Bible to man 'having dominion over the animals' would be more accurately translated from the original text as having 'a duty of care for the animals'. In many Old Testament references the Bible extols the view that animals are worth more than their immediate usefulness to us (Nash, 1990), but this is not reflected in orthodox Jewish society, which places the study of the Mishnah and Talmud over the study of the Bible (Gendin, 1989). Buddhists are strongly encouraged to care for animals, and meditiation is believed to bring affinity to them. The requirement that all adherents to the major religions should care for animals can be used to infer that animals have a *right* to be cared for. Such rights not only are enshrined in religious beliefs but also have been adopted into the legislation of many countries, in terms of prevention of cruelty to animals.

From a moral perspective, it is inconsistent that we adopt different standards for animals according to the benefit that we derive from them. Companion animals usually receive better care than laboratory or farm animals, for whom space is often restricted to maximise output per unit area. Animals in wildlife or safari parks are afforded a similar habitat to the wild, so that the public has the illusion that they are in fact wild. At the bottom end of the care and attention scale, perhaps, are pack and traction animals in developing countries, including cattle for whom work is often excessive. Within the farm animals, different levels of stress may be imposed on the animals according to their type of output. In the case of the dairy cow, which is either lactating or heavily pregnant, or both, for nearly all of its adult life, it is clear that this imposes a metabolic burden that reduces longevity. The average life-span in intensive dairy systems (about five years) is a fraction of the potential of 20 to 25 years, because of the metabolic strain. The high daily output in the early part of lactation, particularly of energy, exploits the cow's ability to catabolise considerable amounts of body fat tissue, which is restored only when milk yield has declined later in the lactation. The constant annual cycle of body fat depletion and restoration stresses the metabolism, and usually the cow succumbs to disease and has to be culled after only two to four lactations. In contrast, cattle for meat production are usually fed a diet that will allow nearly maximum growth, partly because genetic improvement in growth rates has not been as fast as milk production.

Some people believe that the moral right to keep animals on farms depends on the essentiality of the product. Thus it might be more justifiable to farm cattle for the production of food than solely for leather production. It is more difficult to replace cattle food products with other foods than it is to replace leather, since the former are particularly good sources of digestible protein, B vitamins and minerals such as calcium. However, this concept is probably largely derived from a rejection of modern, intensive farming methods rather than a fundamental necessity for the essentiality of animal production. In reality all animal products can be replaced by plant or synthetic products. In some cases this seems entirely justified. The use of large areas of virgin Amazonian forest to produce a beef product for consumption in the USA, which is a country that has its own resources for beef production, is to many people immoral. The global environment is adversely affected by destruction of the rain forest, habitat for endangered forest species is lost and there is extensive debate in the country in question as to whether their natural resources should be used for beef production at the expense of the environment.

In other circumstances cattle production makes a valued and essential contribution to human life. In many developing countries the availability of meat and milk improve the level of human nutrition and they are produced largely from land that is unsuitable for cropping and by-products, that would otherwise be expensive to dispose of, such as straw and agro-industrial wastes. Cattle farming provides useful employment for some of the poorest members of the community and gives them dung, a useful source of fuel, to reduce reliance on wood or fossil fuels. Draft power may also be provided, reducing reliance on tractors and fossil fuel. In these circumstances it is difficult for even the most fervent of animal rights campaigners to advocate the replacement of cattle products with vegetarian options.

Determining the optimum welfare for cattle – evidence from wild cattle

The behaviour of domestic cattle has been extensively studied, but solutions to behavioural problems have been elusive. Excessive licking and sucking behaviour in calves, mounting behaviour in steers, as well as tongue-rolling, prepuce-sucking and other less common stereotypies in steers, persist despite a better understanding of their aetiology than 20 years ago. They contribute to inefficiencies or low-quality production, leading for example in the case of mounting bulls and steers to low-quality meat. Many abnormal behaviours are known to derive from the artificial environment that cattle are kept in, since they are absent in extensively kept cattle. Often they evolve when an animal is thwarted from performing its natural behaviour by deficiencies in its environment. They are particularly common in hot, humid conditions, where the heat stress reduces resistance to environmental deficiencies. Opportunities to modify the environment are always limited, unless productivity is greatly reduced. An understanding of the behavioural repertoire of cattle pre-domestication will indicate which behaviours are innately present in cattle, and allow the environment of domesticated cattle to be most effectively modified to reduce the incidence of problem behaviours.

There are no remaining wild cattle (*Bos aurochs*) that were the progenitors of *Bos taurus* and *indicus* genotypes, the last examples having been slaughtered in Czechoslovakia in the seventeenth century. Detailed information on the behaviour of the progenitors of domestic pig (wild boar), hen (jungle fowl) and sheep (mouflon) is available, as they still exist in the wild. Since such possibilities do not exist with domestic cattle, near relatives are being studied. The Malaysian gaur is well-suited to this task, since cattle evolved in south-east Asia, before spreading across Eurasia until they were domesticated relatively recently in Africa.

The gaur [*Bos (Bibos) gaurus*] is an endangered species that is a wild ancestor of domestic cattle. There have been few studies of their behaviour, despite their importance to understanding the behaviour of domesticated cattle. Those looking after captive gaur cattle in zoos and wildlife parks report that they are more nervous than domesticated cattle when handled by man, however, they do habituate to the presence of humans in the zoo. The behaviour of the leading animal is of great importance in determining the behaviour of the rest of the herd, possibly more so than in domesticated cattle.

Other behaviours appear to be similar – the bull shows flehman behaviour in response to females in oestrus and, for their part, the cows show homosexual mounting during oestrus. In the wild, some sexually mature bulls are integrated with the herd, probably the dominant ones, others living in bachelor groups. The oestrus of the gaur cattle is shorter than that of domestic cattle, which suggests selection by man for extended oestrus in the latter, and artificial breeding techniques developed for domestic cattle are successful in gaur cattle (Godfrey *et al.*, 1991). In contrast to the gaur, feral cattle in Africa have been reported to live in matriarchal groups, with the bulls being evicted to live in bachelor herds when they are sexually mature (Reinhardt & Reinhardt, 1981). The forest-dwelling gaur cattle would find this strategy of little value, because the oestrus mounting display would be of little value in attracting the bulls from afar. In addition, by integrating with them, the bulls will protect the cows and their calves from attack by predators, in particular tigers. The gaur bull is much more fearsome than its domesticated counterpart, the mithun, and is a match for most tigers.

In common with buffaloes, gaur cattle give birth in the half-standing position. Domestic cattle, however, usually lie down, which may be because parturition is more difficult than in wild cattle, either because the calf is bigger or because genetic selection has changed the angle of the pelvis. Rather than being sloping downwards towards the tail, domestic cattle have a much flatter back, which is known to increase calving difficulties. However, a flat back gives better support to the udder, which is much larger in domestic than wild cattle. It also increases the size of the loins, which produce high-value meat.

Gaur cattle usually live mainly in the forest fringes, where there are shrubs and bushes that can be browsed. They find it more difficult to select food in dense tropical rainforest, where they will venture during the middle of the day. High intake rates are required at the beginning and end of the day, because of the quiescent period at night, but more selective feeding and resting in the forest is possible at midday, often near a waterhole. This will also bring them shade in the heat of the day, but interestingly Gupta *et al.* (1999) report that gaur cattle avoid being in the open sunlight even when the temperature is low. Domesticated cattle start to use physiological mechanisms, such as sweating, to lose heat at temperatures as low as 25 to 27°C, and it is appears likely that gaur cattle also have a weak ability to tolerate hot temperatures. Exposure of cattle to warmer temperatures may have adverse effects on their welfare.

The predominance of activity at the forest fringes would have brought the predecessors of gaur cattle into contact with humans practising shifting cultivation in the earliest days of agriculture. Their diet includes browse species, such as bamboo, and tall tropical grasses. Domesticated cattle are often believed to be maladapted to browsing, but will readily do so on forest fringes even if some pasture is available. They are rarely offered the opportunity to browse in modern production systems, but will readily do so if it is provided. It is likely that some browsing would improve cattle nutrition by varying the diet and would in particular provide a good source of minerals, vitamins and rumen-bypass protein compared with grass monocultures. Browse material, in the form of gorse, broom and other shrubs would commonly have been provided for domesticated cattle until 100 years ago, when its unsuitability for mechanised production reduced its popularity in favour of grass. Many browse plants, although now regarded as weeds, can survive in extreme climates and with little additional nutrient supply owing to their deep-rooting habit.

In South-East Asia, gaur cattle have a strong appetite for salt, as do the local domesticated cattle, the mithun (Gupta *et al.*, 1999). This probably facilitated their domestication, since humans attract the cattle back to their compound at night with salt. Modern farmers use the availability of salt as an aid to controlling the movements of their mithun cattle, and the diet of domesticated dairy cattle is also strongly determined by salt contents of the various foods (Chiy & Phillips, 1991).

The behaviour of other relatives of cattle has been studied, but these are too distant phylogenetically or the studies are of insufficient depth to be of major value. In particular the buffalo (*Bubalis bubalis*) has received considerable attention, but it has been subjected to the influence of domestication. Their behaviour is similar to that of the wild gaur and modern domesticated cattle (Odyuo *et al.*,

1995), e.g. they have similar (crepuscular) feeding behaviour patterns (Barrio *et al.*, 2000) and the calves engage in both filial and communal suckling (the latter being more common in female calves) (Murphey *et al.*, 1995; Paranhos da Costa *et al.*, 2000). Some differences in the sexual behaviour of yaks (*Bos grunniens*) are known to exist, when they are compared to cattle, in particular characteristic stomping and tail-swishing behaviours (Sambraus, 1999).

Conclusion

Determining the optimum welfare of cattle first requires that it is accurately measured. This will vary between situations but is connected with their ability to cope with their environment and their feelings over their lifetime. There is a moral imperative to maintain cattle in a high state of welfare, first, to maintain the levels of zoonotic diseases at a minimum, secondly, because moral standards in human society will benefit if animals are kept in good conditions and thirdly, because most modern religions instruct followers to look after their animals well. Evidence from the wild relatives of domesticated cattle is that their behaviour has changed little as a result of human selection, suggesting that intensive housing systems may have deficiencies hitherto largely unrealised.

Chapter 2
The Welfare of Dairy Cows

Introduction

The systems in which dairy cows are kept are diverse, ranging from highly mech-anised systems in which the cattle are kept indoors all year, to extensive systems in which the cattle are outdoors permanently. Production levels are highly vari-able but the level of animal care usually provides at least once or twice daily inspection when the cows are gathered for milk production. The factors influ-encing welfare depend on the system employed, but inadequate nutrition is often a consequence of the high levels of nutrients required for milk production. This will also influence the disease profile, being orientated towards metabolic dis-eases. The milking and housing systems utilised can adversely affect the cow's welfare, as will the social influences afforded by the type of housing. Finally, mutilations by man, such as removal of the tail to stop it having to be cleaned regularly, may prevent normal behaviour and reduce welfare.

Hunger and malnutrition

Hunger is a balance between nutrient demands and consumption. Demands are determined by the requirements for maintenance, production and growth, and the efficiencies with which nutrients are absorbed and metabolised. Usually hunger is determined by energy status, although specific hungers for other nutri-ents commonly in deficit, such as sodium, do exist (Phillips *et al.*, 1999). The domesticated dairy cow has considerably increased nutrient requirements as a result of the increase in milk yield potential (Table 2.1). This increases her need for rest (Munksgaard & Herskin, 2001) and contributes indirectly to the short life that most high-yielding cows have in a dairy herd. The risk of contracting mastitis, lameness, fatty liver disease, hypocalcaemia, acidosis, ketosis and many other diseases increases with milk yield. As a result the mean number of lacta-tions is only three or four in most developed countries, compared with more than ten for feral cows. However, it must not be forgotten that starvation during win-ter months was common in dairy cows until new forage conservation practices allowed food of sufficient quality and quantity to be made available in the twen-tieth century. As recently as the 1950s there was significant mortality of British

Table 2.1 Comparison of milk production in feral and modern domesticated dairy cows

	Feral	Domesticated
Milk production (litres/day)	8–10	30–50
Number of milkings per day	4–6	2–3
Yield per milking (litres)	1–2.5	10–25
Total lactation yield (litres)	<1000	6000–12 000

Adapted from Webster (1995).

dairy cows during winter months due to undernutrition (Garner, 1989). The hay available for cows was of poor quality and concentrate foods were generally not available, being required for human consumption. However, with the increase in use of artificial fertilisers in the latter half of the twentieth century, forage production could be greatly increased. This, together with the development of mechanised conservation and silage feeding techniques, allowed cows to be adequately sustained through the winter. Feeding cows mainly on fermented herbage is not without health risks, which are principally from undesirable micro-organisms, such as *Listeria*, *Enterobacteria*, *Clostridia* and moulds, undesirable chemicals, such as mycotoxins, and excess acidity (Wilkinson, 1999). Some, such as the mycotoxins, can even potentially affect humans consuming milk or meat products from infected cattle.

Improved ability to feed cows in winter has allowed cows to calve in the autumn, producing peak nutrient demands in winter, when the ration can be more accurately formulated than when the cows are at pasture. During the early lactation period, body reserves of fat, protein and minerals, especially calcium, are used to support high milk yields. Webster (1995) has suggested that cows may be persistently hungry at this time, even though they usually have forage available *ad libitum*. This is possible, since intake is limited not by food availability but by the physical capacity of the gastrointestinal tract, and especially the rumen. The rate of removal of the food particles from the rumen is determined by the speed with which it can be digested by micro-organisms. Preliminary results (Cooper *et al.*, 2002) indicate little difference in the extent to which high- and low-yielding cows are prepared to work to obtain extra high-energy food. Theoretically, increasing the nutrient concentration by feeding a ration of high-energy cereals would increase the rate of digestion and allow greater intakes. However, the rumen micro-organisms function at a pH of 6 to 7, and rapid digestion of high-energy foods produces excessive fatty acids as endproducts of digestion. Rumen pH will therefore decline after meals, and the micro-organisms responsible for digestion cannot survive the acidic conditions. The rumen also needs long fibre to support the contractions that mix the contents, and high-energy foods usually have inadequate fibre, resulting in rumen stasis. The primary aim in feeding cattle is to maintain constant and benign conditions in the rumen, which must be considered as a sensitive fermentation vessel, adversely affected by variation in conditions.

Diseases

Production diseases

A failure to provide adequate or suitable nutrients during periods of high milk output leads to a number of common 'production' diseases. Evidently the welfare of cows is adversely affected during clinical disease events, but we have little knowledge of the extent, or impact on welfare, of subclinical disease. For some nutrients, such as calcium, the body has advanced homeostatic mechanisms, and it is likely that there is a sudden failure of these, rather than progressive, prolonged subclinical disease. However, for many other conditions few homeostatic mechanisms exist, usually because there was no need for them pre-domestication. Such is the case for magnesium deficiency, which is common when cows consume young, rapidly growing pasture that has been fertilised with potassium. Potassium inhibits the absorption of magnesium in the rumen, and young, leafy grass has a low magnesium content anyway. The resulting tetany is usually an acute disorder which the cow cannot survive unless magnesium compounds are injected subcutaneously within a few hours.

Bloat is a painful condition that is common in cows fed rapidly digested pasture legumes or cereals. The production of gases by the rumen exceeds their rate of removal by eructation. This may be due to either the presence of a stable foam in the rumen (pasture bloat) or restricted rumen motility (cereal bloat). It is precipitated by the sudden introduction of bloat-inducing foods, especially after a period of restricted feeding, such as during oestrus in the cow. Affected cattle are restless and find lying uncomfortable. Eventually they die of heart failure, or suffocation as a result of inhaling rumen contents.

Lameness

Lameness is probably the most serious disease affecting the welfare of dairy cows kept in cubicle systems, with a prevalence of up to 20% (Clarkson *et al.*, 1996). The annual incidence has been recorded as 35 to 55% in the UK (Clarkson *et al.*, 1996; Kossaibati & Esslemont, 2000), but only 7% in Michigan, USA (Kaneene & Hurd, 1990). Because it impairs an essential behaviour, locomotion, the greater the distance that lame cows have to walk in the management system, the greater impact on welfare. The most serious consequences therefore occur for grazing cows, who are unable to keep up with the rest of the herd in finding the best grazing and will remain as close to the farm buildings as possible to minimise locomotion. Speed of locomotion is reduced, so that if a herdsperson hurries the cows back to the farm buildings for milking, there is clearly a big impact on welfare.

About 90% of all lameness is the result of claw horn lesions, and most occur in the lateral digit of the hind feet soon after calving (Thysen, 1987; Leonard *et al.*, 1996). A cow responds to the pain by minimising the propulsion of the affected limb, reducing her speed of walking, arching her back and lowering her head. The average duration of an episode of lameness is three months (Phillips, 1990a), including the periods of abnormal locomotion before and after clinical lameness, i.e. the forward thrust from the limb is reduced.

Much of the lameness associated with cubicle housing derives from the cow walking on hard concrete covered in slurry. Cows in tie stalls have far fewer problems (Faye & Lescourret, 1989). Laminitis, or inflammation of the horn-producing laminae that present as sole haemorrhages, is a particularly painful and common condition. It is promoted by both the housing conditions and a high-concentrate diet.

A primary cause of claw horn lesions is the reduction in the supportive capacity of the connective tissue of the hoof wall around the time of calving. This results in the pedal bone sinking and/or rotating, putting great stress on the sole. If there are few external pressures on the hoof, for example when cows are housed in straw yards, hoof connective tissue integrity can recover within 12 weeks of calving (Tarlton *et al.*, 2001). However, the shock of regularly stepping on concrete, coupled with the softening of the hoof when the cow stands in slurry, can traumatise the hoof and lead to primary lesions (Tarlton *et al.*, 2002). Primiparous cows are particularly at risk, because they are mixed with older cows and may increase locomotion in escape routines. One form of 'escape' is to stand with the front legs in the cubicle and the hind legs in the passageway, which further increases the pressure on the latter. It is important to keep escape routes clear for cows, especially by preventing blind alleys where subordinate cows may be trapped.

One advantage of concrete surfaces is the high wear rate (Vokey *et al.*, 2001). The growth rate will also be less in cows in straw yards, but the lack of wear can lead to overgrown hooves, backward rotation of the pedal bone and limited contact between the toe and floor. Although such a condition may not initially be painful, the necessary modification of walking behaviour may lead to inactivity and separation from the herd at pasture.

Bad cubicle design may predispose to lameness, as cows spend less time lying in small cubicles, cubicles with a hard surface or cubicles with divisions that impede movement (Horning & Tost, 2001). Hock damage may occur as the animal lies down, and those lying on soft surfaces or in wide cubicles are less likely to experience this problem (Livesey *et al.*, 1998). However, if cubicles are too large cows may attempt to turn around and get stuck, particularly if they are inexperienced at lying in cubicles.

Claw horn lesions may progress to sole ulcers, which are also associated with pedal bone movement, and typically cause severe lameness when they rupture about six weeks after calving. Exploration of the area surrounding the ulcer during treatment may expose the sensitive corium. Claw horn lesions may also damage the 'white line', the name given to the junction between the sole and hoof wall. White line separation can be caused by penetration by stones or fragments of dirt, which may progress even to the sensitive corium. Treatment may involve removal of the hoof wall in extreme cases, with considerable and prolonged pain caused by the injury.

Infectious diseases

Dairy cows do not suffer from many of the traditional range of infectious cattle diseases because they develop immunity when they are youngstock. However, novel pathogens, such as bovine spongiform encephalopathy (BSE), or infectious diseases to which they have not been exposed, such as foot and mouth disease or tuberculosis in the UK, pose a significant threat. The major infectious disease from which cows suffer is mastitis, which may be caused by a variety of pathogens. Some of these are transmitted between cows, but these have been less of a problem in recent years owing to routine use of antibiotics following infection and after the termination of lactation. Non-transmissible environmental pathogens, such as *Escherichia coli*, have become an increasing problem, which is best tackled by improving cleanliness on farms.

The escalating problem of tuberculosis in the UK illustrates the difficulties in permanently controlling infectious diseases in intensive cattle farming. The disease was rampant in the first half of the twentieth century, owing to the lack of control measures and close contact between cattle during housing. Many human deaths followed consumption of infected milk, until pasteurisation began to be widely practised in the 1950s. A compulsory slaughter policy for infected stock and strict control of the badger, the major intermediary host, had almost eradicated the disease by the mid 1970s. However, concern for the welfare of badgers led to a ban on their being culled, and cattle feeding practices that gave badgers access to food, in particular maize, as well as transmission between cattle, have all contrived to allow tuberculosis to increase rapidly in England and Wales. Farmers believe that government should accept responsibility for the control of the disease since it is illegal for them to remove badgers from their farms, but government believes that farmers must accept responsibility for environmental constraints on their farming practices. There are several options for controlling the disease (Table 2.2), which illustrate the difficulty in allocating responsibility for the welfare of intensively farmed cattle between farmers, environmentalists and government officials. No solution is ideal, but government will support only those measures that are ethically acceptable to the public, which excludes wildlife culls, and are not too expensive. Since the number of farmers is decreasing, the government feels responsible to the electorate in these issues and not just to farmers. However, while no solutions can be found that are acceptable to all parties, the welfare of cattle is increasingly threatened by the disease.

Table 2.2 Options for control of tuberculosis in British cattle (Bennett & Cooke, 2001)

Option	Advantages	Disadvantages
Mandatory insurance for farmers against an outbreak	Places responsibility in hands of farmers	High cost to farmers, especially in high-risk areas
Wildlife vaccine	No wildlife cull	High cost of development, seen as invasive by environmentalists
Cattle vaccine	No effect on badgers, gives responsibility to farmers	High cost of development, efficacy may be low, may invalidate herd testing regime
Wildlife elimination measures	Minimise secondary host transmission	Unacceptable to public
Improved biosecurity on farms	Holistic approach, sustainable	Efficacy in doubt while wildlife reservoir exists
More and improved testing on farms, especially at movement	No effect on badgers, responsibility given to farmers	Does not address secondary host transmission, cost
Segregation of cattle and wildlife	Eliminates secondary host transmission	Practicality, high cost
Breeding for resistance in cattle	Acceptable to farmers and public	Efficacy, long time to achieve results, resistant organisms may develop
Create zones with minimal movement between them	Limits spread to low-risk zones, contains the disease	Does not alleviate disease spread in high-risk zones, administration cost

Milking

The development of automatic technology for milk extraction in the twentieth century allowed many more cows to be milked by one herdsperson than when milking was accomplished by hand. *Bos taurus* cows will usually release their milk without a calf, but *Bos indicus* cows need the psychological stimulus of the presence of the calf, suggesting that they may have been subjected to less domestication pressure.

Hand-milking may provide a surrogate stimulus to the cows and the simultaneous provision of a food reward may help them to overcome any reluctance. The removal of milk from heavily lactating cows may offer reward in itself, and they are usually the first to enter the parlour if given the choice. The negative signals to cows that machine milking can provide include being hurried in from pasture by a handler with a dog or motorbike; being controlled in the collecting yard by an electric fence; aggressive treatment from the herdsperson when in the collecting yard or parlour; pain induced by not removing teat cups soon enough; damage to the teat's cardiovascular system by a wrongly set vacuum; danger of slipping on wet concrete floors and close contact with dominant cows. The best parlours allow the cow to enter her stall at will (automated entry parlours), rather than being forced to enter by the herdsperson. Cows develop preferences to enter a specific stall at a specific time and preventing them from doing this can increase their heart rate (Hopster *et al.*, 1998), but it will not reduce their milk production or greatly affect their welfare (Paranhos da Costa & Broom, 2001).

Robotic milking

The recent development of technology to enable teat cups to be automatically attached to a cow has led to the commercial production of fully automated milking units, or milking robots. Such units are now being evaluated world-wide, but especially in Europe. To many members of the public, robotic milking of dairy cows will be an anathema when considering their welfare. However, this may not be true when one compares it to the manually operated milking systems in operation on most farms.

Many aspects of robotic milking can affect the welfare of cows, such as the daily frequency of visits by the cows. The vacuum and pulsation characteristics, which are standardised for all cows in conventional milking parlours, can potentially be tailored to the needs of individual cows in robotic milking systems. Given that in some European countries one-third of dairy farmers are predicted to switch to robotic milking between 2000 and 2015, the technique has the potential to have a major impact on cow welfare. At the start of the millennium, there were just over 500 farms using the system, mostly in Europe, and the next ten years will determine whether the technology has universal application or whether it will be restricted to quite specific circumstances. Will all dairy cows eventually be milked by robots?

The technology is expected to be most readily adopted in areas with small family farms and low availability of inexpensive, hired labour. The ageing population of farmers which usually dominate such conditions would find considerable benefit in reducing their labour input. Such conditions exist in much of Europe and North America, where there are strong economies in non-agricultural sectors, and the technology could help to preserve the family farm in these regions. Large industrial operations are unlikely to use the technology widely because a purely economic assessment would not favour its use.

Theoretically, stockpeople employing robots should have extra time to look after their cows, which it is estimated reduce labour requirements for milking by 30%. A person is still required to fetch cows that do not want to be milked, to attach the cluster to cows if the machine malfunctions and to monitor milk storage and cooling. This may involve night attendance in robotic systems. Economic studies have shown that there is only a potential profit margin from adopting robotic milking if surplus labour can be dispensed with (Arendzen &

Scheppingen, 2000). It may be too optimistic to assume that cows will be more closely monitored in dairy systems with robotic milking, since family farmers adopting the system may choose to use the time released for leisure activities. Undoubtedly, the adoption of robotic milking systems will increase the need for stockpeople to be better trained technically.

An indication that there may be adverse effects of robotic milking on welfare comes from the reluctance of most cows to volunteer for milking more than once or twice a day. This may be because the stress associated with being milked by a robot is greater than the reward of emptying a full udder. Some of the stress may relate to automatic udder cleaning and lack of contact with the herdsperson. On the majority of farms there is a good relationship between the stockperson and the cows, and the direct contact during milking may be valued by both. However, in circumstances where the forcing of cows by the herdsperson or an electronic crowding gate to enter the parlour leads to stress, cows entering a robotic milker may suffer *less* emotional stress.

The cows' reluctance to be milked by a robot makes it usual to offer concentrate feed during milking. This could lead to metabolic disorders if the robot is visited frequently and large amounts of concentrates are consumed at each visit. Cows in negative energy balance may be driven to attend regularly for more food, which will increase milking frequency and yield and thereby exacerbate the negative energy balance. The separation of concentrate and forage feeding in this way could make ration-mixing wagons redundant. However, feeding during milking increases oxytocin production and milk letdown and reduces cortisol production, suggesting less stress to the cows.

An alternative to concentrate feeding to entice cows into the robot is to position the milking unit between the cubicles and the cows' food source, and force the cows to be milked when moving between these two. Cows reduce their frequency of passage between the two systems when this is done, indicating some reluctance to visit the milking robot. The loss of freedom associated with this enforced milking almost certainly reduces their welfare, but possibly no more than in conventional milking systems, where they are usually forcibly milked twice a day.

Because of the high cost of robotic units compared with conventional ones, there is usually only one unit provided for every 40 to 60 cows. This may lead to queues of frustrated cows waiting to be milked at preferred times of the day. However, mean queuing time per milking on commercial farms has been recorded as seven minutes, or 34 minutes per day, which is less than in most conventional milking systems. Some farms use electrified 'cattle drivers' in the robotic units to accelerate cow movement through the unit or associated passages. This will reduce motivation to attend and increase stress.

Mastitis, or inflammation of the mammary gland, is a particularly common cause of poor welfare in modern dairy systems. For several reasons, the incidence of mastitis and the milk parameters associated with this disease, such as the somatic cell count, are usually increased by robotic milking, particularly in the first few months of operation. Perhaps the biggest contributing factor is the sharing of a single cluster by more cows than in conventional semi-automatic milking. Another problem is inadequate or no udder cleaning, with the usual system being wet brushes moving backwards and forwards over the udder. In a conventional parlour, the attendant herdsperson recognises a particularly dirty udder and cleans it more thoroughly. Milking robots cannot always determine which of the four glands has mastitis, in order to divert the milk to a separate container, and there is no possibility to examine a foremilk sample for clots. If a robot fails to detect milk from a cow with mastitis, and the milk enters the bulk tank, the somatic cell count will increase. Failing to detect just 1% of cows with mastitis could increase the bulk milk somatic cell count by more than 50 000 cells/ml. Some incidences of mastitis can be detected from measurements of milk conductivity during milking, but not all. Adding data on milk yield (reduced during mastitis) and temperature (increased during mastitis) can increase the detection sensitivity to 100% and the specificity to 98%, and a fuzzy logic model could increase the specificity to the necessary 100%, allowing abnormal milk to be automatically separated with a high degree of confidence (Hoogeveen & Meijering, 2000). Other possibilities are the automated detection of the enzyme *N*-acetyl-beta-D-glucosaminidase (NAGase), which is released into milk following mammary tissue damage, or near infra-red analysis of milk.

Another potential cause of mastitis in cows milked by robots is the failure of some cows to be milked at the first attempt. They may wait an hour until they try again, with a period of lying on a dirty bed in between. During the first attempt, the teat canal opens as a conditioned reflex, and milk may exude from the teat. This allows bacteria to invade when the cows are lying on dirty bedding.

Some features of robotic milking could potentially reduce the risk of mastitis, but any reduction in somatic cell count compared with conventional milking could be due to the dilution effect of increased milk yield. However, the more regular evacuation of the gland could genuinely reduce bacterial proliferation. In addition, in robotic milking the vacuum level could be individually programmed for each cow and indeed each teat, theoretically allowing the risk of over-milking, teat congestion and teat sinus occlusion to be minimised. This is most likely to be of benefit to cows with conical teats.

Individual management of cows milked by robots offers considerable promise. Ketosis could be detected in cows by acetone sensors at the head of the stall. The monitoring of milk composition could allow major stresses to the cow to be detected, perhaps as changes in protein content. Restriction of the milking frequency of cows in severely negative energy balance could potentially be used to reduce milk yield and hence the metabolic strain on the cow. Furthermore, cows in negative weight balance could be detected automatically by including load sensors in the milking stall or by the monitoring of milk protein concentration. However, if the maximum milking frequency is changed too frequently, it could cause cows to become confused and frustrated. If there is no restriction in milking frequency, cows choosing to be milked frequently may become too thin as a result of increased milk production. Sometimes there are serious difficulties getting cows in calf after a robotic milking system is installed.

Cows may be reluctant to attend a robotic milker voluntarily when they are out at pasture, although if concentrates are offered during milking they can satisfactorily graze at least 350 to 400 m from the robot without the number of visits per day declining (Hoogeveen & Meijering, 2000). The milking robot is not evenly used over the day, as the cows return to be milked in groups, so waiting times can be long and the robot is unused for quite long periods of the day. Pasture will not be well utilised and any reduction in the availability of grazing to cows is likely to reduce their welfare, not least because grazing cows are less likely than housed cows to have health problems.

In summary, the robotic milking systems in use today are likely to reduce the welfare of cows, compared with conventional parlour milking systems. Particular concerns exist over the ability of the robot to recognise quarters that are dirty or infected with mastitis. Enforced attendance is also a cause for concern in some systems. However, there is potential to improve several aspects of cow welfare, by providing for the requirements of individual teats during milking, by reducing any exposure to stressors, particularly when collecting cows for milking, and by relieving the herdsperson of the most time-consuming job on the dairy farm, which will allow him or her to spend extra time managing the herd and looking for individual cows with problems.

Housing

In many parts of the world cattle are housed for at least a part of the year, either because there is no forage available outside or because any forage would be damaged by cattle treading on it. The greatest impact of housing on the welfare of the cattle is on their social structure, since it is necessary to bring them into much closer contact than would be the case if they were outside. Another major effect of housing is on their predisposition to specific diseases, e.g. lameness when they are housed in cubicles (Phillips, 2001). However, cattle can adapt to a variety of housing systems, e.g. they will tolerate being housed individually, or in small or large groups. Space availability can be reduced to little more than that required for the animal to stand up and lie down. A major part of domestication is to facilitate adaptation to housing, as the word suggests. Such changes in the environment often result in abnormal behaviour, some of which is stereotyped, such as tongue-rolling, which develops rapidly in intensively housed cattle with inadequate space and diet. Other behaviours, such as intersucking and excessive licking and grooming, are also indicative of deficiencies in the environment, but are not stereotyped. Sometimes the housing causes a restriction on movement that is not conducive to good welfare, but is for the benefit of the herdsperson. For example, tethered cattle may have a cow trainer (electrified wires) placed above them to ensure that they move backwards when they arch their back to urinate or defecate. The excreta is then conveniently placed in the cubicle passage, rather than on the bedding.

Tethering reduces welfare by restriction of movement (Mueller *et al.*, 1989) and stereotyped licking behaviour (Redbo, 1990). The physiological evidence that the hypothalamo-hypophysial–adrenal axis is stimulated (Ladewig & Smidt, 1989) and T-cell function affected (Pruett *et al.*, 1986) also suggests that tethering reduces the welfare of cattle.

Temperature stress can occur either inside or outside the housing. Heat stress is most common inside because the cattle are protected from cold stress by their considerable heat of digestion. Inadequate ventilation and radiant heat load from a low roof are the most likely causes of heat stress indoors, and outside a lack of shade can increase the radiant heat load sufficiently to cause stress. Cattle are also stressed by driving rain and will seek shelter, particularly avoiding facing the rain.

Stray electricity

Cattle have less resistance to stray electricity than do humans (see Chapter 6). The electricity can arise from faulty equipment grounding, which often occurs in the corrosive environment of the cattle shed, or from a large voltage drop on the farm, which results in the supply being out of phase with the central power source. Electricity is used on the farm to control the movement of cattle, such as electronic crowd gates in the milking parlour, electrified bars in front of self-feed silage or electrified cow trainers to make cows step backwards out of cubicles when they urinate. All of these may produce stray electricity if not properly earthed. The milking machinery itself is rarely the source of stray electricity, but it should be isolated from possible sources and separately grounded. The stray electricity may also derive from off-farm sources, in particular where there are three-phase supplies nearby (Appleman & Gustafson, 1985).

Cows respond to electricity in the parlour by being reluctant to enter the parlour, or quick to leave it. Oxytocin production is delayed where the current is 4 to 8 mA or more, delaying milk letdown. If cows are constantly exposed to electricity in a byre, they initially arch their backs and sway or move from side to side in the cubicle, however, they acclimatise to it within a day. Thus intermittent, irregular shocks are more harmful than continuous shocking. If stray electricity is present in a water trough, cows will lap at the water like a dog rather than immersing their muzzle. The sensitivity of cattle to electricity explains their rapid learning to avoid electric fences (McDonald *et al.*, 1981) and other movement control by electricity. Nevertheless, cattle may become disturbed if controlled by electricity – crowd gates in the parlour collection yard can cause nervousness (Boissy *et al.*, 1998) and at the silage pit avoidance of an electrified bar can restrict intake of self-feed silage.

Social influences

Some aspects of management of cattle have clear effects on welfare, e.g. most diseases adversely affect welfare and the effect is increased with the length and/or severity of the disease. However, the impact of social circumstances is much harder to define. In the presence of a dominant cow, subordinate cows take evasive action, and in a confined space such as a cubicle house many escape attempts take place each day (Potter & Broom, 1990). Overt aggression is rare and an unsuccessful escape attempt is most likely to be met by a ritualised threat display. We should not assume that cows suffer the same stress that humans would under such circumstances. Unless food resources are limiting, there is no evidence that the milk yield of subordinate cows is less than dominant cows, which might be the case if the former are stressed by dominant presence. By contrast the movement of cows between groups reduces milk yield, and high stocking densities in dairy cow buildings can increase milk leucocyte concentrations, suggesting stressful conditions (Arave *et al.*, 1974).

At pasture, dairy cows show evidence of increased vigilance when they are in groups of fewer than eight cows (Rind & Phillips, 1999). Large groups in small paddocks or strip-grazed cows will show more aggression than if they were grazed in a large field. The social influences for grazing cows are therefore a balance between cohesive forces, which are especially strong in small groups, and repulsive forces that help to ensure that all cows have access to adequate pasture.

Competition for resources, such as food, may induce fighting between cows, but even then damage to an individual is rare unless the cows are horned. Competition may be prevented by feeding concentrate at barriers with self-locking yokes, which prevents competition. Both entry and exit from these yokes can now be automated (Halachmi *et al.*, 1998), and in future the welfare benefits of preventing competition between cows at the feed face may favour this system.

Separation of cow and calf will stress some cows, particularly if the separation occurs after a substantial period together. Current practice varies from several weeks to a single day, depending on the price of milk and milk replacer. Initially after separation the cow makes attempts to be reunited with the calf, through increased locomotion and vocalisation and even breaking of separation fences. Feeding and sleep patterns may be altered, rumination reduced and a stress response apparent (from elevated corticosteroids and increased heart rate). Some studies have shown that cows that have had several calves before show less response than primiparous cows (Le Neindre & d'Hour, 1989), but others suggest a greater response (Edwards & Broom, 1982). There is some evidence that cows that are reared in isolation are not as good mothers as cows reared with other calves (Le Neindre *et al.*, 1992). They are slow to start licking their calves but are also less aggressive, demonstrating reduced motivation for social contact, both malevolent and benign.

Tail docking

Tail docking is sometimes routinely practised to reduce the accumulation of faeces around the hindquarters of milking cows. After 7 to 14 days the necrotic tail is usually surgically removed. An alternative is to remove the switch. The tail is used for communication and fly removal, and cows with docked tails have more flies and take alternative action, such as foot stomping and skin twitching to get rid of the flies (Elcher *et al.*, 2001). There is little evidence that the udder of docked cows is cleaner or that they suffer less mastitis, and in the European Union tail docking is banned because it infringes the animal's ability to perform normal behaviour. The effects on calves are considered in Chapter 4.

Chapter 3
The Welfare of Beef Cattle and Draft Oxen

Introduction

Systems used for beef cattle are more diverse than those used for dairy cattle, as the animals can be given the opportunity to grow rapidly, with indoor feeding of high-quality diets, or kept at low stocking rates on rangeland, where growth will be slow. The choice of system is largely determined by the economics of production, although the impact of the system on the animals' welfare is now sometimes considered, particularly if it allows the product to have added value. In Sweden, for example, it is compulsory for cattle to be offered shelter in winter, but they cannot be housed all year without access to pasture. In many European countries, the management of large numbers of cattle is determined by principles laid down by assurance agencies, such as the organic farming regulatory bodies or the Royal Society for Prevention of Cruelty to Animals (RSPCA). At the same time, national and international (EU) regulations have been introduced to provide a minimum standard of welfare for beef cattle, especially for calves reared for veal production. Not only are the physical facilities the subject of legislation, such as pen size, but so too is the provision of adequate fodder. This legislation is directed primarily at veal calf producers, but across the world the low profitability of beef production means that undernutrition is an equally common problem for the welfare of beef cattle. Low profitability arises primarily because of the inherent low output, since cattle are designed to digest low-quality fodder by bacterial fermentation in their rumen, and are usually kept on rough pastureland. Some intensive systems of feeding are used, but only where there is a strong demand for the tender beef that is produced under such systems. Other attempts to increase productivity have met with little success. The once-bred heifer system was developed to increase beef production from the major input, the heifer, which was slaughtered after producing one calf at about 24 months of age. However, in the face of declining beef and milk consumption in many western countries, demand for extra calves is low and the management requirements of the system are too great to justify the marginal increase in revenue.

Undernutrition

In recent years, undernutrition of cattle in the UK has become more common as a result of (1) the low profitability of cattle farming since the bovine spongiform encephalopathy (BSE) epidemic and (2) movement constraints following epidemics such as foot and mouth disease in 2001. In the long term malnutrition (incorrect nutrition), as opposed to undernutrition (underfeeding), is likely to become common in other industrialised countries, as a result of the increase in part-time farming. Part-time cattle owners are not always trained in animal husbandry and consequently may not be aware of the animals' nutritional requirements. In addition government subsidies for agricultural advisory services have been withdrawn in many developed countries, so farmers are less likely to take advice and more likely to feed their cattle too little food or the wrong food.

Different classes of cattle are at varying degrees of risk. In the lactating cow, reduced energy intake from concentrate can be offset by increased catabolism of body fat reserves or by increasing forage intake, but protein reserves are less readily mobilised (Tyrrell *et al.*, 1970; Botts *et al.*, 1979). Protein catabolism during lactation is an indicator of reduced welfare in lactating cows, because it represents loss of an essential body tissue. Forage intake can be reduced for periods of about three weeks by up to 40% of *ad libitum* intake if the forage, but more than this will cause a reduction in milk production, in particular milk protein output, and considerable losses in body weight (Phillips & Leaver, 1985a). Growing cattle do not have the buffer of reducing milk production and are potentially more at risk, especially as profit margins are usually less than for milk production.

In 1998, the UK's State Veterinary Service carried out 6592 inspections of animal welfare on farms (Ministry of Agriculture, Fisheries and Food, 2000), and the RSPCA reported 849 cases of cruelty involving farm animals. Undernutrition and malnutrition of beef cattle, in particular suckler cows, comprised a significant proportion of these incidents. Farmers can be prosecuted under the Agriculture (Miscellaneous Provisions) Act 1968 for failing to provide adequate nutrition, and the penalty is a fine or short jail sentence. The preferred option in cases of prolonged or severe malnutrition is prohibition from keeping animals. This requires prosecution under the 1911 Protection of Animals Act, which prohibits farmers from causing unnecessary suffering as a result of malnutrition. Evidence for malnutrition is usually based on veterinary opinion, which uses a subjective assessment of the animal's condition. Attempts have been made to make assessment of condition more objective and a scoring system from 1 (emaciated) to 5 (obese) has been devised (Edmondsen *et al.* 1989). However, scores are variable between individual veterinarians and a more objective measure of inadequate nutrition is needed.

Droughts

In many parts of the world, the nutritional stress caused by undernutrition arises mainly when a drought occurs, i.e. where the supply of water falls below a critical requirement in an area over a prolonged period. The demand is usually a function of man's activities, and most droughts can be considered man made. In contrast, an area with low rainfall is described as arid, but the ecology of the flora and fauna is adapted to the periodic absence of water. Droughts lead to feed shortages and loss of production principally in grazing stock, and usually have their origin in the rainfall and plant production of the preceding season. In Australia, a declaration of drought is made after a short dry period in the case of high output stock, such as dairy cows, where as little as one month without rain may substantially reduce production, but in the case of beef cattle a drought may extend for several years before a serious loss of productivity is experienced. Thus intensification of pasture and animal production will increase both the risk of drought and the variation in profitability of the enterprise. Drought will also influence the diseases affecting grazing stock, with plant poisoning being common as animals search for fodder, as well as osteomalacia and botulism. Botulism occurs when cattle eat infected bones and can usually be prevented by providing mineral supplements, particularly phosphorus (Blair West *et al.*, 1989) and calcium. The congregation of livestock around small water holes can facilitate the spread of infectious diseases such as tuberculosis and brucellosis.

The impact of droughts can be buffered by feeding supplements to livestock, by sale of stock or their agistment or, in highly intensive systems, by the use of artificial irrigation for livestock crops. Usually grain or hay is used as a supplement, which provides for the energy and protein requirements of the stock. Fodder conservation is an essential part of drought management, but if conditions are too harsh it may be necessary to buy fodder reserves. Grain cannot be suddenly introduced into the ration of undernourished cattle, without running the risk of metabolic upsets. If cattle are adjusted to an all-grain diet, they may still show depraved appetite, e.g. bark and bone chewing, coprophagy and generalised pica. It is important to work out which nutrients are deficient and obtain supplements that are rich in these nutrients, most often protein, energy, sulphur and phosphorus. Urea can be used as an inexpensive source of nitrogen but care must be taken that cattle do not take excessive amounts, which are toxic. Sometimes it is necessary to ration cattle by using blocks or roller balls in drums, which reduce intake by adding a high salt content. This may, however, stimulate demand for water, often in short supply in a drought. Some cattle do not readily compete with others for access to blocks or grain in a trough (Cockwill *et al.*, 2000), and the tolerance of cattle to high sodium concentrations is variable.

In later stages of a drought, it may be necessary to increase the quantities of supplements fed in order that the cattle survive. The effects of drought will be compounded by ill health, particularly that caused by gastrointestinal parasites, which reduce the value of food provided to the cattle. The risks of poisoning become more severe in a drought, as cattle attempt to find additional fodder, similarly their search for water may lead them into dangerous places. In severe winters cattle on rangeland are more likely to consume toxic plants, such as pine needles which induce abortion (Pfister *et al.*, 1998). In severe cold it is usually the absence of forage rather than the low temperatures *per se* which causes stress to cattle (Prescott *et al.*, 1994; Redbo *et al.*, 1996).

Drought management requires considerable skill if the long-term viability of the unit is to be maintained. Overgrazing may satisfy the nutritional require-ments of undernourished cattle temporarily, but in the long term the plant growth capacity is likely to be reduced. Selling unthrifty stock is normally advised for financial reasons, keeping the most valuable breeding stock or those that can gain weight rapidly when conditions improve.

In drought-prone regions, it is important that a drought management strategy is planned in years between droughts. The strategy should include estimates of drought frequency, the cost of supplementation and the financial gain from maintaining cattle growth. Drought frequency has been officially estimated in many regions, since rainfall records have been kept for at least 100 years. For example, on average a major drought will occur in central east Australia every seven years, whereas in the south east of that country it will only occur once every 11 years.

Housing and pasture

Intensification of beef production occurred in industrialised countries towards the end of the twentieth century, largely to increase output through intensive feeding regimes, but also to reduce some costs by housing the cattle. Indoor fat-tening systems that provided cattle with conserved grass or dried cereal grain, or a mixture of the two, gradually replaced systems of fattening cattle on pasture with small amounts of supplementation. The intensification had adverse effects on the welfare of the cattle, since stocking them at high densities led to aggres-sion between animals and health problems, especially lameness and tail tip necrosis on slatted floors and injury in any cattle stocked at a high rate. The main benefit of providing access to pasture is greater space availability, which enables cattle to exercise more fully and reduces the stress of close proximity of other animals. If shelter is provided, it is only used at night in cold or wet conditions (Redbo *et al.*, 1996b). Inside the air is more likely to be contaminated with pathogens or noxious odours, such as ammonia. The action of sunlight on the skin of cattle enables vitamin D to be produced, whereas housed cattle need sup-plements of vitamin D added to the feed. If this is not done, the cattle may devel-op osteoporosis and have reduced fertility.

A sudden change in environment may be more difficult for cattle to cope with than a difficult environment to which they can adapt over time. For example, the transfer of suckled calves to feedlots involves many stresses, particularly adapta-tion to new food types and accommodation (Loerch & Fluharty, 2000). The extensive nature of suckled calf production in most American systems contrasts with the intensive feedlot finishing systems. Some benefit can be derived from introducing a trainer animal, which will encourage new animals to feed and drink (Loerch & Fluharty, 2000). Cattle can adjust to new environments more easily when they are young, and previous experience may considerably influence their satisfaction with their environment.

Overcrowding is common in housed beef cattle. An allowance of 1.5 m^2/finishing beef heifer on slats has been shown to reduce welfare, since growth and lying times were reduced at this density when compared with allowances of up to 3 m^2 (Fisher *et al.*, 1997a). There were no effects on immunity or aggression. In another study with a similar design, cattle stocked at 1.5 m^2/animal lay down for less time than those with 3 m^2/animal, but also performed fewer interactions and had lower baseline cortisol (Fisher *et al.*, 1997b). Cattle stocked at a high rate may be less interactive because of the presence of dominant animals, but these animals may exhibit their authority by mounting subordinate cattle. The buller steer syndrome is recognised mainly in American feedlots, where animals may submit or be forced to accept mounting by other, dominant cattle. If it is sufficiently severe, the mounted animal must be removed or suffer injury or even death. About 2.5% of cattle accepted into feedlots become bullers and mortality rate due to bulling is about 1% (Edwards, 1995). It is therefore a significant welfare problem in feedlot cattle. Bulling activity is more likely to develop in large groups of cattle, over 200 animals, and typically develops after the cattle have been on the lot for about six weeks (Blackshaw *et al.*, 1997). Correction of the problem involves identifying and removing the bullers, avoiding the use of oestrogenic growth promoters and large groups of cattle, and reducing stress by environmental enrichment.

The space allowance for yarded cattle is often less critical than the *quality* of the space, such as floor type. Cattle tend to be cleaner if they are housed on deep straw compared to slats or rubber mats (Lowe *et al.*, 2001), which will affect their value at slaughter. Since cattle spend a significant amount of time grooming each other, which functions partly to keeps their coat clean and free of ectoparasites, it can be assumed that their welfare is reduced if there is significant soiling of the coat. Cattle initially show a marked avoidance of excreta in buildings, but if they are housed there permanently they habituate to its presence (Phillips & Morris, 2001; Phillips *et al.*, 2001).

When conditions are cold outside, cattle reduce their activity levels and lie down more, to reduce evaporative heat losses to the atmosphere. The feeling of being cold is probably rare, even in cattle outside in temperatures as low as −12°C, since shivering is rarely observed (Redbo *et al.*, 1996b). Heat stress is more common, especially where shade is unavailable (Fig. 3.1). Windspeed and relative humidity are also important, but research indicates that cattle are able to cope with quite extreme conditions for short periods (Beverlin *et al.*, 1989).

Stress from flies may be more acute outside than indoors, and the irritation reduces the grazing time and herbage biting rate of cattle. To counteract the irritation, they move their heads, ears, tail and front and hind legs, and skin twitches also increase with the number of flies (Dougherty *et al.*, 1993a,b). In cattle

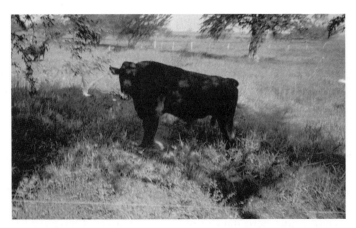

Fig. 3.1 Thermoregulatory behaviour in *Bos indicus* cattle in the tropics. Grazing is avoided in the hottest part of the day and concentrated into the night period.

affected with flies, the front-leg and head and ear movement rates increase as grazing meals progress (Dougherty *et al.*, 1993a,b), suggesting that the level of nuisance caused by the flies increases over time, or that their priority changes form herbage ingestion to fly removal as satiation develops. Other adaptations by the cattle include biting deeper into the sward, perhaps to remove face flies, but also perhaps to increase herbage intake rate so that less time has to be spent grazing, where they are relatively exposed. Another adaptation is to congregate on high ground, where wind may prevent fly infestation.

Ear tags may be used to provide insecticide around the face, but they are normally inserted for identification. The tags used for identification are usually of either metal or polyurethane. Metal tags are more likely to induce a localised reaction than polyurethane ones, with about one half of the animals showing some reaction (Johnston & Edwards, 1996).

Dystokia

Dystokia, or calving difficulty, is a disorder that threatens the viability of both mother and offspring. Fortunately there is opioid-mediated analgesia at parturition, which may be enhanced by ingestion of the afterbirth (Machado *et al.*, 1997). Dystokia is directly linked to genotype, and is most prevalent in beef cattle, since farmers attempt to get large calves from their cows to increase the price that they can sell them for. They therefore often use a large bull on a small cow, which provides the most economic option due to the low maintenance cost of a small cow. The dominant factors in dystokia are the calf size and the area of the pelvic entrance. Breeds that have been selected for muscular hypertrophy, such as the Belgian Blue cattle, are particularly prone to dystokia, especially if there is also a small pelvic entrance (Murray *et al.*, 1999). Breeding goals for sires tend to emphasise the weight of cattle at a certain age, e.g. 400 days, which will increase the fetal growth, causing dystokia unless there is a corresponding increase in the size of the cow carrying the calf. Calving ease could be selectively bred for, since the size of the pelvic opening has a high heritability of 0.3 to 0.7 (Morrison *et al.*, 1986).

Oxen used for traction and other work

Worldwide, oxen are a significant source of draught animal power, even though their use has declined in some parts of the world, because of greater use of tractors and insufficient land to provide animal food. Oxen are preferred to cows, because of their greater strength, even though cows are sometimes favoured for their ability to lactate as well as work. Usually this places too great a demand on the cattle, especially when the only food available is that not required for human consumption. Working cattle are at increased risk of physical injuries, sores and accidents, compared with other cattle. Unlike cattle used for meat or milk production, they are often kept in small groups or individually, congregating only at market places where they may acquire infections. Infectious diseases are likely to reduce work output, and conversely excessive work makes the cattle more prone to infectious diseases (Pearson *et al.*, 1999). Trypanosomasiasis restricts the areas in which cattle can be used for draught purposes.

The nutritional requirements for draught cattle differ from those of growing cattle. High-energy feed is required, since the working energy requirements are high (approximately 1 MJ net energy/h; Vanderlee *et al.*, 1993). Energy requirements can be up to 90% more than maintenance requirements (Fall *et al.*, 1997). Working cattle also sweat a great deal, so additional sodium is required, since sweating depletes blood reserves which are not replenished for several hours after the work has ended (Yadav *et al.*, 2001). Extra water will also be required. Despite these additional nutrient requirements, draught cattle in semi-arid regions are frequently offered by-products, such as cereal crop residues, which have low contents of energy, protein, sodium and water. Alternative feeds include hays and field and roadside grasses, which are usually high in fibre and contain little metabolisable energy. On days when they are used for work, cattle may be in the field working for up to eight hours per day, during which time they cannot eat or ruminate. If they are corralled away from the fields for safety at night, food is often not provided, severely limiting their daily intake. Hence, when cattle are worked for prolonged periods, they usually lose condition unless cereal supplements are provided.

Cattle are also used for pulling carts in many countries and timber in forests in South America. Alternatives include the buffalo for heavy work, but they are less tolerant to heat stress (Pearson, 1989), and for small loads the donkey, which is more drought tolerant than cattle.

Chapter 4
The Welfare of Calves

Perinatal calf behaviour

Environmental influences on the calf start in the womb. For example, calves born to mothers that have been repeatedly transported show a greater response to stress than those born to untransported mothers (Lay *et al.*, 1997). Nutritional influences also start in the womb, for example, the sodium appetite can be conditioned at this time (Mohamed & Phillips, 2001).

At calving, there is a risk of hypoxia, which is increased for large calves in small cows. The bond between cow and calf starts to be formed as the cow licks the calf clean. The licking process stimulates activity in the calf, which encourages teat-searching behaviour. Post-natal behaviour is mainly governed by instinctive motivations, particularly for suckling and hiding in the early post-partum period (Langbein & Raasch, 2000). Suckling motivation directs the calf to find a teat-like object soon after birth, by aiming at a part of the cow's torso shaped thus: Γ, as is provided by the junction between the leg and the trunk. Initially they travel up the vertical leg and then attempt to find a teat at approximately udder height (Broom *et al.*, 1995). Difficulties may arise if the cow has a long pendulous udder, say, if the ligaments are relaxed, or a small udder held closely into the body, as in some young cows. Suckling within six hours gives the calf a source of resistance to infections present in the environment, as well as a source of nutrients, since the cow's blood mixes with milk to allow the calf to obtain the necessary immunoglobulins. The angle of the head while suckling may be important. If the calf is drinking from a bucket in the head down position, the oesophageal groove does not close sufficiently and milk enters the rumen. If the calf drinks from a teat with its head in the horizontal position, the groove closes effectively and milk bypasses the rumen.

The perinatal period of suckled calves is quite different from that of calves weaned early from dairy cows. In the first few days of life, calves at pasture lie passively while their mother obtains food, forming a creche which will often be watched over by a guard cow. Then, over a period of approximately five days, the calves spend less time lying and become more active.

Housing/environment

Calves are often moved to a new environment early in life, and studies of energy expenditure in standing and lying down have shown that they take at least 10 to 12 days to adapt to their new environment (Schrama *et al.*, 1995). Calves that are moved at an early age are up to five times more likely to become ill than calves that are not moved (Webster, 1984). Separation at one day of age can impair social development, with calves separated later, at, say, two weeks of age, having greater response to other calves when they are older and also gaining more weight (Flower & Weary, 2001).

Confinement causes a build-up of motivation for locomotor activity (Jensen & Kyhn, 2000; Jensen, 2001). In a comparison of pens of 56, 66 and 76 cm width, Wilson *et al.* (1999) found that calves in the widest pens spent more time grooming themselves, and those in the narrowest pens had difficulty in changing from a lying to a standing position and in extending their legs whilst recumbent. When not constrained by their pen, pre-ruminant calves normally lie in both the sternally and laterally recumbent positions, unlike older cattle which lie mainly in the sternally recumbent position to avoid passage of fluid from the rumen into the oesophagus. Small pens also reduce the quantity and quality of calves' play behaviour, with highly active play being rare in small pens (Jensen *et al.*, 1998). In group pens some space sharing is possible, since calves will lie close together for warmth or comfort. This leaves much of the pen for locomotion and play, which would be impossible in individual pens. The availability of straw as a substrate for play is important, and the stimulation provided increases the welfare of calves in strawed pens compared with those on slats. Low lighting levels in the calf-house reduce the amount of play and other activities, such as licking objects and feeding (Dannenmann *et al.*, 1985). At low light intensities, calves spend a long time resting. However, other research has shown that calves are more aggressive in the dark and long photoperiods reduce activity, perhaps because the calves are less anxious about their environment (Weiguo & Phillips, 1991). Calves are less sensitive to variation in brightness than are humans (Phillips & Weiguo, 1991), but producers should be aware that high intensity point sources of light, e.g. halogen lights, suspended at low level may stress the calves owing to the glare. Sodium lights or incandescent bulbs are preferable because the wavelength is longer (more yellow/red) than fluorescent, mercury or halogen luminaires, which have more light in the short wavelengths (blue/violet), to which cattle are less sensitive (Phillips & Lomas, 2001).

Individual pens increase the motivation to explore novel environments, compared with group rearing, but calves may be more fearful when isolated in a strange environment (Jensen *et al.*, 1997). Isolation also reduces the social abilities of calves (Fig. 4.1) (Jensen *et al.*, 1999), and they will be dominated by group-reared calves if they are mixed with them. It is better to mix calves from a similar rearing environment, because they are likely to have similar social skills (Veissier *et al.*, 1994). Because isolated calves relate more to their keeper, they

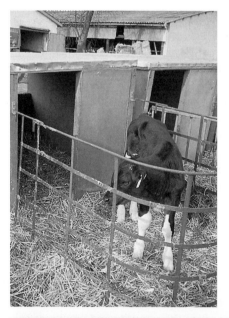

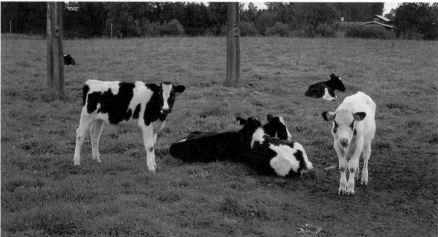

Fig. 4.1 Calves reared in isolation cannot form sibling bonds as they do when reared in an open field.

may be less stressed by handling (Veissier *et al.*, 1998), which in the case of female calves may make them less stressed when they enter the dairy herd (Albright & Stricklin, 1989). However, an increase in milk yield of first lactation cows that had been reared in isolation pre-weaning (Albright & Stricklin, 1989) has not been observed in all experiments (Arave *et al.*, 1992). Calves in individual pens are more likely to develop oral vices, such as tongue-playing, particularly if the pens have solid sides (Seo *et al.*, 1998a,b), but these vices may also derive from inadequate sodium in the diet (Phillips *et al.*, 1999).

Tethering can reduce a calf's lying behaviour as movement is restricted. The later a calf is tethered the greater the effect on the time spent lying (Jensen, 1995). Individual hutches can also provide a stressful environment owing to the isolation, but as with tethering, the calves appear to get used to the stress over time (Macaulay *et al.*, 1995).

The temperature and ventilation relate closely to levels of disease and therefore impact directly on the calf's welfare. Adequate food will ensure that the calf is able to cope with a wide range of temperatures, with an upper critical temperature of 20 to 25°C and lower critical temperature of about 8°C at one week of age (Webster, 1984). For an adequate food supply, the food must be palatable and not too dusty, but not necessarily of high digestibility. The best aerial environment for calves is provided out of doors, as long as cold, damp conditions do not prevail.

Social influences

A potential impact on the welfare of the calf occurs when it is separated from its mother. The responses in the first ten minutes – increased heart rate and vocalisation – are quite mild (Hopster *et al.*, 1995). Feral cattle normally maintain cohesive matriarchal groups, with prolonged bonds formed between cow and calves. Since the bond between the calf and cow extends beyond provision of milk, weaning should be considered as occurring when the cow and calf are separated, which in dairy calves is normally at about one to 14 days of age, not when calves stop receiving milk, normally at about five to seven weeks of age. Calves should not stop receiving milk replacer until they are consuming sufficient solid food, especially concentrate food, i.e. approximately 750 to 1000 g concentrate/day. Beef calves from suckler cows are usually weaned at four to nine months of age, which is still earlier than the natural weaning age in feral cattle. Even when nursing becomes irregular, the mother–calf bond persists throughout the animals' lives in feral cattle herds, and does not wane as new offspring are born (Reinhardt & Reinhardt, 1981). Such bonding is evident in grazing and licking associations. When suckler calves are weaned early, there are combined stresses of separation and loss of natural milk supply. Dissociating these stresses by allowing cow and calf to remain in contact but preventing nursing may reduce the adverse effect on welfare. This can be achieved by keeping them in adjacent fields separated by a fence. Devices can be inserted into the nasal septum which prevent calves suckling, but they are not always effective. When cows and their calves are separated, they spend a long time pacing the field boundaries in an attempt to re-unite, as well as standing and watching each other (Price *et al.*, 2001). Vocalisation is common, but less so if fenceline contact is allowed. Gradually, after two to four days of stressful attempts at contact, cows and calves with fenceline contact begin to utilise the rest of the field area. Loss of weight in the calves following separation, which is a normal consequence of weaning, may be reduced by about half by fenceline contact (Price *et al.*, 2001).

Bonds with peers are most likely to occur with siblings, although some develop with unrelated calves. The earlier calves are weaned, the sooner peer bonds develop, sometimes within a week. Calves in individual pens may have restricted opportunity for interaction with peers. Solid-walled pens offer limited chance of physical contact, but auditory and olfactory communication is still possible. Calves reared in partial isolation spend more time grooming themselves and licking the pen and their neighbours, if they can reach them. The stress of the isolation increases the sodium appetite (Phillips *et al.*, 1999), possibly because of a physiological link, such as the natriorexergenic effect of increased pituitary–adrenal secretion. Failing to provide adequate sodium considerably increases the amount of apparently purposeless oral behaviours, such as licking their buckets, pens and neighbours.

Nutrition

Early in the calf's life, the motivation to suck is very strong. It is maintained after rapidly consuming milk replacer from a bucket or teat (De Passille *et al.*, 1992), which stimulates the release of digestive hormones (De Passille *et al.*, 1993). Slowing the flow of milk replacer fed via a pipe connected to an artificial teat will partly satisfy the calf's need to perform feeding behaviour, and in particular sucking (de Passille, 2001; Loberg & Lidfors, 2001). Controlled sucking devices can, however, cause pituitary abscesses (Fernandes *et al.*, 2000). Automatic feeding devices supplying warm milk to artificial teats enable calves to be group-housed and fed individually from the machine. Enclosing the feeding pen for the calves will lead to longer feeding bouts and more playing with the teat at the end of feeding (Weber & Wechsler, 2001). Failure to satisfy the suckling urge can lead to cross-sucking in group-reared calves, where calves suck each others' body parts, especially the ears, nose, scrotum and navel. This is most common after milk has been consumed, suggesting that it helps to satiate the sucking motivation (Lidfors, 1993). Female calves that cross-suck may develop udder sucking habits as adult cows (sometimes termed intersucking), which can lead to udder damage, mastitis, milk loss and culling of breeding animals. In one Slovakian survey over 5% of cows on large farms had developed this habit (Debreceni & Juhas, 1999), however, a Swiss survey of smaller farms recorded an incidence of just 1.5% (Keil *et al.*, 2001). It has been hypothesised that intersucking persists because it is not prevented, whereas in the situation where cows suckle their calves, the mother's refusal to allow milking at the time of natural weaning would prevent the calf from suckling (Spinka, 1992). Sucking between older calves often starts just after weaning.

Diseases

Calf diarrhoea or scours is commonly caused by *Escherichia coli*, rotaviruses, coronaviruses and Salmonellae species. Loss of fluid is the major welfare risk, although less so now that fluid therapy has become a much more widely accepted treatment. Affected calves lose their appetite. An elevated temperature accompanies many types of infectious diarrhoea, and in the case of salmonellosis the calves may show signs of respiratory distress (Webster, 1984). Feeding of probiotics based on benign bacteria, especially *Lactobacillus acidophilus*, is effective in inhibiting the growth of some bacteria that induce scouring, in particular *Escherichia coli* (Chaves *et al.*, 1999)

Calf pneumonia is largely caused by unsuitable housing conditions, especially inadequate ventilation at times of stress, such as weaning. The diverse range of pathogens causing pneumonia makes it difficult to vaccinate and improved housing is the best cure.

Handling and management

Male castration is mainly performed to reduce the aggressive temperament of bulls. Formerly, when fatty carcases were preferred, it was valuable because it advanced the age at which the cattle started to fatten. Finished cattle could be produced in 18 months, thereby only requiring fodder over one winter, whereas entire bulls would probably need fodder for two winters. Before mechanisation and intensive fertiliser use on pasture made it easier to produce fodder, this was an important consideration. Castration has also proved beneficial in preventing dark cutting, a problem that arises when bulls fight and are stressed before slaughter.

Despite these advantages, the technique is painful for the calves. Surgical removal is the most certain method but may require a local anaesthetic to reduce the pain (Fisher *et al.*, 1996). The pain is intense but it only lasts for a short period. Application of a rubber ring or band produces more prolonged pain, has a longer adverse effect on growth rate, and can leave wounds in older calves (Fisher *et al.*, 2001). A popular alternative is the Burdizzo castrator, which crushes the spermatic cord without damaging the scrotal skin and is less painful than surgical removal.

Dehorning calves prevents them causing injury to other cattle when they are older, particularly if they are in a confined environment, but many breeds are naturally polled. Dehorning is usually achieved by using a hot iron scoop to remove the horn bud. This area, as well as the surrounding tissue, is well innervated (Taschke & Folsch, 1997). The administration of a local anaesthetic lasting about two to four hours prevents any increase in cortisol, but there is a rapid increase after it wears off (McMeekan *et al.*, 1998). Chemical cauterising causes less pain and may not require an anaesthetic, but the solution can run into the animal's eyes, causing great discomfort (Petrie *et al.*, 1996).

For permanent and readily visible marking, cattle are usually branded at about 9 to 12 months of age. This is more stressful if a hot iron is used, rather than by freezing the hair follicles (Schwartzkopf Genswein *et al.*, 1997). Identification of the calves can also be by ear notching, which is less painful (Friend *et al.*, 1994), but because of the limited number of possible markings, it can only be used to distinguish herds, rather than individuals within a herd. Metal or polyurethane tags can be inserted into the ear, but metal ones tend to damage the ear (Johnston & Edwards, 1996), and both will be removed if the cattle get them caught in hedges, etc.

Tail docking of dairy calves is increasingly practised in America as an easy means of preventing the animal having a tail soiled by mud and faeces, which happens when they are kept in dirty conditions. It is performed at about ten days of age by applying a rubber band, in which case the tail either falls off after about 30 days or can be amputated after one week. A hot docking iron can be used, which causes less discomfort than a rubber band. Producers claim that cows with docked tails are cleaner and attract less flies. Swishing the tail is the main method used by calves to remove flies, and the tail is also important for social signalling and to indicate the animal's state. Calves without tails may use other, less successful, methods, such as foot stomping and avoidance of fly-infested areas, to minimise fly numbers. The initial discomfort after docking appears to be mild (Tom *et al.*, 2001), but little is known about whether cattle suffer long-term chronic pain after docking or increased stump sensitivity. The prevention of normal behaviour is considered of sufficient concern for the practice to be banned in some countries.

Veal calves

Veal calves in crates have a lower mortality than those in group pens, but the latter are more able to express their normal patterns of behaviour (Le Neindre, 1993; Plath *et al.*, 1998). Small crates and a dark environment in particular restrict the ability of the veal calf to perform important behaviours adequately, especially lying, grooming and play (see 'Housing/environment' above). An alternative is to leave the calf with its mother until slaughter, but this considerably increases the costs of production. Replacing crates with straw yards also involves a cost, since the efficiency of food conversion is reduced in the latter (Webster, 1984). Iron restriction makes the meat white, which the consumer takes to be an indication that the meat will be tender, although there is little evidence that the taste and texture of 'pink veal' with higher iron levels is worse than 'white veal'. Depleting blood iron status makes calves lethargic. Milk is naturally low in iron, and calves are initially reliant on iron stores in the liver that are present at birth. Calves suckling their dam at pasture will soon get additional iron from pasture, and calves weaned onto solid food will also get adequate iron. The veal producers' aim is to feed sufficient iron to allow normal growth, but to restrict it sufficiently to reduce blood haemoglobin levels. In the EU all calves must have a blood haemoglobin level of at least 4.5 mmol/l, and must receive fibrous food (at least 100 g/day) at two weeks, increasing to 250 g/day at

20 weeks. The provision of fibrous food will assist in achieving adequate haemo-globin levels.

In the long term, better matching of calf production with requirements for beef could end the practice of intensive rearing, particularly if the public can be persuaded that meat of equivalent quality can be reared by other methods. Breeding and feeding dairy cows to have longer lactations will reduce the number of low-value calves produced as a by-product of the dairy industry, which are often reared for veal.

Chapter 5
The Welfare of Cattle During Transport, Marketing and Slaughter

Transport

The traditional practice of driving cattle on foot over long distances to slaughter has now largely been superseded by mechanised transport. Previously drovers moved cattle to market at a rate of about 10 to 15 miles/day and had to protect their stock from excessive hoof wear by shoeing them. Nevertheless the stress on stock was sometimes considerable and losses were often high (Chambers & Mingay, 1966).

Nowadays cattle are transported by road, rail, sea and air. Rail transport is probably best for their welfare, because the animals are attended by a handler and the constant changes in motion direction are reduced. It is, however, generally more expensive than road transport, which is the dominant form of transport for cattle in Europe. In the USA journey times for beef calves are very long (typically 1000 to 3000 km), when they are transported to a feedlot. The distance from the feedlot to the abattoir is, however, usually very short. Road transport involves exposing cattle to a number of potential stressors, including handling by humans (which is especially stressful for extensively reared cattle), mixing with unfamiliar cattle, novel environments, loading onto vehicles and unloading, extreme stimuli (light, sound, vibration, etc.), undernutrition and hyperthermia (Kirkden et al., 2001).

Air transport is fast but expensive, and is usually reserved for excessively long journeys that would be too stressful by road, e.g. cattle sent as aid from Europe to developing countries, or very valuable cattle, such as prize bulls. Continuous access to the animals is essential and the use of humane killers or anaesthetic darts, which would be desirable if the animal becomes highly stressed, is not permitted. Careful consideration should be given to the effects of changes in air pressure and temperature on the cattle.

Mortality during road transport is low for all ages of cattle, compared with other species. Henning (1993) reported a mortality of 0 to 0.01% in adult cattle transported by road in South Africa during the 1980s and 1990s. However, calves and to a lesser extent older cattle often succumb to post-transport respiratory infections and calves may acquire gastrointestinal infections. Sea transportation reduces the cell-mediated immune response, in particular lymphocyte proliferation (Kelley *et al.*, 1981; Blecha *et al.*, 1984). This may be partly due to heat stress, but almost certainly other stressors are influential.

Mortality during sea travel can be greater than during road or air transportation, often because of lack of adequate attention to conditions provided for the cattle. Bruising is frequently observed in cattle following transport, as a result of poor handling techniques, fighting between cattle and injuries incurred during vehicle movement.

Shipping fever

Cattle that suffer prolonged stress during transport are susceptible to respiratory disease within 14 days of arrival. This is usually pneumonic pasteurellosis, caused by infection with *Pasteurella haemolytica* or less commonly *Pasteurella multocida*, and is characterised by pyrexia, dyspnoea and fibrous pneumonia. Primary viral infections, such as infectious bovine rhinotracheitis, may predispose to colonisation of the lungs by pasteurella organisms. In North America, it is the most likely cause of death and approximately 1% of cattle die as a result (Tarrant & Grandin, 2000). During long journeys, there are fewer lymphocytes in blood, which reduces resistance to infection, but a number of studies have shown no relationship between journey length *per se* and the incidence of shipping fever (Kirkden *et al.*, 2001). Other stressors, such as mixing, concurrent weaning and temperature stress, are more likely to be predisposing factors. In beef calves transport often follows weaning, compounding two major stressors. High-concentrate diets fed before transport can reduce the rate of infection, and there is some benefit from providing supplementary nutrients that stimulate the immune system, such as vitamin E and chromium. This will help to counteract the effects of reduced food intake and rumination during transport.

Behaviour during transport

The fact that cattle do not suffer high mortality during transport suggests that they usually cope adequately. However, there are behavioural changes that demonstrate that transport does have adverse effects on welfare. During the journey they lie down less than normal, and they often do not lie down until 15 hours have passed. This may be because they may not be able to get back up after they lie down. If they are highly stocked, they are more likely to stumble and will often remain lying afterwards. Braking is a greater hazard at low stocking densities, whereas cornering is more stressful at high densities (Tarrant & Grandin, 2000). They are most likely to lie down voluntarily if they are in small groups of two or three animals in individual pens. After a journey, cattle will lie down for longer than normal, suggesting that it is a high priority for them to maintain normal lying times.

When standing, cattle usually orientate themselves in a perpendicular or, less commonly, a parallel direction in relation to the direction of travel, but rarely at a diagonal angle (Tarrant & Grandin, 2000). The amount of movement of the animals is largely determined by the type of driving, fast driving on windy roads will cause the animals to have to move regularly to counteract centrifugal forces and rapid acceleration and deceleration. Driving on straight roads at a steady speed appears to be considerably less stressful for the animals. Thus braking, gear changes and cornering should be as gradual as possible. The presence of one highly stressed animal that is moving about a great deal is likely to trigger movements in the other cattle. A slippery floor is also a risk factor, and the frequent urination of stressed cattle exacerbates the problem. At the beginning of the journey cattle defecate and urinate frequently because of the stress. This causes them to lose weight, which can only be recovered after several days of rest. As the journey progresses urination frequency remains high.

Road transport is governed by the strictest legislation in the EU. Cattle should be transported in a vehicle meeting specified standards for all journeys over 50 km in the UK. By EU regulations (Directive 91/628, amended 95/29), if the journey is less than 50 km it cannot take more than eight hours and must be followed by 24 hours' rest. If more than 50 km and in a vehicle of specified standards, the initial journey should not be longer than 14 hours, or nine hours in the case of unweaned calves, with a mid-journey rest of at least one hour during which water should be available. If the rest is more than two hours, it may be necessary to unload the animals to reduce stress, in which case food can be offered as well as water. However, the stress of unloading and reloading during a break may increase the total trauma caused by the journey. Although cattle start eating quickly after unloading, it is several days before glycogen reserves are restored, and it seems likely that a one hour rest off the vehicle is of little value. During the rest, preweaned calves should be offered an electrolyte solution, rather than milk, as the stress may cause scouring. A further maximum journey of 14 hours is allowed following the rest. An extension of two hours to the final journey can be added if the cattle will reach their destination, as long as the vehicle is of high quality. A recent amendment to the EU regulations establishes the need for staging posts in long journeys, at which cattle must be given a 24 hour rest before continuing. There are plans to develop a number of staging posts around the EU, which will be kept in a disease-free state, by regular disinfection and resting of the area.

Standards are specified for vehicles travelling over 50 km. Vehicles should be fitted with a sound roof to protect cattle from the weather if they are travelling long distances. Ventilation is vitally important and air inlets must be provided, and must be opened when the vehicle is stationary. These inlets are usually at the top of the side wall, to prevent draughts, and the aperture depth should be at least 20 cm. These apertures can also be used for inspection of the animals during resting stops. There should be another point of entry to the vehicle for inspection purposes apart from the loading point. This is usually a small door in the side wall.

Loading should be via either a ramp or a lifting platform. Ramps should have a gradient of less than 25°, and should be fitted with battens that are at least 25 mm high and positioned at 20 to 30 cm intervals. Lifting platforms should have side barriers of at least 130 cm for large cattle or 90 cm for young calves. Large gaps between the ramp and the vehicle or the floor should be avoided, otherwise the animals' legs can get trapped. Permanent loading platforms have been constructed on some farms, which take animals gradually to the height of the vehicle and reduce the stress associated with going up a ramp.

Stocking density

There are adverse effects on the welfare of cattle if the stocking density on vehicles is either too low or too high. If too low, they move around more, with potential bruising and stress, unless the journey is particularly smooth. If too high, there is potentially more heat stress, psychological stress from close proximity of other animals, less possibility to regain their stance after sudden vehicle movement and a likelihood that if they fall they will be unable to get back up as other animals will have closed in around them. Therefore on particularly smooth journeys the lower stocking densities are probably preferable, but on normal journeys there will be an optimum density, based on the factors cited above. There are few empirical data on which to base optimum stocking densities, but recommendations from different bodies are broadly similar (Table 5.1). They are usually expressed as maxima or optima, but rarely minima, and are calculated in metabolic live weight, (live weight)$^{0.67}$, or a similar function per m^2. Most commonly used is the maximum stocking density recommended by the UK's Farm Animal Welfare Council, according to the following formula:

$$A = 0.021W^{0.66}$$

where A is the minimum area in m^2 per animal and W is the live weight in kg (Farm Animal Welfare Council, 1991). Using this formula, it can be calculated

Table 5.1 Recommended space allowances and maximum group size for cattle during road transport

	Weight (kg)	Space allowance (m^2)	Maximum group size
Young calves	40–80	0.33	25–30
Old calves	80–150	0.70	15–25
Young steers/heifers	150–300	0.7–1.1	10–15
Older steers	300–700	1.1–1.6	10
Cows	>450	1.3–1.7	5
Bulls	>550	1.7–2.0	5

From Connell (1984).

that adult cattle require 1 m^2 per 360 kg and calves require 1 m^2 per 180 kg. The behavioural reactions of male, female or neutered cattle to transport appear similar, so recommendations are not specific for gender.

Pen size should not be too great or the cattle may aggregate at one end. UK Ministry regulations stipulate that pens should not exceed 2.5 m for calves and 3.7 m for older cattle (Ministry of Agriculture, Fisheries and Food, 1997). Internal divisions should be of an appropriate height – 76 cm for calves and 127 cm for older cattle. Bedding must always be available to provide a soft area for lying, to absorb urine and to insulate the animals in cold conditions. To provide sufficient air space above the cattle, the roof of the vehicle should be at least 5 cm higher than calves and 10 cm above older cattle.

Only fit animals should normally be transported, however, unfit animals may be transported to slaughter providing the journey will not make them unnecessarily suffer as a result of their disability. In the UK, unfit animals cannot be mechanically put onto vehicles for transport (Ministry of Agriculture, Fisheries and Food, 1998), and animals in severe pain should be slaughtered on site. Although a veterinary inspection is not required before moving casualty animals, farmers must complete a declaration with the details of the illness, which accompanies the animal to the slaughterhouse where the suitability of the animal for transportation will be confirmed. Casualty animals should be isolated in the vehicle as long as this does not cause further distress.

The responsibility for the cattle during transport legally lies with two people. The driver of the vehicle is responsible for their immediate safe conduct whilst they are in his or her hands, but the person who consigns the goods, who is often the owner, may also be responsible for their welfare, particularly if there are several modes of transport used in one journey. EU law requires the registration of all commercial transporters of cattle. In the UK the authorisation differs according to the length of journey that the driver is allowed to make (more than eight hours, termed *special* authorisation, or less than eight hours, termed *general* authorisation). Journeys by sea, air or rail require special authorisation, as do any journeys between different member states. The latter also require a route plan, which is authorised by a Divisional Veterinary Manager and signed by someone representing the animals' owner. If route plans are not required, an Animal Transport Certificate is required to specify the name and address of the owner and transporter and basic details of the journey.

Markets

In the UK nearly three million cattle are auctioned annually, including 0.5 million calves. These can be viewed at any time by the public, and as such it is important that standards are high. Weekly markets evolved from the seasonal fairs for the sale of livestock that were driven to them, sometimes over quite a long distance. In the middle of the nineteenth century, weekly markets became favoured by tax laws and permanent sites were established with pens and buildings. Many of the markets were originally situated close to the centres of towns, but have often moved further out because of traffic congestion and the high value of land near to the centre. Over the last 50 years there has also been a decline in the number of markets in the UK from about 1000 to under 200. The decline in the number of abattoirs, as the standards required are increased to EU levels, has resulted in markets fulfilling a role as a centre for collection and distribution of animals, before transport to abattoirs.

Increasingly the use of markets is questioned, not just because of the stress caused to the animals, but also because of the potential for disease transmission, which became evident during the 2001 foot and mouth outbreak in the UK. Cattle which go through markets, rather than travelling direct to an abattoir, are more likely to suffer bruising (Hoffman *et al.*, 1998), which will downgrade the carcase and is direct evidence that auction markets are damaging the welfare of cattle.

The time pressures put on staff in markets may encourage them to mistreat cattle to accelerate animal movement, but it is in no-one's interest to mistreat the animals severely as they may become more difficult to move. Training programmes have been developed, which instruct market personnel in handling and welfare of stock in their care. Electronic auctions have become commonplace in North America, mainly because distances that animals would have to be transported to a live market are large. They are beginning to be used in Europe, but more for animal welfare and health reasons.

The standards of animal welfare in markets have for some time been a focus of attention, and there is also considerable concern that the number of movements that an animal makes during its lifetime should be reduced. In the UK, welfare standards are legislated under The Market Sales and Lairs Order 1925 and Amendments, The Welfare of Animals in Markets Order 1990 and Amendment and the Welfare of Animals (Transport) Order 1997.

A voluntary code of practice was introduced by the Livestock Auctioneers Association in 1996 (Livestock Auctioneers Association, 1996). This makes a number of recommendations to maintain welfare at markets. Each market should have an Animal Health and Welfare Officer, who is responsible for the health, hygiene and welfare of stock, including preparation of the premises for the sale, loading and unloading of animals, penning, food and water supply to the animals and removal of animals. A deputy may be appointed with responsibility for specific classes of stock in large markets. The name and contact details should be prominently displayed in the market. This appointment does not absolve the market managers or auctioneers from their duty to animal welfare. During the sale of an animal at a market, its ownership and the responsibility for its welfare pass from the person who brought it to the market, to the auctioneer and finally to the purchaser or his representative. It is also recommended that markets are attended by a veterinary surgeon. If this is not possible, arrangements should be made for one to attend at short notice. All incidents have to be recorded and this can be used as evidence by the state veterinary service or local authorities in dealing with a persistent problem. Pens for dairy cows and calves should be covered, and hygienic conditions should be maintained in all pens, with provision of bedding, especially for calves. The time that the animals spend in the pens should be restricted to a minimum. Isolation pens should be provided for sick animals and the sale of sick animals is prohibited. Livestock weighbridges should be suitably designed to prevent injury to the stock. Sale rings should have suitable floors and straw or other material spread on them to prevent slipping.

Markets are inspected by personnel from local authorities in the agriculture department. These people also hold meetings of interested bodies, organise training for market personnel and ensure that veterinary staff are available. The local authorities are responsible for taking action if welfare infringements occur in markets within their area. It is recommended that annual market liaison meetings are held between the market operators, local authorities and the state veterinary service. It is also recommended by the UK's Livestock Auctioneers Association that water should be provided so that animals do not become thirsty. Especially at risk are lactating animals during hot weather. Water should be provided to cattle during a long stay, in particular those staying overnight (as required by legislation). Food should be provided every 12 hours. In the past there has been some resistance by the buyers to the provision of water because of the increase in the animal's weight. Hygiene should also be attended to as soon as possible after the market, with adequate disinfection of all pens. Cows should be milked at the normal times, and the temptation to delay so that the cows are displayed with turgid udders should be resisted. The size of an udder is in any case not a good indicator of milk yield.

Livestock are either sold in their pens or through sales rings, where the animals are brought to the buyers. Sales are invariably by auction, and there is no doubt that the markets perform an important social function for farmers, many of whom live in isolated areas. Most purchases are by farmers themselves, or agents who purchase on behalf of farmers or abattoirs. Much of the detail of requirements for abattoir lairage applies to market pens. Cattle should not be overstocked, mixing should be avoided, and electric goads should only be used if absolutely necessary and applied only to the hindquarters. The use of sticks with points or nails in them is prohibited and when a stick is used, it should be as an extension to the handler's arm, not as a weapon. Cattle should not be moved by twisting their tail, and broken tails provide evidence of this. Similarly calves should not be kicked, dragged by a neck tie, lifted by their tails or punched. Calves cannot be auctioned under seven days of age or with a wet navel. Farmers' dogs can also distress cattle and should be effectively controlled.

Much can be done to improve the design of new markets to improve the welfare of cattle being sold there. Permanent loading and unloading ramps can be provided, as well as passageways for more efficient movement of animals around the market. Lairage and pens must be provided with water and shade. Floors should be non-slip with grooved concrete, and in areas of heavy animal traffic, such as in an auction ring, the floor should have a covering of sand, straw or wood shavings. The auction ring should be central in the market, to minimise animal traffic. Smooth flow of animals should receive detailed planning, with no projections or sharp turns that might injure animals. Regular removal of urine and faeces must be allowed for and there should be contingency plans for dealing with escaped and injured cattle.

There is also a voluntary code of practice for livestock auctioneers that controls the buyers' rights, for example that cows will not have been the subject of embryo transfer or a caesarian operation unless stated in the programme (Livestock Auctioneers Association, 1998). The UK government also issues guidelines in the form of Codes of Practice for the Welfare of Animals in Livestock 1998.

Slaughter

Every year about two million cattle are slaughtered in the UK through about 400 abattoirs. The number of abattoirs licensed to EU standards is small, leading to long journeys. When they arrive the cattle may be held in lairage to allow them to recover, or they may go direct to slaughter.

Lairage

In terms of animal welfare, the quality of the lairage is of major importance. Lairage allows the slaughterhouse to receive animals at all times and to plan the killing efficiently without needing to slaughter as soon as animals arrive. It also allows animals an opportunity to rest, which may improve meat quality. If, however, the lairage is inadequate and animals have to be mixed, the stress induced may reduce meat quality, especially when bulls are slaughtered.

In the UK, it is recommended that loose cattle should have at least 2.3 to 2.8 m^2 each, tied cattle 3.3 m^2 each and calves (up to six months) at least 0.7 m^2. In addition all cattle should have enough space to stand up, lie down and turn around. Walls must be high enough to prevent animals climbing over them and be easily cleaned. They are usually solid sided to reduce stress to the animals. Draught-free ventilation and slip-free floors are important for the animals' welfare. An animal that slips or damages itself on protruding objects may bruise itself, leading to reduced carcase revenue. Lighting must be provided for inspection, but should be dimmed at night.

Water and conserved fodder is normally provided, but the latter may only be in the form of straw put in the pen for bedding. In the UK, animals that are to be slaughtered within 12 hours do not have to have food provided.

Movement to stunning

The route to the stunning area should be clear. Animals will always move more easily if they go from a dimly lit area to a well lit one, round gentle bends rather than sharp corners, and slightly uphill rather than downhill. Other distractions to moving cattle include sparkling reflections on a wet floor, air hissing, high-pitched noise, air draughts blowing towards approaching animals and poor maintenance of facilities, such as worn-out or slick floors that cause animals to fall (Grandin, 1996). An abattoir survey in Canada found that 21% of plants had slick floors that would cause animals to slip and fall, and 27% had high-pitched motor noise or hissing air that caused animals to baulk, and air draughts were a problem in 10% of plants (Grandin, 1996).

Encouragement to cattle to move should preferably be given by a stick used as an extension to the handler's arm, not as a weapon. A purpose-built electric goad can only be applied to the hindquarter muscles in the UK if the shocks are for no more than two seconds, are well spaced out and there is room for the animal to move forward [The Welfare of Animals (Slaughter and Killing) Regulations, 1995]. Even then cattle will often vocalise after the shock as a sign of distress and this can be used as a sign of poor welfare (Grandin, 1998). The route to the stunning crush should be clear and direct. Cattle may baulk at the site of the crush, showing signs of alarm and fear, perhaps followed by submission if excessively challenged, e.g. with frequent use of the electronic goad. The goad is of little value after an animal has gone down, as it will only exacerbate the non-compliance, whereas retreat by the handler will eventually cause the animal to stand.

The stunning and slaughter processes

The cattle first enter a crush for stunning, which usually has solid sides, one of which can be released to allow the animal to roll out of the crush after stunning. The sides are usually narrower at the bottom of the pen than the top, so that if the animal goes down before stunning it does not fall to the floor but gets wedged in. This makes it easier for it to stand again. Fixed head restraints are not usually used because they cause considerable distress to the animals.

Cattle are stunned with either a captive bolt or a non-penetrating concussion stunner. Occasionally a free bullet is used. The captive bolt is retractable and should travel into the brain at 73 m/s, creating sufficient intracranial pressure to make the animal unconscious. Lower speeds and less effective stunning may occur if the machine is not regularly cleaned (Gregory, 1998). There are unconfirmed reports that up to 7% of cattle are ineffectively stunned, with 3% needing to be stunned twice (Hornsby, 1990). The gun is fired by a trigger or upon contact. It is noisy, so disturbing cattle in line for stunning. The concussion stunner is a bolt with a mushroom-shaped head that is fired in the same way as the captive bolt. In some countries it is forbidden as it is often ineffective and heavy haemorrhaging of the nose is common. Following stunning, the animals are generally unconscious within 10 to 12 seconds.

Young cattle may be stunned electrically but this only results in their being unconscious for about 18 seconds (Anil *et al.*, 1995). Both calves and adult cattle are then hoisted and stuck with a knife, whose function is to sever the brachiocephalic trunk. Visually evoked responses are extinguished within five seconds.

Religious slaughter

Halal, Shechita and Jhatka methods of slaughter are practised by Muslims, Jews and Sikhs, respectively (Gregory, 1998). In the UK all religious slaughter must be conducted in a licensed slaughterhouse, and local authorities license the slaughtermen. Slaughtermen are given extensive training for Jewish but not Muslim slaughter. Stunning is not usually practised as it is believed that the animals should be conscious at the time of death. However, some countries, most notably those in Scandinavia, require stunning for all cattle. Death is caused by severing the major blood vessels in the neck with a knife, and by decapitation in the Jhatka method. Muslim slaughterers must invoke the name of Allah before the event. Blood must be thoroughly drained after death as both Muslims and Jews are forbidden from eating blood, a custom which originally reduced disease risk in the hot countries where these traditions evolved. Cattle are stuck in Halal slaughter but in Shechita slaughter there is a cut through the abdominal wall and diaphragm. Then a Jewish inspector places his arm into the chest cavity to inspect the animal's condition. This can occur when technically the animal is still alive.

Dark cutting

This is of major concern for meat quality, but is also indicative of a welfare problem. Cattle that are stressed pre-slaughter are prone to excessive depletion of their muscle glycogen stores, which leads to a high pH, particularly in the hindquarters, and dark, firm dry meat with poor organoleptic properties. If the energy demand is too great, it is met by anaerobic metabolism of carbohydrate reserves, potentiated by adrenergic activation, with less lactic acid production. The resulting high pH reduces shelf-life, because bacterial growth is facilitated, and the meat is dark as less myoglobin is oxygenated (Warriss, 1990). With reduced glycogen reserves, bacteria use glucose and amino acids on the surface of the meat for substrates. The putrefactive amines generated give the meat its characteristic spoiled odour. Resting of the cattle following stress may be of little value, since it takes three days or more to restore glycogen levels. It is therefore better to slaughter stress-susceptible cattle on arrival at the slaughterhouse, rather than holding them overnight. Where the latter is inevitable, the risk of dark cutting increases significantly.

Glycogen reserves in the liver and muscles are depleted both by the heavy muscular work, and often by long-term inanition. The condition is most common in young bulls, in which mounting is more likely than in steers and heifers, and particularly occurs after bulls have been stressed by mixing and/or a difficult journey. About 20 years ago a survey showed that the proportion of animals classified as 'dark cutters' was 11 to 15% for young bulls, 6 to 10% for cows and 1 to 5% for steers and heifers, with the value of the carcase being reduced by about 10% (Tarrant, 1981). Steers that have been mixed and regrouped several times pre-slaughter also show dark cutting, as do heifers in oestrus. Mixing stress-susceptible cattle such as bulls (Kenny & Tarrant, 1987a), deprivation of energy intake pre-slaughter and high temperatures (Immonen *et al.*, 2000) will all increase the risk of dark cutting. Particular care should be taken with horned cattle, which should not be mixed unless they have been reared together. The amount of fighting pre-slaughter closely correlates with the post-slaughter muscle pH. Fighting is most common between young bulls, but even then it is rare in well-fed and rested animals. The bulls are most likely to be aggressive when they are mixed in lairage. Mounting of subordinate cattle is common, leading directly to glycogen depletion (Le Neindre *et al.*, 1996), but can be prevented by hanging electrified chains just above the animal's back. An animal's experience has a major influence, with cattle that are used to close confinement and stress having a less pronounced reaction to the stresses imposed in the period up to slaughter than those reared in extensive conditions. In any event, several hours of stress are required to produce dark-cutting in well-fed cattle. The condition can be avoided by keeping bulls separate before slaughter or by slaughtering immediately on arrival at the abattoir.

Double-muscled cattle are particularly susceptible to stress (Monin, 1981). They are more easily exhausted during exercise and develop metabolic acidosis more readily, through reduced lung size and less capacity of the organs that utilise lactic acid – heart, liver, kidney, etc.

Chapter 6
Environmental Perception and Cognition

Introduction

An animal's behaviour is its reactions to stimuli, which are largely determined by its perception of the internal and external environment. The internal environment is created mainly by endogenous rhythms, which generate motivation but are influenced by exogenous circumstances. The external environment is perceived through sensory faculties, especially the five classical senses of sight, taste, hearing, olfaction and touch. Other environmental phenomena are perceived, such as gravitational forces and the weather, and, though generally of less importance, may at times strongly influence behaviour. Also, cattle sense man-made forces, such as electricity and perhaps electromagnetism.

Signals are produced by the sensory receptors, which are often contained in specialised organs. The signals are then processed by the brain to produce information that can be acted upon and remembered if necessary. Cattle differ considerably from humans in both their sensory and processing capacities, and a more detailed knowledge of this information and the use to which it is put is essential if we are to understand their interaction with their environment.

Vision

Some of the major senses are used relatively infrequently, but vision is involved to some extent in the perception of most stimuli and is, as in humans, the dominant sense in many situations (Blaschke *et al.*, 1984) and responsible for approximately 50% of total sensory information. Aspects of visual information processing can be estimated by optometric measurements (e.g. radius of curvature and refractive power of the eye), by measuring neural activity in the visual cortex of the brain or by investigating the behaviour of the animal psychophysically.

Animals obtain visual information in stages. Initially a primal sketch is formed from the retinal images; then from this is extracted the relevant information, such as depth, motion, shape, size and shadow, which is processed to form a stereoscopic image. Finally there is abstraction in combination with cognitive memory to produce information that can be stored and acted upon. In farm animals, the first stage – primal sketch formation – is probably similar to that in humans because eye structure is similar.

Colour vision

Cattle have both rod and cone receptors, with two to three rods per cone in the fovea and five to six near the papilla. This suggests a good mechanism for dichromatic colour vision and it has been confirmed psychophysically that cattle can distinguish different colours (Gilbert & Arave, 1986; Riol *et al.*, 1989; Phillips & Lomas, 2001), especially those in long wavelengths (yellow, orange and red). The ability for animals like cattle that were once prey to perceive red accurately and respond rapidly may reflect its survival value when a member of the herd was attacked and blood appeared. This feature of cattle vision may be utilised when bullfighters provide a red stimuli for the bull to charge, since red stimulates increased activity (Phillips & Lomas, 2001). Colour discrimination may also be useful in food selection – green food is more attractive than red food (Uetake & Kudo 1994), and cattle appear to retain their memory for colours for long periods (Porzig & Laube 1977). Cattle have difficulty in distinguishing the shorter wavelengths, blue, grey and green (Riol *et al.*, 1989).

Image quality

In common with many other mammals, there is evidence that cattle may be myopic (Rohler, 1962). Basic shape discrimination is possible, for example between squares, circles, triangles and single or double lines (Baldwin, 1981). However, visual acuity is less than 1/50th of that possible in humans, with estimates varying from 12 to 24 arc minutes. From a distance of 1.5 m, cattle can only detect a white circle of diameter 1 cm or more, when it is within a black circle of diameter 36 cm (Rehkamper & Gorlach, 1998). Their pupil is ovoid, which gives them better acuity in a vertical plane (Rehkamper *et al.* 2000), because the edge of the pupil is used to enhance the sharpness of the image on the retina, and changes in the shape of the pupillary cleft will be mainly in the vertical plane. Altering the refractive index in the vertical plane of the eye (Pierscionek, 1994) might help to focus the image, but cattle probably have little ability to change the shape of their lens (accommodation), even though it is pliable. The image is probably more effectively perceived in the peripheral regions of the retina than in humans. However, cattle also have a 'visual streak' – an elongated area of high ganglion cell density in the horizontal plane of the retina. This will help to identify predators on the horizon. Since cattle spend much of their time grazing, when the pupillary cleft is not parallel to the horizon but 20 to 30° below it, the eliptical shape may function to create a sharp image of vertical objects on the horizon. Visual acuity may be better for moving objects than static ones.

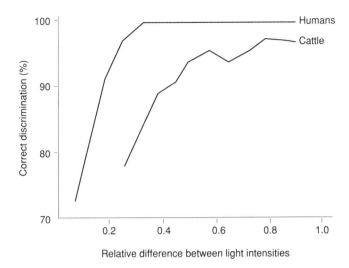

Fig. 6.1   Light intensity discrimination abilities of humans and cattle (Phillips & Weiguo, 1991).

Cattle are able to discriminate objects of different light intensity, but not as well as humans (Fig. 6.1) (Phillips & Weiguo, 1991). They may use this to select dark green herbage, which has a better nutritional value.

Field of vision and stereopsis

Eyes are positioned on the side of the head to give a wide field of vision, about 330°, which is good for predator awareness. The limited overlap of ruminant eyes, only 30 to 50° compared to 140° in man, means that stereoscopic vision is probably limited at short distances, depending on the position of the fovea (Fig. 6.2). However, other means are employed to judge distance: moving objects can be positioned by overlap of monocular cues (parallax), and memory of object size will allow distance to be estimated. Recognition of danger is probably easier if the subject is moving and can be recognised and related to previous experience.

Photoperiodism

In addition to receiving and conveying information on visual images, photoperiodism is used to set the internal clock. Perception of photoperiod is relative rather than absolute, since there are residual effects of photoperiod when it is artificially manipulated. Cattle produce a physiological response to a long day when a six hour day is supplemented with a burst of light for 15 to 60 minutes in the middle of the dark period, demonstrating that they have a photosensitive period about 15 to 18 hours after dawn. Although diurnal rhythms are evident in the absence of photoperiodic cues, the light:dark cycle is responsible for the fine control of the clock.

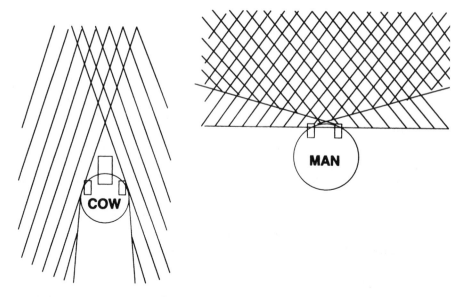

Fig. 6.2 The human and bovine visual fields showing the area of binocular overlap where stereoscopic vision is possible.

In cattle the length of the light cycle also affects reproduction (to match peak intake requirement of offspring to peak feed availability) and production. Cattle probably perceive both rate of change and actual photoperiod. Productivity is reduced when cows are in a declining, short daylength. Extending daylength can improve a poor environment for cattle, leading to less aggression and locomotion (Weiguo & Phillips, 1991), which may be related to a feedback of prolactin on the hypothalamus, causing neurons to increase dopamine synthesis (Zinn *et al.*, 1989). Cattle will work for a light reward, and their preference is for a daylength of approximately 16 hours (Baldwin & Start, 1981), which has also been shown to give the highest productivity compared with 10 or 24 hour daylengths.

Hearing

Although hearing is suspected to be less important to cattle than vision, it is of particular importance in intraspecies communication. Vocal communication in cattle is much less complex than in humans, although it does extend to recognisable syllables (see Chapter 9).

Auditory powers can be determined from an animal's behaviour, its head size and morphology of the pinnae. Compared to other mammals, cattle have better hearing at low frequencies and worse hearing at high frequencies. The high-frequency hearing limit is generally related to the interaural distance, if it is large, such as in elephants, the high-frequency hearing limit is low. Cattle have a similar interaural distance to that of humans but a greater high-frequency hearing limit (Fig. 6.3) (Heffner & Masterton, 1990). This may relate to the need for cattle to be able to hear small predators, such as vampire bats *(Desmodus rotundus),* that use high-frequency vocalisations. On hearing the call of the vampire bat, cattle will flee and disperse to an open area where bats are unlikely to attack (Delpietro, 1989). High-pitched sounds, such as from parlour machinery, may disturb cattle but not be audible to man.

The optimum frequency (where sound can be heard at the lowest amplitude) occurs at 1 to 4 kHz in humans and 8 kHz in cattle (Fig. 6.4), and here the intensity threshold is lowest at about −11 decibels (Heffner & Heffner, 1983). This optimum frequency is usually reserved for the overtones of high-frequency alarm calls, which in cattle reach 8 kHz. Below this intensity the hearing threshold increases, i.e. the sound has to be louder to be heard, and the minimum frequency that can be detected by humans and cattle is similar at 20 to 25 Hz. Above 8 kHz hearing threshold increases again, and the maximum intensity that can be perceived is 35 kHz in cattle but only 20 kHz in humans.

A second aspect of hearing – binaural localisation – relates to the animal's ability to position a sound accurately, in the same way that stereopsis enables the distance of a visual stimulus to be determined. Many species, particularly those that evolved as predators, are able to locate the direction of a sound accurately in the vertical plane. They are generally less able to judge sound direction in the horizontal plane or to judge the distance that the sound has travelled before it reaches them. There are two mechanisms that can be used for sound localisation

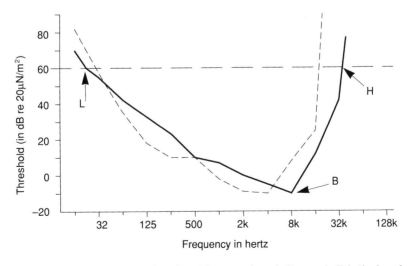

Fig. 6.3 Hearing curve in cattle (——) and humans (– – –). For cattle B is the best hearing frequency, H is the high frequency hearing limit and L is the low-frequency hearing limit (Heffner & Mastarton, 1990).

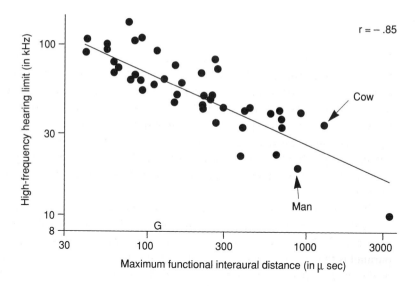

Fig. 6.4 Relation between maximum functional interaural distance (interaural distance/speed of sound) and the highest audible frequency (at 60 db SPL) for more than 40 mammals with complete behavioural audiograms (Heffner & Masterton, 1990).

in the vertical plane: first, differences in the phase of the sound as it arrives at the two ears, which is used to locate low-frequency tones; and secondly, differences in the frequency of the sound between the two ears, which serves better to locate high-frequency tones. Both cattle and man might be expected to have good sound localisation abilities because of their large interaural distance (Fig. 6.4). However, whereas humans use both mechanisms to be able to accurately locate a sound to within 1°, cattle use mainly intensity difference cues and can only locate a sound to within 30°. From an evolutionary perspective, it was important for predators such as humans to pinpoint accurately the direction of their prey, whereas prey animals, such as cattle, need only an approximate idea of where danger lies before fleeing. Some animals, such as man, that have a fovea and good visual acuity in the centre of their field of vision, need to reinforce this with accurate sound localisation. Cattle, with their broad field of best vision (about 130° compared with 1° in man) and their retinal cell concentration, do not need this degree of accuracy. The extents of binocular vision and binaural localisation powers are probably also linked physiologically.

Auditory stimuli such as music may encourage dairy cows to approach voluntary milking systems (Uetake *et al.*, 1997), although definitive evidence is not yet available. Cattle can be trained to advance to a milking parlour or a feeding site in response to an auditory stimulus (Albright *et al.*, 1966), and there is anecdotal evidence that dairy cows produce more milk when music is played to them at milking time (Evans, 1990).

Olfaction

In common with most other vertebrates, cattle are able to detect odours from inanimate and animate objects and utilise the information to modify their reproductive, ingestive or social behaviour. The detection of odours has been studied less than other primary senses, but they are clearly of major significance to cattle, which evolved as prey animals needing durable, covert signalling. Olfactory signals are used particularly in intraspecies communication, where they synchronise reproduction, act as territorial markers and signal the presence of predators. Other possible messages from odours include aggression, hunger and anxiety.

The first stage in odour perception is when the odour enters the oronasal cavity by the mouth or nasal orifices. This chemically stimulates olfactory receptor neurons (ORNs), which terminate in cilia that are bathed in mucus. Acting in parallel is the chemosensitive trigeminal pathway, whose neurons also terminate in the nasal cavity. Neurons in this pathway are activated by many of the same chemical stimuli that activate ORNs, but the trigeminal system is particularly specialised in detecting irritants.

The third major site of odour reception in cattle, in addition to the olfactory and nasal trigeminal free nerve endings, is the vomeronasal organ, which is absent in adult humans. It is situated in the roof of the mouth and consists of blind tubular diverticula, lined with olfactory epithelium. Vomeronasal organ neurons are not ciliated but end in microvilli, which are particularly sensitive to hydrated low-volatile compounds. These are common in urine and are used for social and sexual communication, particularly the detection of oestrous females by the male. The reception of odours by the vomeronasal organ is also used for reinforcement and the maintenance of sexual interest during copulation. Air is sampled via the buccal cavity and the nose, although the nostrils are partially closed by the curling of the lip in this behaviour. The characteristic flehman expression, in which the head is directed upwards with the mouth ajar, the tongue flat and the upper lips curled back (Fig. 6.5), is thought to aid odour sampling in ruminants by allowing air to contact the roof of the mouth during inhalation. Flehman is also believed to act for appeasement, being the antithesis of the threat display.

Pheromones are a specialised group of chemical attractants produced by animals to stimulate other animals. They are present in all body fluids including sweat, and there are many different types in cattle, including alcohols, diols, alkanes, ethers, diethers, ketones, primary amines and aromatic alkanes. The oestrous pheromones are mainly released from the body surface, particularly the hindquarters and genital region, rather than in urine, faeces or vaginal mucus (Blazquez *et al.*, 1988). Cows in oestrus spend much time sniffing and licking the anovaginal areas of other cows. Bulls respond to odours produced by teaser bulls even more than to pheromones identified in the blood of oestrous cows (Presicce *et al.*, 1993).

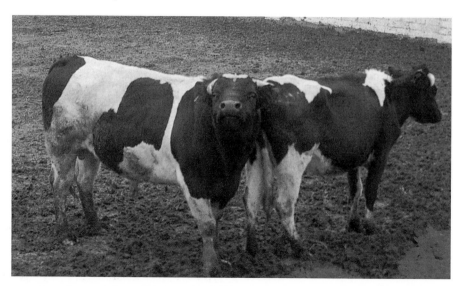

Fig. 6.5   Flehman expression in a bull guarding a cow.

Pheromones also convey fear, and cattle respond to the pheromones produced by fearful conspecifics by increasing cortisol production and stopping activities that might expose them to perceived dangers, such as feeding (Boissy *et al.*, 1998). Fear pheromones are present in the blood (Terlouw *et al.*, 1998) and also in other body fluids, such as urine. Cattle are also sensitive to the odours of potential predators, such as dogs, spending more time sniffing the air and in cautious movement (Terlouw *et al.*, 1998).

Comparative mammalian olfaction

Other ungulates use scent marking more extensively than cattle – the dikdik builds dung heaps and rubs its forehead on them to increase its scent, and the pronghorn urinates before defecating to amplify the scent. Deer have tarsal and sudoriferous scent glands in their head to mark their territory. Sheep are reputed to be able to track conspecifics in mountain territory, presumably by detecting tarsal gland secretions. Bulls paw and dig their horns into the ground, then throw the soil over their withers, which may amplify their scent. In deer smell is also important in diet selection, but in cattle smell is probably unimportant when they graze a uniform pasture with a limited range of botanical species, because repeated exposure to odours reduces sensitivity as the number of vacant receptor sites diminishes. In humans odour perception may be impaired not so much by the sensory apparatus as by the lack of detailed information processing by the brain. Much of this is due to lack of training, because we focus on developing other sensory abilities. If challenged, humans can identify their own odours, synchronise menstrual cycles using body odours and recognise their mothers' odour at five days of age.

Chemical sensitivity

The chemical sensitivity of cattle ranges from being able to detect very weak solutions of sodium salts (10^{-4} M solutions of sodium bicarbonate) up to large hydrocarbon molecules and steroids (Bell & Sly, 1983). In comparison with man, a microsmatic animal, cattle are macrosmatic, being able to detect much smaller differences in odour concentration. Despite possessing two nostrils, there is little evidence that mammals can accurately localise odours (Leveteau & Daval, 1981).

Taste

Chemoreception by taste (gustation) has been extensively studied in man and cattle. Generally four primary tastes are identifiable and can be correlated to physiological requirements: sweetness for energy supply, saltiness to control electrolyte balance, bitterness to avoid toxins and tannins which reduce the nutritional value of the plant, and acidity to regulate pH. There may also be separate metallic and monosodium glutamate tastes, but probably all tastes derive from combinations of these four primary tastes. The receptors are located in specific areas of the tongue, and differ in their taste discrimination, sensitivity and positioning on the tongue between cattle and man. In cattle and man the salt taste is on the tip of the tongue. In man the sweet taste is also located there, but in cattle it is at the base of the tongue (Hard *et al.*, 1989). This difference may relate to the longer time that food is masticated (releasing soluble carbohydrates) in the middle to rear section of the buccal cavity in cattle.

Several compounds that taste sweet to man, e.g. monellin and thaumatin, do not to cattle. Cattle generally experience a greater sweet taste from monosaccharides than disaccharides, with the most potent sweeteners being glycine, Na-saccharin and xylintol. When presented with NaCl, xylintol enhances the salt taste, acting as a flavour enhancer. Tastes can also be antagonistic, for example the taste of the potent sweetener thaumatin can be reduced by NaCl (Chiy & Phillips, 1999b). The bovine tongue is not very receptive to quinine, which has a strong, bitter taste in humans, but many concentrate food components, such as shea nut meal, cherko (dried coffee grounds) and cocoa bean meal, appear to be unpalatable because of their bitter flavour. Both salty and bitter tastes have the potential to reduce the rate of intake of concentrate food, whereas a sweet taste can enhance it (Chiy & Phillips, 1999b). Cattle self-adapt to a salty taste over time, i.e. any reduction in palatability diminishes. At low concentrations, the addition of salt to the diet of cattle increases its palatability, with differences in concentration of as little as 1 g Na/kg dry matter (DM) being readily perceived (Phillips *et al.*, 1999). Cattle will tolerate medium concentrations (up to 6 to 11 g Na/kg DM, depending on their sodium status), but higher concentrations will diminish intake.

There are also no distinct water receptors in cattle as there are in man, but mechanoreceptors in the posterior part of the bovine tongue are responsive to material flow and can detect water passage. Thermoreceptors are also present in the tongue. The regurgitated bolus provides a mechanism for chemoreception of rumen conditions, especially acidity, but it is not known to what extent it is used.

The sense of taste develops at an early age in ruminants, as early as mid pregnancy in the sheep fetus, and the maternal diet can affect the dietary preferences of the offspring. Taste perception and discrimination thresholds change with advancing age. In cattle the discrimination threshold to sucrose is less for calves than adult cows. In sheep the intensity of salt flavour ascribed to a standard NaCl solution increases fourfold from the fetus to adulthood, whereas that to KCl decreases by about 30%. Adult cattle prefer pure water to a concentrated salt solution but calves do not, suggesting that a similar increase in NaCl perception with age occurs in cattle. KCl has a less potent salt flavour than NaCl for cattle. The appetite for sodium is particularly acute in sodium-deprived cattle, who show excessive licking behaviour in an attempt to get supplementary sodium (Phillips *et al.*, 1999).

Cattle can be conditioned to avoid poisonous plants by dosing them with LiCl at the same time as the plants are consumed, which causes gastrointestinal discomfort. LiCl can safely be used to form conditioned aversions in suckling cows, who are often at risk of poisoning, since LiCl is not expressed in milk, thereby preventing any avoidance of their mother's milk by the suckling calves (Ralphs, 1999).

Epidermal receptors

The skin contains a number of sensory receptors, mechanoreceptors to detect movement and force, thermoreceptors to detect temperature and nociceptors to detect damaging pathological conditions, such as inflammation. Humans have increased sensitivity in the hands, especially the fingertips, which effectively become sampling tools in exploratory situations. Cattle frequently use their extended mouth for this purpose.

Nociception and pain

Cattle probably have similar mechanisms for sensing pain to humans (Iggo, 1984; Livingstone *et al.*, 1992). The emotional response to noxious stimuli increases with the magnitude and duration of the stimuli (Stephens & Jones, 1975). It is also increased in isolated cattle, hence the presence of herdmates reduces the emotional response. The overt responses to pain are not as great in cattle as in man, because cattle evolved as prey animals and man as a predator. It is disadvantageous for a prey animal to indicate that it is in pain, as it may be singled out for attacks. In contrast, higher-order predators such as man are more likely to benefit from an overt pain response, particularly high-frequency vocalisation (an alarm call) to attract assistance and divert the animal from an excessive (shock) reaction.

Pain suppression may be mediated through endogenously secreted opioids. The analgesic opioids raise the threshold for pain perception and act on the same part of the brain as morphine. One such agent – β-endorphin, an endogenous morphine-like substance – permits passive reception of highly noxious stimuli in both cattle and man, with little perception of pain, preventing a damaging adrenal reaction and in cattle the attraction of predators.

A further reason for the reduced pain response in cattle may be that, although there can be little doubt that they do feel pain, the cerebral capacity to process information from nociceptors and produce painful sensations from it may be less than in humans (Iggo, 1984). The cerebral cortex that processes sensory stimuli is much more developed in man than in cattle. This does not necessarily mean that cattle feel less pain than humans, but may indicate that they suffer less psychologically from the long-term consequences of pain – anxiety, depression, etc.

The perception of pain can be diminished or eliminated by the use of anaesthetics (Graf & Senn, 1999). This will only be effective where the pain is short term, such as that caused by dehorning, where a cornual nerve block will reduce the cortisol and heart rate response to hot iron cauterisation (Grondahl Nielsen & Simonsen, 1999). However, calves show evidence of pain after the analgesic activity has diminished, even if applied to give eight hours' protection (McMeekan *et al.*, 1998). Parturition is a potential time of increased pain, but pain thresholds increase close to parturition and following parturition the ingestion of amniotic fluid enhances an opioid-mediated analgesia (Machado *et al.* 1997). Substances with analgesic properties, such as morphine, can be demonstrated to increase the nociceptive threshold (determined by the movement of the foot following the application of a thermal stimulus) (Machado *et al.*, 1998). Endorphins may reduce sensitivity to pain, and such self-administration of analgesics can occur during stressful events such as isolation (Rushen *et al.*, 1999a).

Perception of temperature

Cattle perceive thermal information in the form of extreme ambient temperatures, relative humidity or wind speed (or a combination of these) (Beaver *et al.*, 1996), which are detected by thermoreceptors, skin dryness (particularly in the throat and nasal passages) and mechanoreceptors, respectively. The optimum temperature is usually referred to as the comfort or thermoneutral zone, above and below which cattle have to work physiologically to sustain their core body temperature. They have to learn the importance of being in an optimum temperature (Beaver & Olson, 1997), and young cattle are more likely to use areas where the ambient temperature is below the comfort zone than older cattle. Older cattle learn to use favourable microclimates and exploit exposed areas at times when ambient temperatures are increased. Cold temperatures rarely stress cattle (Beverlin *et al.*, 1989), since the lower critical temperature of adult cows is –23°C (Houseal & Olson, 1995), and at sub-zero temperatures the availability of fodder is more of a problem than the temperature (Prescott *et al.*, 1994). However, they are prone to heat stress, especially if they have a high metabolic rate because of high productivity and/or they consume a high fibre diet which produces considerable internal heat of digestion. Initial responses to high temperatures include increased respiration rate, which occurs as low as 21°C, but further increases in temperature, above 25°C, reduce food intake and hence the heat of digestion.

Perception of temperature, as with most other stimuli, is relative rather than absolute. Response to localised thermal loading of one part of the body is reduced if the ambient temperature is low (Veissier *et al.*, 2000).

There are genetic differences in the susceptibility of cattle to thermal load, which may derive from differences in perception, but are more likely to derive from differences in endogenous heat production and heat dissipation. Holstein-Friesian cattle are particularly prone to heat stress, compared to *Bos indicus* cattle, but mixed groups may follow the less resistant cattle in reducing grazing time (Jan & Nichelmann 1993).

Perception of electric and magnetic fields

Cattle can readily detect low level electric currents, which often exist in parlours where the wet environment and connection of machinery to their udder make the cattle prone to stray voltage. Most cows will alter their behaviour to a 3 mA current, which corresponds to 0.7 V, and some will respond to a 1 mA current or 0.2 V (Henke Drenkard *et al.*, 1985). The resistance to the passage of electricity is only about 250 to 400 Ω, as a result of their direct contact with the floor at four points. The resistance provided by humans is two to ten times as great, depending on footwear, etc. As a result, the level of current that will disturb cows is much less than for humans. At low levels of current, 2 to 3 mA, a cow's heart rate is elevated by about three beats per minute (bpm), at 10 mA this increases to +17 bpm and at 13 mA it increases to +30 bpm, with severe behavioural responses. Mild behavioural responses include flinching and vocalisation, progressing to a startled response and avoidance behaviour. The stress caused to cows by stray voltage makes it desirable to impose a legal maximum. In terms of voltage, about 1 to 2 V will elicit a response from the majority of cows, therefore stray voltage should be less than 0.35 V, which will be perceived by less than 10% of cows (Appleman & Gustafson, 1985).

There is circumstantial evidence that the behaviour of cattle is affected by strong electromagnetic fields, such as exist around TV and radio transmitters (Loscher & Kas, 1998). Humans can detect the presence of low-frequency electric fields remotely, via hairs on the body (Odagiri-Shimizu & Shimizu, 1999) and are especially sensitive when atmospheric humidity is high. Cattle may use the hairs on their muzzle for the same purpose.

Perception of humans

Cattle may accept their stockperson as the head of their hierarchy, or animals at the top of the hierarchy may perceive them as a threat. The rearing environment in the first three months of life is important in forming subsequent attitudes to humans – those reared in extensive conditions are more likely to be afraid of humans and aggressive towards them (Boivin & Le Neindre, 1994). There is also a genetic component, with calves from some breeds and genotypes being more afraid of humans. Cattle habituate to the presence of humans and the positive reinforcement that they may provide in the form of petting or stroking, otherwise known as gentling (Boivin & Garel, 1998). They are more easily handled during lactation following gentling during the transition period. Nevertheless, nearly 20% of the variation in milk yield is believed to be due to fear of humans (Breuer *et al.*, 2000). The sound of the human voice, particularly when raised, is especially likely to induce fear (Waynert *et al.*, 1999).

Chapter 7
Acquisition of Behaviour and the Use of Selective Breeding to Improve Welfare

Innate or learnt?

The behaviour of cattle is determined both by instinct and experience, although the contribution of each is often disputed. One way to resolve this is to look at the behaviour of animals isolated from the relevant environmental influences at birth. This is of dubious validity for some behaviours, e.g. vocalisation, which can be influenced when animals experience their mother's call *in utero*. Even so, there is no doubt that some behaviours, particularly those needed immediately after birth, are almost entirely innate (fully developed and complete at first appearance). Examples of these are suckling and standing and those rhythmical behaviours which are fundamental to the life process (and tend to be under the control of the autonomic nervous system), such as breathing and defecation. Rearing calves in isolation produces socially maladjusted adult cows – less dominant, more nervous, less interactive with other cows and having poor mothering ability (Warwick *et al.*, 1977).

Learning evolves from a motivation to acquire information through experience. It is fastest in young cattle, but they also forget most rapidly (Kovalcikova & Kovalcik, 1984). For example, the rudiments of sexual behaviour are inherited and possibly so is the motivation, but the successful operator has to learn the art of courtship display and mounting. Complex behaviours usually have an element of learning involved, particularly those, such as sexual behaviour, which are not used in early life. Inexperienced bulls therefore show a high degree of unsuccessful mounting, often onto a cow's front end or side. Mastering the mounting procedures takes place not only through practice as adults but also during juvenile play.

Some behaviours are acquired solely through learning, including many of the activities that cattle are required to perform when under the control of man, e.g. operating an out-of-parlour feeding device. These activities have to be learnt, because genetic selection for these behaviours has not occurred in the limited time that cattle have been kept in intensive husbandry. They may be learnt directly from the stockperson, as when calves are trained to drink milk from buckets, or from fellow herdmates, which is increasingly necessary as herds increase in size and the time for human contact between man and individual animals is limited. This is not to say that man has had no influence on the genetic control of cattle behaviour. Culling of animals with difficult temperaments has almost certainly contributed to the docility of cows today, and the improved reproductive performance of cows exhibiting a strong oestrus has probably enhanced this characteristic (Baker & Seidel, 1975).

Methods of learning

Operant conditioning

This form of learning evolves when an animal obtains a desirable (reward) status if a certain exploratory action is taken. It is effectively trial and error learning, and the animal must experience the reward repeatedly before the behaviour is learnt. For example, a cow learns to use an out-of-parlour feeder by putting her head into the feeder, after which feed is delivered into the trough. Such inquisitiveness enables cattle to take advantage of new opportunities arising in the environment. Operant conditioning is the most common form of learning in cattle since they are not timid animals and will readily explore new situations. The mechanism can be a powerful tool for researchers to learn about environmental perception.

Classical conditioning

This form of conditioning is distinct from trial and error learning in that it involves the formation of an association between an unrelated 'neutral' stimulus and a response. The response is 'conditioned' once this association is formed. Most learning in farm animals is initially by trial and error, but the response is maintained through the formation of associations between neutral stimuli and the response. Cattle kept in confinement are usually in a precise rhythm of behaviour patterns and they soon learn to distinguish the sequence of events that precedes the direct stimulation of a response. For example, a wagon delivering feed in a cattle shed normally elicits immediate feeding behaviour, but may be preceded by the sight or sound of someone starting a tractor, putting feed into the feeder wagon or simply opening the door to the shed. These neutral stimuli are then more likely to elicit the feeding response than the later conditioned stimulus, particularly in a competitive situation where the first cows to the feeding barrier get the most or best feed. Animals use the simplest and most reliable stimuli to elicit a response. If they had to interpret all the signals before they responded, it would be a waste of their energy and they would be slow to act. So, they only use a small number of stimuli and often only one aspect of each. The bright red colour of the tractor that will feed them may be sufficient if this is the only time they encounter it. Dairy cows are thought to be initially operantly

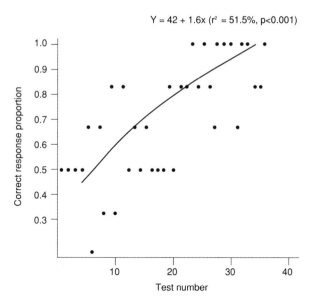

Fig. 7.1 Learning curve of calves during the training period of a light intensity discrimination test.

conditioned to letdown their milk, as they find that allowing the cluster to be put on their udder releases the pressure. Soon, however, the response becomes classically conditioned and the cows use conditioned stimuli, such as entry to the collecting yard, to trigger milk letdown.

Conditioned learning can be a powerful tool to learn about the discrimination powers of animals. For instance, calves placed at the entrance to two chambers, one of which had a brighter light source than the other, were able to learn how to indicate the brighter of two chambers to receive a feed reward (Phillips & Weiguo, 1991) (Fig. 7.1). Their discrimination ability can be determined by varying the difference between the lights, and compared to other species. It takes a long time to train cattle to perform such activities, in this case 40 tests each, partly because there is a long time between tests while cattle are moved in and out of the test arena. The information obtained must be combined with anatomical knowledge and behavioural observation to get a more complete idea of discrimination power.

Conditioned learning can also be used to train cattle to indicate their preferences, and the strength of (or motivation for) these preferences is shown by pushing a lever. The lever is usually mounted about 1 m from the floor, or alternatively the animal may break a beam passing between two photoelectric cells. The animal can receive such rewards as feed or heat. It may be difficult to distinguish a definite preference from the animal playing with the activator, but this may be overcome by comparing the activation of the lever or beam with a dummy lever or beam, which produces no response. Alternatively the number of lever presses required to elicit the response can be increased (fixed interval schedule) or the period of time that elapses between lever pressing and the response increased (fixed ratio schedule). Introducing a cost to the animal (work for the fixed ratio schedule, time for the fixed interval schedule) allows the researcher to determine the extent to which the animal is motivated to receive the reward. Using a fixed ratio schedule, it has been possible to prove that high-yielding cows are not prepared to work harder than low-yielding cows to obtain a concentrate food reward (M. Cooper, personal communication).

Insight learning

The more complex an animal's behaviour, the more it needs to store stimuli–response details and use these to control behaviour. Most higher-order animals can put together a sequence of these response patterns to produce a required response. For example, a cow may go through an elaborate procedure of following and bullying a subordinate cow at a concentrate feeder in order to steal her portion of the feed. The complexity of the procedure gives an indication of the intelligence of the animals, but it is also related to the degree of exploratory behaviour they perform. More nervous and less exploratory cattle are slower to learn conditioned responses.

Investigatory behaviour

Investigatory behaviour is at the centre of much of learning. It is most common in the young calf, but this is likely to be partly because the number of new stimuli is very high at this time, and as the calf gets accustomed to its environment, less exploratory behaviour is produced.

The posture of cattle exploring the environment displays the degree of confidence that they have in the response. A confident approach is one where the head is not greatly extended (Fig 7.2), whereas an unconfident approach allows for a more rapid retreat by extending the head (containing the sensory organs) further and keeping a greater distance between the stimulus and the means of retreat, the legs (Fig. 7.3).

Tests of learning ability in cattle have been numerous, including multiple choice selection (Gardner, 1937), training to do specific tasks (Breland & Breland, 1966) and even performance in mazes (Kilgour, 1981). Perhaps not surprisingly, Kilgour found that cattle performed better than cats and opossums in a maze since they readily explore new areas and move into open spaces.

Breeding for improved welfare

Anthropogenic changes in the cattle genotype have been the result of selection since the start of domestication, 8000 to 10 000 years ago. Recently, increases in the rate at which changes in genotype can be achieved suggest that it may be possible to adapt cattle to intensive management systems by selective breeding.

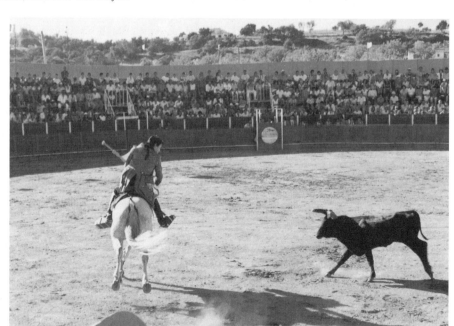

Fig. 7.2 Confident approach by a young bull, with legs thrusting forward and head retracted.

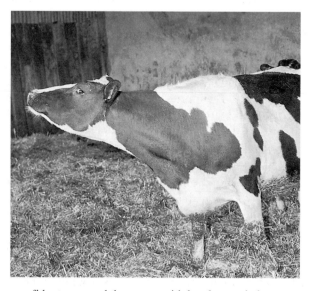

Fig. 7.3 An unconfident approach by a cow, with head extended.

The financial objective assumed by most geneticists, if not always by breeders (Owen, 1989), has had some adverse effects on cattle welfare. Double-muscling traits have been favoured, whereas in the wild, and even many farming systems, they would not have been perpetuated because of the frequent need for Caesarian delivery of the calf. Leg disorders, such as osteochondrosis, have become common in beef cattle selected for rapid growth and kept in confined environments. Cattle have been bred for systems that concentrate on one aspect of production, e.g. growth or milk production, which forces them to accommodate the high output in this area by modifying performance in other ways. So, if cows are bred to produce large quantities of milk, their offspring will not grow well for the production of meat. Frequently the capacity to reproduce is compromised, with high-yielding dairy cows being more likely to show anoestrus (Esteban *et al.*, 1994). Some argue that an animal's 'fitness' can only improve as a result of selection for production, and even that disease susceptibility must be reduced as a result of breeding for increased financial return. However, livestock managers are increasingly able to circumvent deficiencies in the animals' behaviour and function created by intensive breeding. For example, the reproductive cycle of cows can be controlled by administering exogenous hormones (Roche, 1989).

Ethical considerations of the relationship between animal breeding and animal welfare

We now have the ability to alter drastically the genetic constitution of entire cattle populations in a few years. If we wish to use this power to manipulate the genome of cattle, not for economic gain but to improve their welfare, we must decide whether it is ethically correct to make these changes.

There are now well-established views on the attitudes people adopt with respect to animal care (DeGrazia, 1996; Sandøe *et al.*, 1997), and these can be extended to the manipulation of the animal genome for the purpose of improving animal welfare. The most extreme views are held by animal rights supporters and those with utilitarian beliefs. In brief, the former believe that all animals have the same rights as humans (Ruh, 1989), which would prevent any genetic intervention by man. The opposing, utilitarian, view would be that welfare should be included in breeding programmes only if total suffering is reduced. If, however, breeding for improved animal welfare reduced human welfare because there was less food available, or the improvement in animal welfare was offset by a reduction in the welfare of the human attendants, and the net effect was an increase in suffering, utilitarian theory would not support such action. The latter consequence is perhaps unlikely, but the former is a realistic possibility with the expansion of world population and increased demand for food.

Others would argue that we must not change animal types so much that they are essentially a new species. This puts an artificial boundary on genetic manipulation. If we create an animal, such as a dairy cow, that cannot reproduce naturally we have effectively created a new species. Genotypic diversity is the species' insurance against being threatened by disease epidemics or changed circumstances that challenge the species' adaptation to its (economic) environment. The recent BSE outbreak in the UK illustrates the vulnerability of our farm animals, and may have been encouraged by the lack of genotypic diversity in the UK dairy cattle population. Although BSE is not simply inherited (Wilesmith *et al.*, 1988; Wijeratne & Curnow, 1990), it is highly likely that there is an inherited susceptibility to the disease (Bradley, 1993), which is most widespread in British Friesian cattle. Ethically, therefore, it is at least as important to consider the long-term welfare of the species, in terms of its survival as a domesticated animal, as well as the suitability for most economic production in the prevailing systems of production.

If we assume the right to manipulate animals we must include the welfare of future generations as well. It is logical that the welfare of the species as a whole is at least as important as individuals within the species. Barnard and Hurst (1996) emphasise the expendability of individuals and attack our obsession with 'individual preservationism'. The imposition of a *species* boundary, however, is questionable, since it is no more than the collective expression of the genome in a group of interbreeding animals. In defining selection criteria for cattle we might choose to place more emphasis on preserving genetic diversity within the species. This still identifies the risk to the genotype as being of greater importance than the risk to individuals, and would permit, for example, a challenge to an individual cow's welfare if it had to be transported long distances to participate in genetic preservation research or practice. Animal rights theory would not sanction adverse effects on the welfare of one individual for the benefit of others.

Further insight into the ethics of including welfare in cattle breeding objectives can be gained by trying to understand how humans acquired the strong interspecies empathy that is at the centre of our current concern for animal welfare. Caring for other species is not unique to humans; many animals in symbiotic or commensal relationships with other species have to protect the other species in their relationship (Wiese, 1996). Our own empathetic feelings are not generalised to all species – they do not normally extend much to potentially dangerous species such as snakes or spiders. Indeed these often create phobias, which are known to have a genetic component (Kendler *et al.*, 1992). However, the ability of humans to interact with and manage a large number of animal species for our own benefit indicates why we show empathy to so much of the animal kingdom. Those animals that give us the most benefit evoke the greatest empathy, particularly farm animals and companion animals. An ability to recognise, and ameliorate where possible, the suffering of cattle in their charge would have benefited humans throughout the long history of dependency on them. Thus, the early recognition and treatment of diseases in early domesticated cattle would have enhanced the survival rate of both the animals and humans which depended on them.

Breeding for environmental tolerance

Many of the current welfare problems in farm animals relate to the fact that the environment in which they are kept is quite unlike the one in which they evolved. Hence their behavioural needs are particularly unsuited to intensive housing conditions. Vices develop, such as tongue rolling in steers (Karatzias *et al.*, 1995), as a result of the thwarting of natural behaviours. There is considerable evidence that susceptibility to abnormal behaviour is under genetic control (Feddersen-Petersen, 1991; Watt & Seller, 1993), and in particular that the sensitisation of dopamine receptors is under the control of genes that convert extracellular stimuli into long-term changes in neuronal activity.

The possibility exists to breed animals that do not perform abnormal behaviours (Craig & Muir, 1996), but it is not certain that in all cases their welfare is greater than that of those performing the deleterious behaviours. It is possible that animals that do not exhibit the abnormal behaviour are those that do not find the environment frustrating, assuming that the animals' perception of the environment varies with their genetic makeup. However, the abnormal behaviour may be providing a release from the frustration of the abnormal environment, and performing the behaviour, therefore, improves the animal's welfare. The behaviour of domestic cattle is characterised by behavioural plasticity in comparison with their wild counterparts, which could include the capacity to perform abnormal behaviours to dissipate the motivational forces that are thwarted in intensive management systems (Paul *et al.*, 1995).

As well as behavioural modification, it may be possible to breed cattle that can cope better with the high output achieved by breeding efforts since 1950. Thus cattle with greater forage digestion capacity or improved resistance to output-related diseases could be important breeding objectives in the future.

Heritabilities of behaviour traits

Few experiments have been conducted to estimate the genetic, as opposed to environmental effects on behaviour traits (Table 7.1). The inheritance of feeding behaviour was first studied scientifically by Hancock (1950) using monozygotic twin dairy cows. This work suggested a strong genetic component to grazing behaviour, although environmental effects could not be totally disregarded. Later research (Macha & Olsarova, 1986), however, has shown weak inheritance of grazing behaviour.

Grazing behaviour and feeding behaviour with conserved feeds appear not to be highly correlated, because the ingestive behaviour of cattle offered conserved feeds is highly heritable but grazing time is not (Mokhov, 1983; Baehr *et al.*, 1984; Wassmuth & Alps, 2000). Probably there has been less natural selection for feeding on conserved fodder than for long grazing times. This may be because cows are short of time to consume sufficient grazed herbage, but not to eat sufficient conserved feeds because of the higher rate of ingestion. There have always been obvious advantages for cattle that are prepared to graze for a long

Table 7.1   Heritability estimates of behavioural traits. Heritability range is from 0.01 (weakly inherited) to 0.3+ (strongly inherited)

Personality		
O'Bleness *et al.* (1960)	Temperament	0.40 ± 0.09
New Zealand Dairy Board (1961)	Temperament	0.06
Beilharz *et al.* (1966)	Dominance	0.44
Dickson *et al.* (1970)	Temperament	0.53
Shrode and Hammock (1971)	Temperament	0.40 ± 0.30
Brown (1974)	Maternal protective temperament	0.32 (Hereford) 0.17 (Angus)
Mishra *et al.* (1975)	Temperament	0.19
Persson (1978)	Temperament	0.12–0.18 0.16–0.45 0.24
Salcido and Eugenio (1979)	Temperament	0.04
Wickham (1979)	Temperament	0.11
Stricklin *et al.* (1980)	Temperament	0.48 ± 0.29
Sato (1981)	Temperament	0.45–0.67
Agyemang *et al.* (1982)	Disposition (degree of trouble to herdsman)	0.03
Fordyce *et al.* (1982)	Movement in crush	0.25 ± 0.20
	Movement in race	0.17 ± 0.21
	Movement in crush plus head restraint	0.67 ± 0.26
	Audible respiration in crush	0.20 ± 0.16
	Audible respiration in race	0.57 ± 0.22
Mokhov (1983)	Cattle encounters	0.52
	Cattle aggressive interactions	0.88
Baehr *et al.* (1984)	Quiet behaviour	0.75 ± 0.38
	Fast movement	0.61 ± 0.38
Fordyce and Goddard (1984)	Temperament in crush	0.0–0.10[a]
	Vigour of movement	0.0
	Audible respiration	0.0
	Kicking	0.0
	Bellowing	0.09
	Kneeling down	0.10
Hearnshaw and Morris (1984)	Temperament	0.03 ± 0.28 *(Bos taurus)* 0.46 ± 0.37 *(Bos indicus)*
Buddenberg *et al.* (1986)	Maternal behaviour (protection of calf from humans)	0.06 ± 0.01
Le Neindre *et al.* (1996)	Ease of handling	0.22
Burrow and Corbett (1999)	Flight speed	0.38–0.45
	Flight speed score	0.08
	Crush score	0.30
Ingestive behaviour		
Mokhov (1983)	Forage feeding duration	0.68
	Rumination duration	0.59
Baehr *et al.* (1984)	Visits to concentrate dispenser	0.61 ± 0.27
Macha and Olsarova (1986)	Grazing time per day	0.003 ± 0.026

Continued opposite.

Table 7.1   (*Continued.*)

Santha *et al.* (1988)	Rumination time per day	0.15
	Rumination bout length	0.20
Mendoza-Ordones *et al.* (1988)	Drinking rate	0.43
	Gulps per second	0.68
	Intake per gulp	0.52
Winder *et al.* (1995)	Rangeland diet selection	0.51–0.87
Wassmuth and Alps (2000)	Forage feeding time	0.40
Reproductive behaviour		
Rottensten and Touchberry (1957)	Oestrus intensity	0.21
Blockey *et al.* (1978)	Serving capacity	0.59 ± 0.16
Mialon *et al.* (2000)	Calving to first oestrus interval	0.12

[a]Significant dam–daughter correlations, suggesting a non-genetic maternal effect.

time, at the expense of other behaviours such as resting, and there has probably been natural selection for this trait. Therefore selection for grazing time could have occurred gradually over many millennia, whereas cattle have been given conserved feeds by man for only a very limited period. Selection on rangeland is more heritable, and may relate to the different strategies adopted by different families (Winder *et al.*, 1995). Some may need to be more vigilant and select small quantities of high-quality feed, whereas others may feel safe to graze for long periods and consume large quantities of low-quality material.

The other major behavioural characteristic to be examined for genetic influence is personality. This has been measured both as the behavioural response of cows with calves to approach by humans and as the behaviour of cattle in a confinement crush. The response of a cow with calf to humans has a low to moderate heritability and a low genetic correlation with production characteristics. Temperament in the crush has generally been found to have a variable heritability of 0 to 0.4. However, greater heritabilities have been found when cattle are highly challenged in the crush by imposition of a head restraint. Greater heritabilities have also been found in *Bos indicus* cattle, which are generally more difficult to handle than *Bos taurus*. This suggests that an extreme nervous reaction or 'fit' in the crush is more highly heritable than the normal range of reactions seen during mild stress in the crush. Undoubtedly there has been prolonged selection by humans for resistance to milking stress, but possibly not for a major stress reaction such as in a crush. Repeatability of temperament scores in the crush has generally been high, suggesting that measurement technique is not a problem, although the different aspects of temperament – movement, respiration, bellowing, kicking – that have been recorded to represent temperament might account for some of the variations in results.

Despite some inconsistencies, the heritability of many behaviours is high, particularly those not selected for before or during domestication. A low heritability for reproductive behaviour is expected, since it is related to reproductive potential and has been extensively selected for in the past. Similarly we would expect docility to have been selected for during the process of domestication and still to be selected for today. In contrast, behaviours associated with the use of man-made equipment, such as concentrate dispensers, have not been selected for and tend to have a high heritability. A few behavioural traits have also been linked to major genes, such as fearfulness in double-muscled cattle, but most are multigene traits.

Breeding for resistance to transmissible diseases

Transmissible diseases provide one of the most obvious challenges to cattle welfare. Although much progress has been made recently in controlling infectious diseases, such as mastitis, by routine use of drug therapy and even prophylaxis, it is acknowledged that the efficacy of these measures is rapidly diminishing as the disease organisms mutate to evolve resistance (Axford *et al.*, 1999). Since cattle vary in their susceptibility to disease, it is likely that selective breeding could reduce the disease incidence.

It is clear that there are no genes conferring universal resistance to diseases (Bumstead *et al.*, 1991), and it is necessary to identify areas of the host resistance that are deficient in a particular environment. The animal's immunity is made up of two components: innate and acquired immunity. The degree of specificity of innate immunity is often unclear and there is little hope of improving the specificity of the acquired immunity, since the genetic coding possibilities for T-cell or immunoglobulin variants are already greater than the cellular capacity. The acquired immunity specificity is governed by three gene complexes, which code for the histocompatibility antigens, T-cell receptors and B-cell immunoglobulin receptors (Doenhoff & Davies, 1991). Although there is some scope for enhancing the quantity and quality of immune responses (Edfors-Lilja, 1996), selection for individual responses, such as antibody production, tends to lead to negative effects on other responses, such as macrophage activity (Biozzi *et al.*, 1984). However, selection for combined responses is possible and has been shown to produce an improvement in general immune capacity and possibly higher growth rates in pigs (Edfors-Lilja, 1996). Progress is slow mainly because the genetic basis for immune responses in farm livestock is poorly understood. For example, it is known that some quantitative trait loci have considerable influence, but it is unclear whether this is caused by single or multiple mutations at a single locus or mutations at several linked loci.

A major problem with attempting to enhance the immune response is that disease organisms constantly change to present new challenges to the animal. The animal's defence mechanisms and reproductive strategy of regular genotype changes have evolved to keep the disease challenge under control. Indeed if it were not for new diseases and environmental challenges, reproduction might never have evolved as a means of manipulating the size and genotype of a population. Rarely in the wild are new strains of disease organisms able to have the same impact that they can have in farm livestock. This is first because of the close contact between farm livestock and good conditions for the survival of disease organisms. Housing increases the disease challenge, and stocking density in the house largely determines the strength of the challenge, with only minor possibilities for reducing the contamination risk through ventilation (Webster, 1984). Secondly, the limited cattle genotype that is emerging from recent focusing of production on the Holstein-Friesian breed reduces the potential rate of selection of resistant animals to new disease challenges.

We can attempt to improve artificially on natural selection as a means of optimising the disease resistance of cattle, but we should not underestimate the difficulties involved. It is not simply a matter of increasing the output of the host defence mechanisms. These are already designed to produce the optimum response (Doenhoff & Davies, 1991), which minimises the cost to the animal while at the same time keeping the disease organism under control. In this respect stable host–parasite relationships have evolved that are symbiotic. If host resistance is enhanced the virulence of the disease organism is correspondingly increased. For parasites and viruses in particular, the organism is most successful when it minimises the host damage and a commensal relationship ensues. Adaptations are expensive as the reproductive outcome is uncertain and the metabolic resources of the individual may be used up (Barnard & Hurst, 1996).

The greatest potential for genetic selection to enhance disease resistance is probably in circumstances where cattle are kept in environments that are far removed from that in which they evolved and to which they have not yet had time to adapt. Some of the greatest challenges are to be found in developing countries. Considerable progress has been made, e.g. in identifying cattle that are resistant to trypanosomiasis in Africa. This disease is the greatest constraint to the productivity of recently imported cattle in Africa (Murray *et al.*, 1991). Over several thousand years breeds of local cattle, such as the N'Dama and West African Shorthorn, evolved their own resistance, but these are not as productive as modern European cattle. Wildlife are carriers and do not suffer severe clinical symptoms, but they do provide a constant reservoir of disease organisms, rendering eradication of the disease impossible. If quantitative trait loci for trypanotolerance can be identified, it should be possible to transfer the relevant regions of the genome to more productive cattle and produce novel genotypes with favourable disease resistance and production characteristics. The major challenge, however, is to understand the physiological basis for trypanotolerance, because it is only this understanding that can reduce the virulence of the disease in the long term. Clearly the trypanosome haemoprotozoans are capable of commensal relationships in some cattle and wild animal genotypes that should be the objective of current breeding programmes for high output cattle. Reliance on trypanocidal drugs and vector control has diminishing effectiveness, which is prompting considerable interest in disease-resistant stock.

There are many difficulties in attempting to achieve enhanced disease resistance status of farm livestock. One is that the prevalence of most diseases in any farm livestock population is low, and the potential for selection by traditional breeding methods is limited. Persistent diseases such as bovine tuberculosis present a growing threat, yet breeding for resistance offers little potential because of the low prevalence in the population. The use of markers and indirect selection methods is receiving increasing attention (Muller & Brem, 1996).

A further difficulty is the multifactorial nature of the challenge. Disease resistance is rarely controlled by a single gene and polygenic traits are not well understood (Wakelin, 1991). Major gene effects are usually deleterious for farm animals and it is increasingly evident that manipulation of disease resistance will usually involve multiple loci. Fortunately the technology for doing this is advancing very rapidly. Early techniques of microinjection were risky because of the lack of control of the outcome, but embryo stem cell integration can now produce gene clones more reliably. The use of marker loci potentially makes the whole genome accessible and the development of genetic maps, together with advanced statistical techniques, will make it possible to identify the genes that contribute to disease resistance (Womack, 1996). Transgenic manipulation for enhancing disease resistance suffers from the major drawback that only a limited genetic pool will be preserved if transgenic cattle are extensively multiplied. The disadvantages of a limited foundation stock could to some extent be overcome by cryopreservation of gametes, but there may be ethical objections to the widespread adoption of the practice (Ballou, 1992).

Another difficulty with breeding for disease resistance is that increasing resistance to one disease may reduce the productive efficiency of the animal, because of negative genetic correlations between these traits. For example, because the prevalence of mastitis increases with milk yield (Emanuelson, 1988; Eriksson, 1991), breeding cattle for mastitis resistance will reduce milk yields unless this is included as a trait in the selection index, in which case progress in either trait will be retarded. There is also some, limited evidence that some genes conferring susceptibility to a certain disease may also code for fitness in the host (Doenhoff & Davies, 1991), suggesting that certain disease organisms may confer resistance to other, more pathogenic organisms. However, if cattle acquire a disease which weakens a particular organ, it is likely to increase susceptibility to other diseases targeting that organ. Hence cattle will be predisposed to tuberculosis by other diseases, such as pneumonia, that target the pulmonary system.

Breeding for resistance to mastitis in dairy cows

Bacterial diseases have been increasingly treated by administering antibiotics, and it is not surprising, because of their rapid multiplication rate, that resistance to the antibiotics is found soon after they are routinely used on farms (e.g. resistance to antibiotics used to treat mastitis in dairy cows) (Bryson & Thomson, 1976; Berghash *et al.*, 1983). Routine administration of antibiotics at cessation of lactation results in more pathogenic organisms colonising the mammary gland during lactation, particularly those that are abundant in the environment of the cow, such as *Escherichia coli* (Schukken *et al.*, 1989). Host resistance could be improved by breeding dairy cows for low somatic cell concentrations in milk (Bramely, 1978; Coffey *et al.*, 1986). However, since the somatic cell concentrations are both the biological marker and a part of the host defence mechanism, there is concern that host resistance will decline if cows are bred with too low somatic cell concentrations. As evidence for this, when somatic cell concentrations are high owing to a recent infection, the susceptibility to reinfection is low (Bramely, 1978). However, somatic cell concentrations are positively genetically correlated with the rate of infection, suggesting that some progress against mastitis could be achieved by using appropriate sires (Coffey *et al.*, 1986).

There is evidence that selection for improved udder shape and function will reduce mastitis prevalence (Rogers *et al.*, 1991). Selection for less pendulous udders with shorter teats (Politiek, 1981) and narrower teat canals (Seykora & McDaniel, 1985) is recommended and is essentially reversing some of the unwelcome effects of breeding for high milk yields (Fernandez *et al.*, 1995). Modern milking systems have the capacity to automatically identify fast and slow milking cows, which could be incorporated into selection criteria. The advantages of rapid milk ejection in reducing milking times will probably diminish when robotic milking systems allow cows to be milked unattended.

Prophylactic measures of treating farm livestock with probiotics rather than antibiotics have often failed to bring the expected benefits (e.g. Greene *et al.*, 1991). This may reflect a lack of knowledge of the most effective bacteria in providing protection, the precise site of action and the optimal dose. The opportunity remains to breed livestock that are colonised commensally rather than parasitically.

The consequences for animal welfare of traditional breeding practices

In view of the difficulties of defining and incorporating animal welfare into breeding objectives for farm animals, it is necessary to consider the impact of traditional breeding practices on animal welfare.

The consequences of breeding for increased feed conversion efficiency

Increased feed conversion efficiency is likely to be a major directive of cattle farmers in the future. This may result in the selection of animals with increasingly low activity rates to reduce maintenance requirements. In the future the intensification of livestock farming is likely to mitigate against grazing systems. Maintenance energy requirements are typically increased by 10 to 20%, compared with housed feeding (National Research Council, 1978; Agricultural and Food Research Council, 1993). Housing will also be encouraged by increased possibilities for mechanisation of dairying systems, e.g. robotic milking, by the continuing escalation of labour costs, and by the greater efficiency of harvesting herbage by machine than by the grazing animal (Phillips, 1988). However, intensively housed dairy cows have a greater incidence of several diseases, most notably mastitis, than those with access to pasture (Krohn & Rasmussen, 1992).

The dairy farming industry has largely escaped the attention of more radical pressure groups, probably because grazing animals are anthropomorphically viewed as contented. Nutritionally the grazing dairy cow may be far from contented, because the intake of grazed pasture is often insufficient for high-yielding cows (Phillips, 1989). High-yielding cows have to spend up to one half of the day grazing, which may cause stress in itself. Greater control of the nutrient supply is afforded by housed feeding, but it can be at the expense of the welfare of the cow, so far as her physical environment is concerned. The optimum for cow welfare is probably a system based on grazing but with forage supplements to allow adequate nutrient intakes (Phillips & Leaver, 1985b).

In the face of increased attractiveness of year-round housing to intensive cattle farmers to minimise labour requirements and facilitate mechanisation, it will be necessary to breed cattle that will tolerate intensive housing conditions (including factors such as hoof health, mastitis resistance and less aggression between cows).

A multifactorial approach to the consequences for animal welfare of traditional breeding objectives

Traditional breeding objectives have an impact on animal welfare in a complex manner (Table 7.2). The following description illustrates the approach, but it should be noted that this can lead to errors, or too rigid an interpretation of the use of animal welfare measures.

Increasing growth rate in cattle for meat production can lead to increased diseases such as leg disorders and dystokia. It reduces longevity because an animal can be slaughtered at the same weight at a younger age. It may reduce reproductive fitness by the effects on dystokia, for example. Breeding for greater food conversion efficiency will either increase growth rate, decrease food intake or both. The effects on welfare are, therefore, likely to be similar to growth rate.

Table 7.2   Matrix illustrating the effects of breeding for production on various measures of cattle welfare

| Breeding objectives | Welfare indicators | | | | | |
	Behaviour	Disease	Mental satisfaction	Production rate	Longevity	Reproductive fitness
Growth rate	?/–	– –	–	+ +	– –	–
Food conversion efficiency	–	+	–	+ +	– –	–
Carcase conformation	?	+/–	?	+	+	–
Reproductive capacity	–	–	– –	+		+ + +
Milk yield	–	–	–	+	–	–

+, Positive effects (number indicates intensity); –, negative effects (number indicates intensity); ?, variable effects.

Carcase conformation: it has been common in recent years to selectively breed animals with a low level of fat cover, which reverses earlier trends in cattle breeding at least. Body composition has a strong genetic base (Owen, 1990) and has implications for most welfare indicators. Breeds such as the Belgian Blue have a high frequency of double muscling, and it is highly likely that the responsible genes will be transferred to other breeds (Charlier *et al.*, 1995). Double muscling is associated with a greater risk of dystokia, which reduces reproductive fitness.

Breeding for increased reproductive capacity and milk yield will have adverse effects on animal welfare if the modification is not accompanied by improved nutrition to support the increased output.

Chapter 8
Play Behaviour

What is play?

Play behaviour is difficult to define and it is even unclear whether it is a single behaviour, with a common goal and motivation. Play behaviours can be defined as structural transformations and functional rehearsals or generalisations of behaviours or behavioural sequences (Fagen, 1981). There is no attempt to identify a common objective for play. Therefore, 'play' refers to activities with definable characteristics, but most of these differ from other behaviours only in scale (Loizos, 1966).

Common components of play are exaggerated or repeated versions of other behaviours, particularly those used infrequently such as fighting, fleeing and copulation that are used for survival. The sequence of the components of the behaviour may be re-ordered or incomplete and usually lacks the consummatory phase. Play is often preceded and accompanied by signals that the behaviour is play, and typically playmates interchange roles frequently.

Typical manifestations in cattle are:

(1) *Mock fleeing*. Running, trotting, cantering and galloping, often with tail elevated.

(2) *Mock aggression*.
   - Bucking with both hind feet jerked up posteriorly and often to one side with an accompanied lateral twist of the hindquarters.
   - Kicking with one or both hind feet, often at moving objects.
   - Head butting playmate, stockperson or other objects, goring and head-pushing movements.
   - Prancing and mock challenges, with head lowered or shaken from side to side, often accompanied by snorting.
   - Vocalisation, varying in type with the degree of excitement. Most vocalisations are normally of low amplitude and frequency (Kiley, 1972).

(3) *Mock copulation*. Mounting other playmates, inanimate objects and even stockmen, sometimes with pelvic thrusts. A large proportion of mounts are disorientated – head to head, head to side, intention mounts and solicitation. Mock copulation is not accompanied by erection of the penis or vaginal intromission.

(4) *Environmental exploration.* Investigation of novel objects in the environment, in particular to determine their reactivity – patterns of movement, noise, etc.

Some age effects are evident in cattle play. The first forms of play are usually solitary and are usually mock fleeing, in particular running, gambolling and jumping. Calves may also be involved in play with adults at an early age. The mother is an important stimulant to play, since in her presence the calf will feel safe to emerge from the creche and engage in play. At a later age, play is usually between peers, and it involves social interactions more frequently, particularly head pushing, mounting and other associative behaviour (Vitale *et al.*, 1986). Camargue cattle have also been observed to horn bushes and hummocks during play (Schloeth, 1961).

Gender effects are also evident – male calves more often initiate and are the recipients of play than female calves, and they are more often the protagonists. They take part particularly in combative and social play. There is circadian variation too, which shows that play is most common in mid morning and mid afternoon, and rare at night (Vitale *et al.*, 1986). The frequency of play in housed cattle is positively correlated with light intensity, which could be due to psychosomatic stimulation (Dannenmann *et al.*, 1985). Play is often thwarted in housed calves due to inadequate space, but is common in grazing calves (Fig. 8.1). Calves that are unable to play may find it difficult to adapt to new circumstances and they are emotionally immature and shy. After a period of play deprivation, such as during confinement, animals compensate with extra play, suggesting that this is an essential behaviour. However, play can be 'switched off', since it ceases during periods of inclement weather.

Functions of play

Play contains components of many behaviours but may arise from a single motivation. Because of its multicomponent nature, it is difficult to ascribe a single function to play. Early theories of play function were sometimes negative, regarding it as useless, perhaps a vestigial behaviour from some period of evolution. Indeed it has even been cynically referred to as the 'wastepaper basket of imperfectly understood animal behaviour' (Loizos, 1966). We should, however, acknowledge that play itself is still poorly understood. For instance, it may be indistinguishable from stereotypic behaviour in some circumstances. These early ideas coincided temporally with the Victorian belief that 'children should be seen and not heard', thus denigrating play in both animals and man as a worthless activity. This belief was not without some logic, however, as play is normally restricted to well-fed animals and was seen by some as a means of dispersing excess energy. Although some of this energy could be stored in mature animals as fat tissue, in the juvenile this is not physiologically so common. In the absence of normal releasers, other methods have to be found of dissipating the energy,

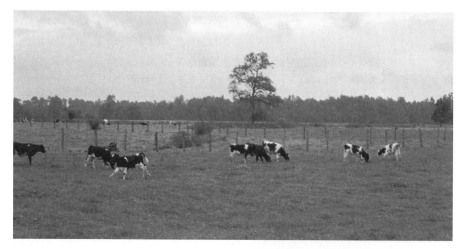

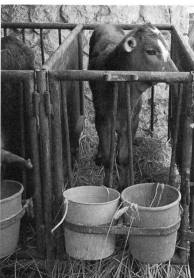

Fig. 8.1 Penned calves have little opportunity for play (right) but in the grazing situation it is common (above).

and in this respect it is relevant that well-fed animals play more frequently than poorly fed ones (Brownlee, 1954). Some protagonists of the energy dissipation theory believe that play may be a vestigial behaviour from reptilian ancestry. In reptiles neonatal activity is of adaptive value, since food must be quickly found. After evolution to mammals, however, neonatal activity was of less value, since food was provided by the mother and, rather than reset all the biological mechanisms in place for neonatal play, locomotor–rotational play, comprising locomotion, rotation of the body and leaping, evolved as a means of redirecting the behaviour (Fagen, 1981). However, this theory ignores the value of more complex forms of play.

The energy dissipation theory therefore fails to acknowledge a biological value of play *per se*. That there must be such a value is suggested by the fact that animals demonstrate motivation for play (Hinde, 1970). After prolonged confinement, the incidence of locomotor play increases (Jensen, 2001). Animals engaging in play risk injury, predation, as well as loss of time and energy. Natural selection models often prescribe against play behaviour, so the benefits must be considerable. Nevertheless, play clearly has a lower priority than behaviours essential for body maintenance – feeding, drinking and sleeping. Highly productive dairy cattle, which spend up to two-thirds of their time in ingestive behaviour (grazing and ruminating) alone, play very little in comparison with calves that spend only one-tenth to one-quarter of their time in ingestive behaviour. One reason may be that the cows' need for physical training would be low on account of the large amount of time spent actively grazing.

The widely supported physical training theory proposes that play serves to exercise body function, in particular the muscles associated with infrequently used survival functions such as flight, agonistic behaviour and reproduction. These muscle groups are then strengthened by vasodilation and the survival function is enhanced. There is every reason to believe that wild cattle engaging in physical play increase their strength, endurance and survival skills. In addition, there may be sensorimotor training, through stimulation of the vestibular apparatus, which houses the inner ear sense organ. In support of the motor training theory, we find combat play more common in male than female calves, in preparation for the greater role that combat normally played in adult male wild cattle. Locomotor rotation movements are useful in predator avoidance and are commonly seen in cattle. Apart from muscular and sensor training, many aspects of body form and function respond to training. Bone, connective tissue, the circulatory, respiratory and endocrine systems and even the central nervous system all respond to activity and may be entrained by play behaviour. In addition olfactory communication may be facilitated by play, and training of response systems may occur.

Further evidence of the necessity of physical training comes from the existence of prenatal 'play'. Extensive movement of the calf fetus, especially rotation and movement in the immediate prenatal period, suggests muscular training for the post-natal period. A curious behaviour is the regular practice movements towards the birth canal in the last trimester of pregnancy, which uses muscles that are not particularly required in the post-natal period. Nervous reflexes are also practised, since veterinarians searching for life in a fetus will often pinch the nose or a hoof, through the rectal wall, in the hope of finding a movement response (Jackson, 1995). Such movements usually exist, although there are clearly somnolent periods when calves do not respond (P. Jackson, personal communication). Practice breathing also occurs, even though the calf swallows amniotic fluid. Anoxic calves become hyperactive *in utero*, although this is presumably in an attempt to obtain oxygen rather than play.

The physical training theory of play has difficulty in explaining 'intellectual' play, a calf playing with a gate latch in a pen, for example, or the random, rather illogical nature of play if it is purely for exercise. Another theory, therefore, is that play serves to increase and stimulate learning. Cattle can learn about environmental features through play, and novel environments stimulate play. Cattle also learn their position in the dominance hierarchy through play, which prevents damaging aggressive interactions later on. Again the rather irrational nature of play is hard to explain if this is the main aim. Play also helps juvenile cattle to learn behavioural patterns and responses and thus serves as practice for adult function. However, only limited improvement of play characteristics is usually seen from the time the calf first starts playing, which may be a few hours after birth. Also, play is not confined to juveniles: adult cows, for example, can take delight in charging round a field when the stockperson is attempting to collect them for milking. Less time is devoted by adults to play than juveniles, except where the mother assists in juvenile play. Play is always by mutual agreement, usually between two animals, although group and solo play is observed. A mother's rejection of play advances by her offspring when they get older probably arises from her need to rest. As the calf develops, the cow encourages her calf to form peer bonds in order that she can prepare for further reproduction. Mutual play between peers usually benefits both partners equally; there is no evidence that one partner is damaging the survival potential of the other. Mutual pauses, role reversal and the absence of damaging fighting all serve to ensure mutual benefit.

In prey animals such as cattle, play may also serve to keep the young together through social facilitation. The sight of two calves playing frequently acts as the stimulus for a third to join in. Isolated calves are more at risk from predation. Play may also go one stage further by strengthening social bonds to increase the cohesion of the herd and act as a catalyst for social facilitation.

A possible function of play that is not frequently considered is the psychological reward. However, the frequency of play is broadly correlated with the degree of cerebralisation in animals. Animals with a high degree of cerebralisation, especially primates, also perform more intellectually challenging forms of play. The size of the brain in ungulates is not entirely relative to body size, being larger than in rodents or insects but smaller than in the higher mammals (MacPhail, 1982). Fagen (1981) believes that there is a hierarchy of play, with simple forms, such as solo locomotor rotation and play fighting, predominating in lower order animals. Higher order animals do use the simple forms, but they also develop complex forms, such as reciprocal chasing, games of tag and king-of-the-castle, and involvement of females in social play. Cattle show quite considerable amounts of play, in comparison with other higher mammals, but probably not as much as caprines, such as sheep or goats. Usually 1 to 10% of the day is devoted to play in juveniles.

Play is encouraged by novel stimuli and in particular by tasks which are just beyond the immediate intellectual capacity of the animal. Cattle appear, for example, to gain satisfaction from playing with a latch on a door until they can open it. A state of psychological and physical well-being is a requisite for play.

Fine, sunny weather stimulates play, and increased light perception has been associated with endorphin release in the brain. Sick animals do not play, but this may be because energy reserves are conserved to combat the disease. There is therefore convincing evidence that animals receive psychological rewards from some forms of play, but it is difficult to judge whether these rewards are the objective of play, as most physically useful tasks involve some psychological reward. In addition, performing intellectually challenging tasks could increase cognitive powers, which again could have survival value.

Some researchers consider repetitive, stereotyped behaviours, such as tongue-rolling in steers, as play. Such behaviours do not function to train the animal, either physically or mentally, but animals performing such behaviours regularly appear to be able to avoid self-damage in environments where the normal behaviour of the animal cannot be performed (Wiepkema *et al.*, 1987). The behaviour appears to have a de-arousal function which reduces sympathetic nervous activity (Seo *et al.*, 1998b). Tongue-playing is particularly common in penned veal calves (Wilson *et al.*, 1999), and can be performed for up to 15% of the time (Sato *et al.*, 1994). It may relate to the deficiencies of the diet more than the lack of space or companionship. In particular, the absence of the ability to suckle stimulates tongue-playing (Seo *et al.*, 1998a).

Play is therefore a multicomponent behaviour with almost certainly more than one objective. As such we may be wrong in ascribing one term to it, and think-ing of it as one behaviour only. This, however, is a problem which probably only reductionist research into neuroendocrine control can answer.

Chapter 9
Social Behaviour

Introduction

Animals are generally classified as solitary, aggregated or social. Social animals employ communicative behaviour that transcends sexual union, and aggregated animals maintain a lower interindividual distance than equidistant spacing in the environment, but without communication other than sexual. Cattle are social animals in the fullest sense of the word, with complex communication channels and allelomimicry exhibited in many behaviours.

In order to truly understand the social behaviour of domesticated cattle, the reasons for the cohesive forces that existed in non-domesticated cattle must be appreciated. Forming a herd reduced the risk of predation by leaving large areas of grazing land devoid of cattle and reducing the chance of a predator seeing the animals or picking up a trail. Predation was probably also reduced by the rapid flight of large numbers of animals in random directions, thereby confusing the predator. The effectiveness of tasks such as surveillance would be increased in a herd, but under conditions of low pasture availability the interanimal distance would have been increased to ensure effective coverage of the total area. Also the opportunity for members of a herd to learn survival tactics was increased through social facilitation (Dumont & Boissy, 1999).

In addition to these factors favouring herding in wild cattle, domesticated cattle have shorter interanimal distances than other grazing ungulates (Lewis, 1978), which is probably due to selection by man for ease of herding over thousands of years. Domestication has allowed man to control cattle for productive purposes. To obtain full control man must usually displace the top-ranking animal in the dominance order. This is readily accomplished by most competent herdsmen with a herd of cows, but it is difficult, for example, in a herd of bulls, which are naturally more aggressive and stronger than cows. A herdsman may form a 'social pact' with bulls, and even top-ranking cows, whereby both tolerate each other's presence, but agree to minimise contact that could result in aggressive interaction. If regular close contact with bulls is unavoidable, strong expression of human dominance is required. For example, Fulani tribesmen are noted for their aggressive attitude to bulls from birth because the management system necessitates frequent close contact with all their cattle. Dominance of all the cattle by the tribesmen is a necessity, rather than a social pact, and this can only be achieved by aggressive control of the bulls from birth (Lott & Hart, 1977).

In wild Gaur cattle, which are one of the few remaining wild cattle genotypes, living in the forest regions of south-east Asia, social grouping allows all types of cattle to be members of the herd, adult males and females, juveniles and adolescents. In feral cattle, herd social organisation usually takes the form of matriarchal groups, consisting of mother and offspring, and bachelor groups of bulls, grazing separately (Reinhardt & Reinhardt, 1981). Dominant bulls join the matriarchal group when there are oestrous cows, which is the reason for their signalling by mounting behaviour. This difference between feral cattle in extensive grazing and forest-dwelling wild cattle may derive from the difficulty of signalling by a mounting display to bulls in the forest.

In domesticated cattle these natural groupings are replaced by groups of cows and growing cattle, usually divided into similar age and single sex groups after about six months of age. Bulls kept for reproduction may be solitarily confined for much of their life, or they may be run with a herd of cows or even rotated between herds. These changes in the social structure from the natural groupings and the intensive husbandry methods used increase social tension. In the case of growing male cattle, the stress caused to bulls by close confinement may make them difficult to manage safely without danger to the stockperson, and castration is often performed to improve their temperament by reducing aggression.

Social interactions

Social interactions form the communicative medium for social information transfer. They are an initial part of environmental *exploration*, which is followed by *recognition* of environmental cues. Once position in society is established, regular *communication* is used to maintain status and assess environmental changes. Finally *bonding* occurs between the animal and the features of its environment.

Exploratory behaviour

Exploration is the exhibition of investigation behaviour towards other animals (usually herdmates) or inanimate objects, and is maximised in yearling cattle (Fig. 9.1) (Murphey *et al.*, 1981). In the immediate post-natal period exploration is directed primarily towards the dam and not to the environment, as adequate defensive behaviour has not yet been established, e.g. fleeing. This is mainly to establish suckling behaviour in the calf (Das *et al.*, 2000). Innate maternal behaviour by the cow causes her to lick the calf and eat the placenta. There then usually follows a refractory period, when cattle are fearful of novel stimuli, such as unfamiliar calves, and which is more pronounced in calves that are reared individually as opposed to in groups (Jensen *et al.*, 1997). After being attracted

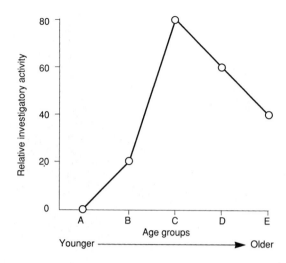

Fig. 9.1   Investigatory behaviour in different classes of cattle. A, preweaned calves; B, weaned calves; C, yearling heifers; D, two-year-old heifers; E, adult milking cows (Murphey *et al.*, 1981).

principally to its dam, the calf will develop attraction to its environment and peers. In general the more complex the environment, the more exploratory behaviour is displayed (Kenny & Tarrant, 1987b). This period of exploration eventually declines but can be re-initiated if the animal moves to a new environment or is placed with a new group of cattle. Exploratory approaches usually occur with the head extended and legs sloping forwards, which most effectively advances the sensory apparatus on the head towards the subject of investigation but enables a rapid retreat to take place if necessary.

Recognition

Recognition of herdmates allows social interactions to be conducted without the need for repeated dominance establishment. It is mainly achieved by vision, although sound is also important for maternal–juvenile recognition. Olfactory confirmation takes place at close quarters, but the visual and vocal cues provide the primary recognition responses and are additive (in line with Seitz's law of heterogeneous summation of stimuli) (Soffie & Zayan, 1977). There is some degree of specificity, allowing recognition of the sight or sound of an individual herdsperson for example (Murphey & Moura-Duarte, 1983). However, little is known about the scope of the recognition memory of cattle. It has been suggested that cows can recognise 50 to 70 herdmates (Fraser & Broom, 1990), and if this is true it could explain why larger herds than this tend to be subdivided. A cow is able to recognise her calf after only a few minutes of contact post partum. The exploratory licking by the cow reinforces the bond and aids subsequent recognition by the addition of salivary pheromones to the calf's coat (Fig. 9.2).

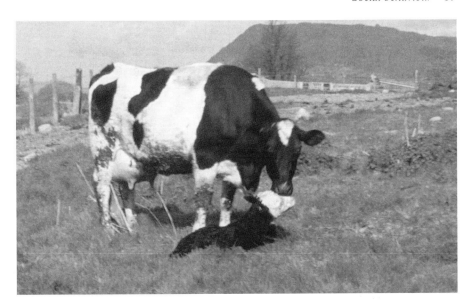

Fig. 9.2   Licking by the mother reinforces the maternal bond.

Later, the calf probably recognises its mother by her coat markings, vocalisation and odour (Murphey *et al.*, 1990). Watts and Stookey (2000) considered that it is not clear that the cow can recognise its calf by its vocalisation, but the calf can definitely recognise its mother's call, which may relate to calves' need to respond when called, but not to draw attention to themselves by calling.

Communication

As prey animals, non-domesticated cattle would have been discouraged from excessive use of intraspecial communication that attracted the attention of predators. However, domestic cattle have lost some of these inhibitions, especially as adequate communication is of vital importance in an intensively managed gregarious species.

Visual communication

Visual signals are one of the main methods used by cattle to communicate, particularly to indicate aggressive and reproductive states. They are also vital in food procurement, and cattle respond more to visual cues than auditory ones.

In the case of aggression, the signals confirm and reinforce the recognition or dominant position of participating animals. Threats are given which represent an intention to attack. In bulls this takes the form of lowering the head, drawing the chin towards the body and inclining the horns to the opponent (Fig. 9.3), with intention to charge actions such as pawing the ground. Other threat activities include head shaking and neck and head rubbing on the ground (Fig. 9.4), which is not visual communication but to mark the ground with salivary pheromones.

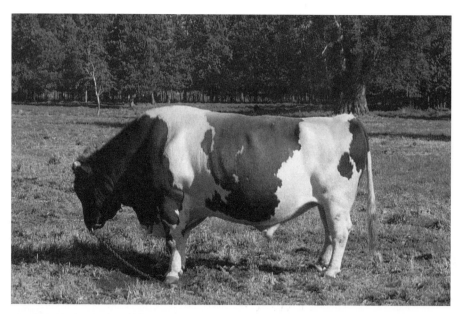

Fig 9.3 Threat posture in the bull.

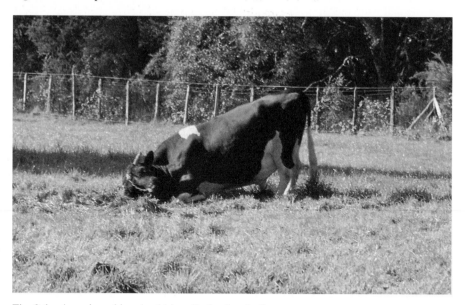

Fig. 9.4 A neck and head rubbing display in a bull.

These activities during the threat display indicate the intention to pursue and execute a direct physical and violent attack on the other animal. In cows the threat is less forceful and generally involves a head swing towards the opponent. Submission is usually indicated by lowering the head and turning away, as if to retreat. Actual retreat indicates a greater degree of submission. The objective of the submissive display is to indicate acceptance of the dominance of the opponent, by lowering/belittling parts or all of the body and suggesting retreat.

Reproductive display is similar in the bull to the threat display, but in the cow reproductive receptivity is indicated to bulls, other cows (to initiate the formation of a sexually active group) and not least to man, by homosexual mounting and standing to be mounted. Some indication of appeasement is necessary and flehman is believed to fulfil this function as an antithesis to the threat display. The cow exhibiting the standing reflex is receptive, not necessarily the mounting cow. The body elevation provided by homosexual mounting would have been particularly useful to cows grazing in tall, open grassland, where the bulls would form a separate herd some distance away. Mounting cows, although not necessarily receptive, are usually approaching receptivity so their activity is not entirely altruistic, as they themselves may benefit from the presence of a fertile bull. In domesticated cattle, where the bull is normally removed from the herd, such homosexual mounting is of great benefit to the herdsman to indicate the right time to bring in a bull or to use artificial insemination.

The tail is an important signalling device in cattle, although it also functions in locomotion and to remove flies (Kiley-Worthington, 1976). It is usually held horizontal during defecation and urination to avoid the hindquarters being soiled. Tail movements are either dorso-ventral or lateral. The head and tail tend to make dorso-ventral movements in synchrony, so that for example, both the head and tail are elevated during an exploratory position. Accompanied by postural tonus and prick ears, this position will solicit orientation and approach by other cattle. It indicates preparation for locomotion and full use of the sensors to investigate the source of the stimulus. Tails are also elevated during oestrus display, fighting, threats, greeting, suckling and homosexual activities in both male and female. Conversely, when the tail is held between the legs, the animal is often cold or frightened or may have been chased. Figure 9.5 illustrates the possible postures for cattle with different dorso-ventral tail positions, and the situations eliciting such signals.

Lateral movements of the tail are often for fly removal, but can be a response to more general cutaneous irritation, such as rubbing, or stimulation, such as of the vulva or penis during sexual behaviour. Tail wagging is also common when cattle experience minor irritation, and especially when their behavioural needs are thwarted. Cows will wag their tail as a threat to a calf, if they are about to kick. Threats by other cattle may be met by tail wagging, which will cease if fighting ensues.

Facial expressions are probably of less importance than in many other mammals for many reasons. From an anatomical point of view, the facial musculature is less well developed, also the need for complex mood display, which occurs in advanced societies of primates for example, is probably not needed and, finally, the distance between animals would often preclude the use of facial gestures as signals. However, there are subtle signals that are used and others may become recognised with further research. The flehman expression, in which the

(a)   (b)   (c)

(d)   (e)

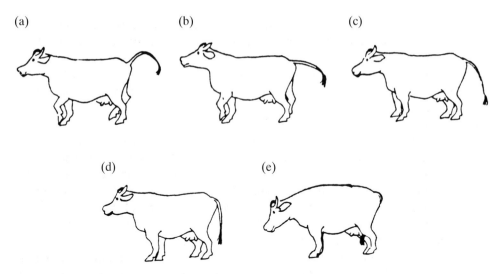

Fig. 9.5 Dorso-ventral tail positions and the associated postures (Kiley-Worthington, 1976). The situations eliciting these postures are for: (a) cantering/galloping/approach/avoidance; (b) urination/trotting/fighting; (c) walking/defecation/sexual approach by female (oestrus display); (d) standing/pain/sickness/drowsiness; (e) fear/being chased/defensive threat/submission.

head and neck are extended upwards, the lips are curled back (Fig. 9.6) and air is sampled through a partially opened mouth, functions to allow air to pass to the vomeronasal organ. The size of the eye's white surrounding the pupil increases with the degree of frustration or surprise in cattle, and in humans retracting the eyelids (which increases the proportion of white in the eye) is a also sign of surprise (Ekman, 1979). This gesture may be common in many mammals, and functions to increase environmental monitoring. Cattle often perform routine behaviours, such as eating, ruminating or lying, with their eyes half closed, which may reduce visual signals to an essential minimum. The pinna of the ears too may be involved in expressive behaviour, but this has not been studied, the only known movements being in response to acoustic signals or flies. Other bodily signals have

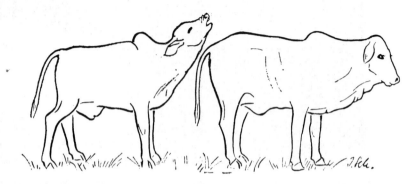

Fig. 9.6 Flehman in *Bos indicus* (Reinhardt, 1983b).

also been the subject of limited study. The defecation of fearful cattle, as well as other mammals, could function as a signal to other animals to flee, but it could also function to evacuate the gut. Tail position during sexual activity, threat and grooming animals is elevated, but the significance of this is unknown. In sick, cold or frightened animals it is withdrawn between the legs, which may conserve heat.

Olfactory communication

Olfactory sensitivity is greater in cattle compared with man (see Chapter 6), and it is therefore likely that it is relatively more important in social communication. The chemical messengers used for intraspecial social communication and also for interspecial communication are called pheromones. They are secreted by interdigital, infraorbital, inguinal, sebaceous and salivary glands and are particularly concentrated in the perineal region. They are also present in milk, urine and the other body secretions.

As described in Chapter 6, odours are received through both the nose and the vomeronasal organ in cattle. The vomeronasal organ is particularly involved in receiving pheromones that control aggressive behaviour and the oestrous cycle of cows. Bulls can detect a change in the pheromonal secretions of cows up to four days before the day of oestrus (French *et al.*, 1989). On the day of oestrus the main olfactory system of nasal detection is operative and the flehman expression is not always used. The ability of bulls to predict oestrus in cows relates to their tendency in wild herds to 'guard' cows as oestrus approaches. In domestic herds where there is no competition between bulls this does not occur. To test for cows' odours bulls sample the urine of potential oestrous cows and mark the ground with pheromones by rubbing their head and neck on the ground. Homosexual cow relationships appear to be stimulated by sniffing and licking, particularly in the perineal regions (Fig. 9.7). Other animals, such as dogs, cats and rats, can also detect the oestrous odours of cows, but they are not able to distinguish pre-oestrous odours from those produced at other stages in the cycle in the way that bulls can.

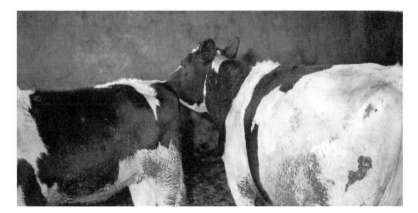

Fig. 9.7 An oestrous cow sniffs the anovaginal area of another oestrous cow to test for pheromones.

Tactile communication

Tactile communication is mainly used in aggressive encounters, grooming and sexual behaviour.

Aggressive encounters

In aggression the main forms of tactile interaction are charging, head pushing, butting and occasionally kicking. Mounting can be said to have both aggressive and sexual functions (Klemm *et al.*, 1983). Charging is used primarily by bulls, and the approach is rapid and accompanied by lowering of the head, often using the horns as a weapon. Head pushing is characterised by locking of horns in horned breeds and by contact between foreheads. Heads are lowered to exert maximum force and a rigid stance is adopted (Fig. 9.8). Each animal attempts to overpower/outmanoeuvre its opponent and gain access to butt the vulnerable flank or udder area. Often the losing combatant will wheel around in an attempt to prevent access to the flank area (Fig. 9.9). Violent butting at the end of the bout is usually avoided: the purpose of the fight is to establish dominance and only the 'threat' of injury is used. This type of fighting is common in bulls and cows, whereas steers more commonly indulge in butting, aggressive riding and kicking (Hinch & Lynch, 1987). Butting involves a characteristic upswing of the head usually to either the head or flanks of the other animals. The force of the movement varies from a mild push to a severe blow. Bunting is a similar action (the term is more often used to refer to the repeated pushing of the udder by a suckling calf to stimulate milk letdown).

The variation in aggressive tendencies between individuals has long been the subject of debate, not least as we try to explain our own self-destructive inclinations. Lorenz (1966) argues in favour of an endogenous supply of aggression, which, when supplemented with environmental triggers, necessitates release through agonistic acts (Fig. 9.10). The relative absence of aggression in wild/semi-wild cattle herds with adequate resources suggests that in cattle, environmental stimuli are more important than endogenous cues. Individual variation in aggressive tendencies in competitive situations may relate to, first, variation in pain perception, secondly, individuals' determination to maintain access

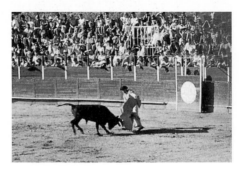

Fig. 9.8 The charge by a bull, with a characteristic lowered head, exposure of the horns and erect tail.

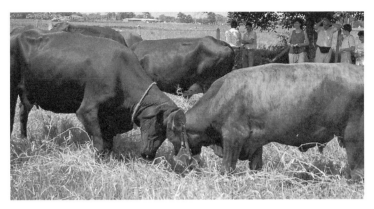

Fig. 9.9 Head-to-head contact in cattle, where they engage in circular movement, each attempting to force a retreat by the other through overpowering them, or to gain access to their vulnerable flanks.

to resources and, thirdly, position in the dominance order. High-ranking individuals show more aggression than low-ranking ones (Collis, 1976; Wierenga *et al.*, 1990), but this may arise from the need to maintain status rather than any genetic disposition.

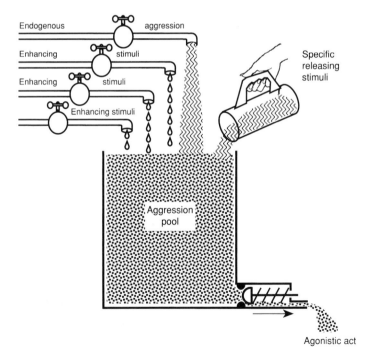

Fig. 9.10 Lorenz's hydraulic model of aggression (Lorenz, 1996).

Grooming

Grooming is primarily a body care activity but it has nutritional, communicative and psychological functions. Self-grooming is widely believed to function as a displacement activity (Dannenmann *et al.*, 1985; Jensen, 1995) and is characterised by licking activities (Fig. 9.11), but rubbing of the head (Fig. 9.12) and neck (Fig. 9.13) is also common. Allogrooming (grooming others) acts as an affiliative behaviour (Wood, 1977; Reinhardt & Reinhardt, 1981), and is mainly characterised by one animal licking the head and neck regions of other animals (Fig. 9.14) that are in a similar or slightly subordinate position in the dominance order. All animals in a herd are groomed but only about three-quarters of the animals in a herd do the grooming (Sato, 1984). As preferred partners are often kin, allogrooming may thus function not only to maintain dominance position

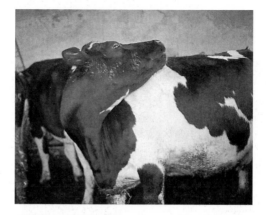

Fig. 9.11   Self-grooming by a dairy cow.

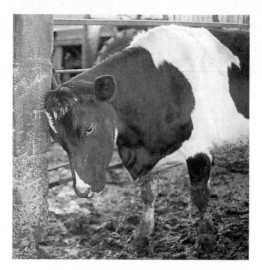

Fig. 9.12   Head rubbing by a dairy cow against the corner of a wall.

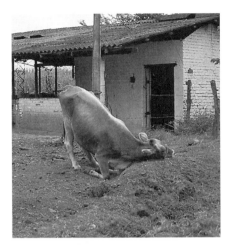

Fig. 9.13 Neck rubbing on the ground.

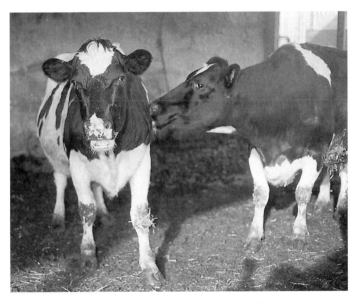

Fig. 9.14 Allogrooming in two dairy cows, involving mainly licking of the forequarters of a cow by another.

but also to reinforce family bonds and those between adult cattle. Fraser and Broom (1990) also attribute dopaminergic functions to allogrooming, suggesting that since the hormone prolactin is known to be associated with grooming and also dopaminergic activity, grooming may, via prolactin, cause opiate induction and self-narcotisation. The fact that allogrooming is increased in more intensive environments, where stereotypies are often performed for self-narcotisation, supports this hypothesis.

Sexual interactions

Sexual encounters, both homosexual and heterosexual, are the third kind of tactile communication. Chin pressing on a cow's back by a bull or another cow tests for the rigid back stance and whether she will be receptive to mounting.

Allogrooming activity by members of a sexually active group (SAG) increases during oestrus, but in this instance the same attention is paid to the anovaginal area as to the head and neck. Immediately prior to coitus, direct tactile stimulation of the vulval area by nudging by the bull is common.

Vocal communication

As gregarious grazing animals, cattle make more use of vocalisation for communication than solitary animals would, although it is used less than by true forest-dwelling species such as jungle fowl, where vocal communication is more effective than other communicative methods. The absence of predators in most farm situations probably explains why cattle, and in particular calves, are more vocal than other grazing prey animals. In the social context vocalisation is used for recognition and eliciting contact, as well as greetings, threats and fear display. Vocalisation has been associated with arousal in several studies (Von Borell & Ladewig, 1992; Lidfors, 1996; Zimmerman & Koene, 1998).

Specific cattle calls cannot be identified and their range of vocalisation forms a continuum, but certain types of call are commonly associated with specific behaviours or emotional states. In particular, as the animal becomes more excited the length, amplitude and pitch of the calls increase. With calves, the calls during isolation are of lower frequency and carry further than during branding, perhaps suggesting greater stress (Watts & Stookey, 1999).

Cattle calls may be classified according to several characteristics (Kiley, 1972).

The syllables

Five main syllables are used (best represented by *m*, *en*, *en*, *h* and *uh*), although these are not mutually exclusive. The '*m*' syllable is produced with the mouth shut and the sound emitted through the nostrils. '*En*' is produced with the mouth open, and most of the sound emitted from the mouth rather than the nose. The glottal lips may be tightened as the pitch increases. The '*en*' sound is usually a sudden increase in frequency and amplitude from the '*en*' sound and is the same phenomenon as overblowing a wind instrument. The '*h*' sound is produced with an open or closing mouth as the diaphragm and lips relax after the '*en*' sound. Finally the '*uh*' sound is produced during rapid inspiration. These five syllables are combined into six major calls, again not mutually exclusive: *mm*, *men(h)*, *(m)enh*, *menenh* and two see-saw calls, *(m)(en) enh* and *menenhuh* (Table 9.1).

Amplitude

This is generally less for calls such as *mm*, where the mouth is closed, and is greater for the '*en*' than '*en*' sound.

Table 9.1 Description of the characteristics of cattle calls

	Call					
	mm	*men(h)*	*(m)enh*	*menenh*[a]	*(m)(en)enh*[b]	*menenhuh*[b]
Duration (s)	1–3	0.5–4.1	1.0–2.8	0.8–3.5	0.7–2.3	1.3–2.9
Repetition	Variable	Up to 10 times	Variable	Up to 10 times	1–20 times	1–10 times
Amplitude						
m	Low–medium	Low–medium	–	Medium	Medium	Medium
en		Medium–high	High	Medium–high	–	High
en/h	–	–	–	High	High	High
h		Low–medium	High	Medium	Medium	High
uh						Medium–high
Pitch (Hz)						
m	50–125	50–125	–	75–100	75–125	75–125
en		125–300	125–250	100–250	Rising	Rising
en				500–800	175–500	250–750
h				100 falling	Falling	Falling
uh						1000–1250
Tonality						
m	High	Medium–high	–	Medium–high	High	Medium
en		Medium–high	Medium–high	Medium–high	Medium	Low–medium
en				Medium–high	Medium–high	Low–high
h		Low	Low	Low	–	Low
uh					Low	Low–high

After Kiley (1972)
[a] May preceded see-saw calls.
[b] See-saw calls.

Pitch

This is generally increased as amplitude increases. The fundamental tones are typically 50 to 1000 Hz but the overtones can reach 4 to 8 kHz in the *en* syllable, which is near the hearing limit in man but within that for cattle (see Chapter 6). In the loudest calls the pitch alternates between high and low in much the same way that human singers sustain a note by alternation of the pitch (vibrato). The pitch of a call also indicates social status in that the freedom to vocalise at a higher pitch is reserved for more dominant animals (Hall *et al.*, 1988).

Tonality

This is the musical quality of the sound as determined by the variation in frequency of the note. The fundamental tone is the lowest frequency sound, and there are also overtones which are multiples of the fundamental but less audible.

Length

Length refers to both the duration of each call and its frequency of repetition. Most calls are one to three seconds in length, this being restricted by the maximum duration of expiration. Cattle in a more excited state are more likely to repeat a call.

Message

This is interpreted by Kiley (1972) from anecdotal evidence, since little research has been conducted on the meaning and identity of different cattle calls. She believes that the *mm* call indicates a mild level of excitement as when a familiar herdmate or herdsperson approaches, during anticipation of a pleasurable event such as milking or feeding, or during courtship. It is also used by bulls guarding oestrous cows and for recognition purposes, since the long wavelength of the sound facilitates intra-aural localisation.

The *men(h)* call indicates a state of slightly increased excitement and is commonly referred to as a 'moo' or, in old English, 'low'. It may be uttered in situations of mild frustration as when cattle are waiting for food, are isolated from the rest of the herd or are mildly fearful. It is the commonest of all cattle calls in most herd situations.

In the *(m)enh* call the degree of excitement and tension is heightened, such as when a cow has her calf removed, when cattle are very hungry and often by bulls during the threat display. The *menenh* call is an extension of this where the animal is in its greatest state of excitement and is often colloquially referred to as a 'holler' or 'roar'.

The two see-saw calls are primarily produced by bulls in an excited state and by the change in frequency they emphasise the excited state of the caller. They are also part of the dominance display and may inhibit other bulls from agonistic acts (Fig. 9.15).

Cattle calls change as the animal ages and calling by all cattle, especially bulls, is strongly socially facilitated. Bulls tend to vocalise more than cows and steers

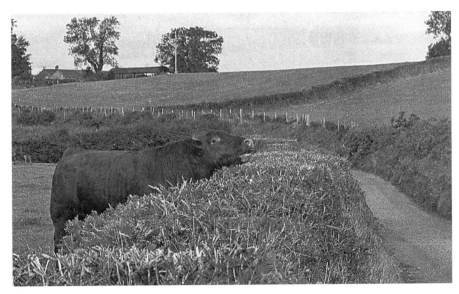

Fig. 9.15 A bull uses high-amplitude, open-mouthed vocalisation to attract the attention of cows.

and are particularly vocal in spring and summer (Hinch *et al.*, 1982b) (Figs 9.16 and 9.17). Cows and calves in the wild vocalise more in winter, possibly because of the low availability of food at this time. In domestic circumstances, calves normally use vocal communication primarily for indicating pain and distress, such as around feeding time or at weaning. Grandin (1998, 2001) has suggested that the frequency of vocalisation can be used as an indicator of cattle welfare at slaughter plants, even though it cannot be definitely said that vocalising individuals within any one plant are suffering more than those that do not vocalise (Watts &

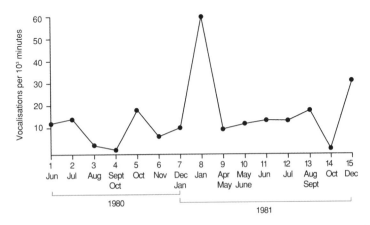

Fig. 9.16 Cow vocalisations expressed as number of vocalisations per thousand minutes of observation time (Hall *et al.*, 1988).

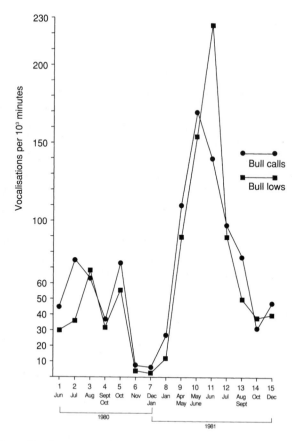

Fig. 9.17 Bull vocalisations expressed as number of vocalisations per thousand minutes of observation time (Hall *et al.*, 1988).

Stookey, 2000). This has been used effectively in practice and may help to influence slaughter practice (Grandin, 2000).

Cattle can recognise calls by individual conspecifics, and it is likely that they attribute meaning to specific calls, but this has not been demonstrated yet. They may do the same for human communication as they can learn to come in from pasture for milking when called (Albright *et al.*, 1966) and calves can learn individual names (Watts & Stookey, 2000). The sound of humans shouting is particularly alarming for cattle, as assessed by changes in heart rate (Waynert *et al.*, 1999).

The possibility that calls might differ during oestrus, or that bulls may stimulate oestrus expression by calling, remain unexplored (Watts & Stookey, 2000). Calves in individual pens may even alter their arousal state at feeding by frequent calling, since such regular vocalisation does not occur in the field. Calves are normally singletons and so do not need to attract the attention of their mother, which animals in large litters may have to.

Intraspecial bonding

Mother–filial bonding

In cattle it is the female parent, rather than the male, which normally becomes bonded to the offspring. This bonding develops soon after birth and, given the opportunity, will persist as a matriarchal family group (Reinhardt & Reinhardt, 1981). The initial bonding, which is termed imprinting, has the following characteristics. It develops during the sensitive period, which for a precocious animal such as *Bos taurus* occurs in the immediate post-natal period. It is permanent and irreversible, but its strength will depend on the extent of other imprinted bonds which the dam has. A cow with twins therefore develops a weaker bond with each calf than a cow with a single calf, and this encourages the twins to form sibling bonds (Price *et al.*, 1986). Within a semi-wild herd of cows and calves the bond between dam and daughter will persist as the dominant social force (Reinhardt & Reinhardt, 1981), and the males disperse to form bachelor groups. Equal preference is generally given by the dam to her offspring, regardless of their age and sex.

Multiparous cows form stronger bonds than primiparous cows through greater contact and contact-seeking behaviour with their calves, and they are more disturbed by separation (Price *et al.*, 1986). Primiparous cows show more abnormal maternal behaviour but spend longer suckling their calves than multiparous cows, perhaps because the milk flow rate is less. The creation of a strong maternal–filial bond is therefore a learnt characteristic, although much of the stimulation by the calf is innate. Intensely selected dairy breeds such as the Holstein-Friesian show weak dam–filial bonding. They are more easily cross-fostered and removal of the calf for artificial rearing has little effect on its temperament, whereas in less developed breeds such as the Salers (Le Neindre, 1989 a,b) artificial rearing reduces the social adaptability of the calves. In all breeds, artificially rearing calves in isolation reduces their social adaptability compared with group-reared calves and results in their occupying lower positions in the dominance order in later life. Isolation rearing is often advocated to reduce between-calf contact and hence disease spread, at a time when the animals are very susceptible to infection. It stresses the calf, but this seems to condition the animal to accept stress in adulthood and may encourage a good relationship between the stockperson and the cattle rather than strong bonding between cattle.

Thus, it can be seen that cattle are socially adaptable, and in the absence of a preferred social partner they strengthen the bonds with other partners. For the young calf the dam is the preferred social partner, followed by kin, other peers and lastly other species such as humans.

Imprinting tends to occur within species, but is not confined to certain classes of individuals (Thorpe, 1963). However the bond is created at a time when the calf is naturally drawn to the dam by suckling motivation and the chances of other bonds being created during the period of primary socialisation are small. The imprinting bond is preserved by grooming, both during and after suckling, but other forms of communication like vocalisation must be important, since calves that are muzzled to prevent suckling and grooming still develop a bond with their dams. The bond, and in particular suckling, maintains the post-partum anoestrus in the cows for about eight weeks to prevent early rebreeding.

The benefits of a strong mother–filial bond are many, particularly in wild cattle. For the dam, the need to perpetuate the family line is paramount (Dawkins, 1976). For the calf the initial reward is in the form of protection: the afterbirth and other residues are consumed by the dam to minimise the risk of predation, and nutrition is provided in the form of milk. Early licking of the perineal region stimulates the functioning of the gastrointestinal tract and excretion (Kovalcik *et al.*, 1980). Later the calves learn dietary and other habits from their dams (Provenza & Balph, 1987) and acquire a stable position in the herd structure.

Peer bonding

The first evidence of peer relationships usually comes in the calf's first or second week of life. The dam may leave her calf in a 'creche' of other calves whilst she grazes nearby. Often she remains within sight of the calves. If she does not, as may occur in extensive grazing conditions, another cow may keep watch over the nursery. Creches are more often formed under extensive grazing conditions, where the cows need to leave the calves to cover the area effectively. Typically the calves spend two to five hours per day in the creche and leave it when they need to begin grazing, after about 10 to 15 weeks. Under intensive grazing conditions calves usually stay with their dams or may play with peers whilst their dams graze.

Juvenile–juvenile bonds are more likely to occur between siblings, because sibling calves are brought into frequent contact with each other through their mother. The bonds are maintained through play and grazing associations, not by allogrooming, as is the case with adult cattle. The formation of the bonds is irrespective of the sex of the calves, but male–male bonds are likely to be broken earlier than female–female. Sex differences which relate to adult function appear in their play: males indulge more in play mounting, which enables them to learn correct orientation and timing of this behaviour. This enhances their performance, as adult males and bulls that have not had the opportunity to practise are not so reproductively able (Silver & Price, 1986). Homosexual mounting may persist in groups of intensively housed adult bulls, and some subordinate bulls may be excessively ridden as a form of aggression by the dominant bulls. Usually, however, it is the bulls with more masculine conformation that are ridden more and show more aggressive behaviour.

In adult cows, peer bonds are preserved by allogrooming and grazing and less by play. Allogrooming is generally unidirectional, i.e. only one partner grooms, whereas most grazing partnerships are bidirectional, i.e. both animals prefer to graze with each other (Reinhardt & Reinhardt, 1981). Only about 20% of partnerships are common to both grazing and grooming associations, so different partners are usually chosen for the two activities. Not all adult cows, however, develop associations, as some prefer to remain solitary.

Interspecial bonding

The intensification of agriculture during the last 50 years has led to increased emphasis on single species animal farming, without the complexities of mixed species. During this period less emphasis has been placed on efficient utilisation of natural resources, which is often greater in mixed farming systems, and more emphasis has been on labour efficiency, which often necessitates single species farming if high output is to be achieved. Cattle and sheep were traditionally recognised as good grazing partners (Fig. 9.18), and cattle and goats have similar advantages of pasture utilisation complementarity. Normally the two species graze separately in species groups, but there is considerable overlap in areas utilised. This preserves intraspecific social cohesion and minimises interspecific conflict. Similarly cattle and deer rarely interact, the latter being afraid of cattle (Mattiello *et al.*, 1997). In competitive situations horses dominate cattle, which in turn dominate sheep (Arnold, 1984). Dominance also plays a role in cattle acquiring diseases, as dominant individuals are more likely to approach wildlife, whereas the subordinate cattle are usually shy in doing so. In New Zealand it has been found that this approach of dominant cattle to possums apparently predisposes them to tuberculosis, which is common in the possum (Sauter & Morris, 1995).

In extensive grazing conditions protection of small ruminants from predators can be achieved by bonding them to the cattle at an early age. In the Americas the coyote and the puma still cause an appreciable risk of predation of both adult

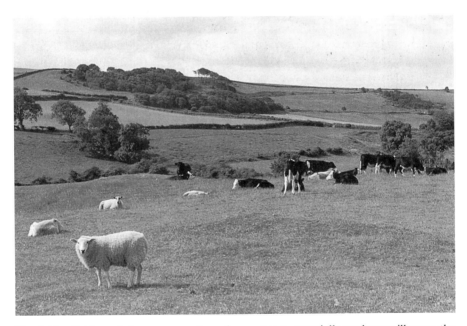

Fig. 9.18   Cattle and sheep are good grazing partners, especially as sheep will graze the areas around cattle faeces and vice versa.

and juvenile sheep and goats, despite the increasing loss of the predators' natural habitat. This may prevent farmers keeping sheep or goats, particularly near forests or in silvo-pastoral systems. Domesticated dogs or horse patrols can be used for protection but are not very effective at night. Systems of protection have been developed of bonding the small ruminants to cattle, usually heifers. Normally this can be achieved by penning young sheep or goats with the cattle for about 60 days, although a longer period is necessary if the cattle show aggressive tendencies to the young animals. When the bond is formed interspecific distance is reduced. During an attack protection is achieved by the sheep positioning themselves amongst the cattle (Anderson *et al.*, 1988), whereas non-bonded sheep would move away from the cattle. Calves may also be at risk of predation in extensive circumstances, and possible protectors include dogs, donkeys and llamas (Smith *et al.*, 2000).

Social organisation

Social hierarchies

In all intensively managed stock a strict hierarchy develops to determine priority of access to resources. The existence of a hierarchy reduces aggression by eliminating the need for repeated agonistic encounters to determine priority, thus ensuring that scarce resources are rapidly and easily given to the strongest and fittest animals. The hierarchy is not the same for all resources (Dickson *et al.*, 1967), because some individuals attribute more importance to certain resources and will fight harder to gain access to them. Separate hierarchies can be demonstrated for access to feed, space, sexual partners and milking, although several of these show close correlation. The order of greatest concern in intensive husbandry situations is usually the hierarchy for space priority, which is usually referred to as the dominance order.

Dominance order

This hierarchy has been variously described as a hook, bunt, peck, rank, aggressive or competitive order, social rank or dominance status. It usually indicates priority of access to space (Potter & Broom, 1987), because it is measured by observing agonistic interactions between cattle when space availability is reduced, e.g. in a passageway or other confined area. Space allocation, and more particularly the preservation of personal space, is at the heart of the social organisation of cattle. It may be contested indoors, such as when subordinate cows try to feed away from the dominant cows at a feeding face (Manson & Appleby, 1990), or outdoors, such as when aggression increases in response to the provision of a food supplement for grazing cattle (Clutton Brock *et al.*, 1976). In a group of cows at risk of fly infestation, dominant cows are more often to be seen in the centre of subgroups, demonstrating their priority of access to high-quality space (Kabuga, 1993). Some regular exchange of animals from the centre to the periphery of a subgroup takes place in these circumstances, probably as a result of jostling for central positions. In the grazing situation adequate space is normally assured, but priority of access to the best grazing may form the basis of the herd hierarchy, which could explain why dominant cows have sometimes been found to produce more milk than subordinate cows in grazing systems (Reinhardt, 1973). Other hierarchies, e.g. order of entry into the milking parlour, are less keenly contested than access to space.

As the dominance order becomes established in a herd, the aggression becomes ritualised, and this is more common in cattle than other ungulates. Little more than a swing of the head may be needed to confirm status by the dominant animal and a slight avoidance movement by the subordinate animal. Allogrooming confirms dominant status, and acceptance of a conspecific's superiority is at least partly controlled by pheromones. Sato *et al.* (1990) described the function of licking as possibly being a reduction of tension. They suggested that licking is independent of social dominance, but still being licked more could indicate a greater social competence. Animals close in the dominance order need to confirm status more regularly, and changes in order may occur in 25% of the herd annually. Kin are most likely to engage in allogrooming, suggesting that it also functions to cement family ties (Sato *et al.*, 1993).

Older members of the herd with an established position initiate less aggression, because experience in the herd conveys social advantage and may frustrate the rank ambitions of younger members. Younger members must constantly challenge older members to elevate their position in the hierarchy. The prime determinants of dominance are age or lactation number (Schein & Fohrman, 1955; Beilharz *et al.*, 1966; Brantas, 1968; Sambraus, 1979; Beilharz & Zeeb, 1982), weight and size (Schein & Fohrman, 1955; Brantas, 1968; Sambraus, 1979; Stricklin *et al.*, 1980), with age often being the most important (O'Connell *et al.*, 1989). The relationship with age demonstrates the advantage of experience, but not familiarity (Schein & Fohrman, 1955). Brantas (1968) identified chest girth and body length as key characteristics contributing to the relationship between live weight and dominance. Although weight and size are correlated with age, the social skills necessary for gaining a high rank need to be learnt. This usually occurs as juveniles during play, and animals reared in spatial isolation are usually dominated by animals reared in groups (Broom & Leaver, 1978).

In addition to experience and physical ability, a third factor, emotionality or fear, determines dominance and varies in importance in different individuals. Of the three factors, it is likely that physical ability is most important in a highly competitive situation, as animals learn to overcome their fear to obtain priority of access, and the benefits of experience are less of an advantage if agonistic encounters are frequent and young members can rapidly learn the art of social elevation. Under these circumstances young members of the herd can increase their status faster than in less competitive situations. In competitive situations more complex relationships are formed, and the order may develop from simple linearity to include triangular and even more complex relationships (Fig. 9.19).

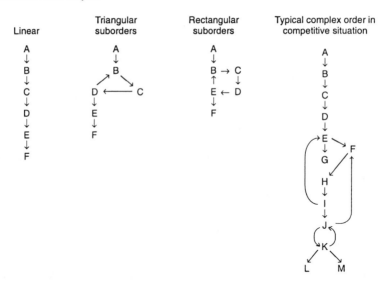

Fig. 9.19 Dominance orders, with triangular and rectangular suborders (Beilharz & Mylrea, 1963a,b).

In complex dairy systems over 40% of pairs of cows can be observed to displace each other at different times (Wierenga, 1990), suggesting non-linear dominance orders.

Physiological status will affect an animal's position in the dominance order. Cows in oestrus have elevated status to enable them to obtain access to a partner, but pregnant cows have reduced status to limit the risk of damaging aggressive encounters (Beilharz & Mylrea, 1963a,b).

The dominance hierarchy is particularly important in intensive husbandry because there is little opportunity for low-ranking individuals to escape. They constantly have to move about so as to avoid high-ranking individuals (Arave *et al.*, 1974) and this creates stress. Spatial priority also relates to access to lying areas, in particular cubicles. Preferred cubicles – those in the centre of a line or those with enclosed fronts that offer more privacy – will be occupied by high-ranking cows at preferred times. Low-ranking cows are left to occupy these at other times or to take less preferred cubicles. The spatial memory of cattle is good (Bailey *et al.*, 1989), which facilitates the enforcement of hierarchical access to cubicles.

Dominance and milk production

Dominant cows will produce more milk than subordinates if there is limited supply of food (Albright & Arave, 1997). Some authors have found a low positive correlation between milk yield and dominance (Beilharz *et al.*, 1966; Dickson *et al.*, 1967, 1970; Soffie *et al.*, 1976), but others have found stronger, statistically significant positive relationships (Schein & Fohrman, 1955; Reinhardt, 1973; Sambraus *et al.*, 1979). Grazing cattle utilise their dominance more when herbage is available *ad libitum*, since there is greater diversity, and a dominant individual with priority of access to food can graze the best quality of herbage (Barroso *et al.*, 2000). The digestibility of herbage chosen by cattle is approximately 150 to 200 g/kg dry matter greater than the herbage on offer (Le Du *et al.*, 1981). Dominant goats (Lovari & Rosto, 1985) and deer (Thoules, 1990) are more efficient grazers than their subordinate counterparts, the latter displaying more or longer head lifts during grazing, presumed to relate to vigilance for the presence of dominant animals, and a slower rate of biting forage as a result. Cattle probably also show this pattern (Phillips & Rind, 2002a). The greater milk yields of dominant than subordinate grazing cows has been observed experimentally (Reinhardt, 1973) and may also relate to their faster feeding rates (Phillips & Rind, 2002a). Subordinate cows could seek to obtain improved grazing away from the herd, but the desire for this would be counteracted by the cohesive forces that encourage the cows to stay together for protection. There is therefore an optimum interindividual distance for grazing cows, determined mainly by group size (Rind & Phillips, 1999), and the concept of an 'ideal free distribution' of animals at pasture (Milinski & Parker, 1991) probably does not apply to grazing cattle because of the cohesive, anti-predator forces.

Feeding order

Rank determined by competitive cattle feeding behaviour is closely correlated with rank determined by spatial encounters (Rutter *et al.*, 1987), suggesting that both food and space are of similar importance. However, some compensation for having a low priority of access is possible in the case of feed restriction. When feed is spatially distributed or feeding barriers are designed so that high-ranking individuals cannot prevent low-ranking ones from feeding, there is little need for a feeding order. In the case of conserved forages offered at a feeding barrier, dominant animals will usually eat at preferred times and subordinates at less preferred times, unless there is space for all to eat at once. An allowance of 15 cm manger space per animal is adequate for beef and dairy cattle to obtain *ad libitum* intake, but increasing the trough size or the density of the diet may reduce competition for food (Ingrand, 2000). It has been estimated that cattle of 17 to 21 months need 47 cm to allow uninhibited expression of feeding behaviour (Longenbach *et al.*, 1999).

If forage availability is restricted, the rate of eating of conserved feeds will be increased to a certain extent, but not enough to allow the dominant cows to eat a great deal more than subordinate cows. This is because the rate of intake of forage is inherently slow, and all cows therefore eat for most of the allocated time. Position in a feed priority order may become more important if concentrate feeds are offered in restricted amounts. Cattle usually prefer concentrates to forage, and considerable aggression may result as dominant cows attempt to get more than their share. Individual feeders have therefore been devised which restrict the concentrate allowance to a programmable quantity every few hours. For lactating cows these may be placed in the milking parlour to allow intakes of up to approximately 5 kg per milking. Artificial milk replacer can be similarly rationed mechanically for calves. If grazing animals are fed supplements at pasture, the proportion of animals not consuming supplement is increased by limited trough space, small supplement allowance and neophobia to feed or feed delivery devices. Thus increasing trough space will increase the variation in intake between animals (Bowman & Sowell, 1997).

Grazing cows do not appear to exhibit a feeding order of initiation of grazing based on dominance, but separating dominant and subordinate grazing cows reduces milk production (Phillips & Rind, 2002a). This may be because dominant grazing cows eat more when subordinate cows are present, which has also been found with housed cows (Olofsson & Wiktorsson, 2001). Order of initiation of grazing may be based on yield and the cows' nutritional requirements, since high-yielding cows begin grazing earlier than low-yielding cows in the first grazing bout of the day (Rind & Phillips, 1999). This suggests that high-yielding cows have a greater hunger in the early morning than low-yielding cows.

Access to milking machines

Access to milking machines in a parlour may be a priority resource, as a result of their potential to relieve udder pressure, and the opportunity to obtain food in the parlour and after milking. However, milking order, or the order of presentation of the cows for milking, is only weakly related to the dominance order (Dickson *et al.*, 1967; Reinhardt, 1973; Soffie *et al.*, 1976). There is some tendency for more dominant cows to enter the milking parlour earlier but it is more likely to be the higher yielding cows. There is a positive correlation between milk yield and milking order (Gadbury, 1975; Rathore, 1982), which is believed to derive from the greater reward to a high-yielding cow of relief of udder pressure during milking, compared with a low-yielding cow.

The reward that entering the parlour offers to a cow depends on the frequency of milking, the milk yield of the cow and the provision of concentrates. If cows are milked just twice a day and the intervals are uneven, e.g. 16 hours overnight, 8 hours during the day, then high-yielding cows will suffer from high udder pressure before morning milking and will experience a greater reward than low-yielding cows. If one milking is omitted, as for example might happen following the breakdown of an automatic milking plant, cows show signs of discomfort, such as early and more frequent urination (Stefanowska *et al.*, 2000). Cows with subclinical or clinical mastitis are more reluctant to enter the parlour, as milking may cause discomfort (Rathore, 1982). If concentrates are offered in the parlour, cows with priority of access for food will tend to enter early. At a given stage of lactation high-yielding cows are likely to be more hungry than low-yielding ones because of their more rapid removal of fermentation end products. However, early lactation cows may be less hungry than late lactation cows because the gut is involuted.

Maintaining the same order of entry into the milking parlour does not seem to be of major or lasting importance to cows. It is not related to the peer associations and can be readily rearranged through training. Although some rearrangement of order is readily tolerated, cows do prefer to be milked at approximately the same time each day. In a block calving herd the order is not clearly defined when the cows are in early lactation but becomes more ordered in mid to late lactation.

Cows exhibit a side preference in the milking parlour, and the consistent choice of one side in the milking parlour is evidence of formation of a routine (Hopster *et al.*, 1998). Such behavioural lateralisation might be associated with specific immunological and neuroendocrine parameters, but may also be learnt avoidance of a potentially aversive situation. Grandin *et al.* (1994) showed that cattle generally tend to stay in a routine once they have learnt one side to be aversive in a Y-maze even when the aversive and normal side are being switched. This suggests that coping strategies could be interpreted as differences in the need for predictability and control (Hansen & Damgaard, 1993).

Sexual partner priority

In many modern husbandry systems, natural reproduction is superseded by artificial insemination using specially selected male sperm-lines, or less commonly by embryo transfer, using selected male and female genotypes. In less intensive systems bulls are used, but the male:female ratio is much lower than would naturally be the case. It is only in large, extensively managed herds, usually kept for beef production, that several bulls may be run together, and in these circumstances there is a possibility of priority of access to sexual partners being gained by dominant bulls. In such circumstances dominance, and in particular age, will determine which bulls serve most of the cows. In one herd with four bulls aged two to ten years, over two-thirds of the cows were served by one bull, the oldest one (Blockey, 1978). Dominance was perpetuated by the top male refusing other males access to the sexually active group of females. Only when four or more cows were in heat simultaneously were other bulls able to serve the cows. If there were fewer cows, attempts to copulate by the subordinate bulls were interrupted. The mere presence of the dominant bull in an adjacent pen will reduce the attention paid by a young bull to a female (Lopez *et al.*, 1999). The aggregation of receptive females into a sexually active group helps the dominant male to maximise the inheritance of his genes and is therefore an evolutionarily useful behaviour. As reproductive priority is so closely linked to genetic inheritance, it is to be expected that strong dominance effects will be present in the fight to gain access to receptive females. Natural selection therefore requires that the most dominant bull serves cows to his capacity before other bulls are given opportunities. Unfortunately the most dominant bull is not necessarily the most fertile and the herd reproductive rate can be compromised.

Dominance also influences the manifestation of oestrous behaviours between cows (Orihuela, 2000). Small, subordinate cows, particularly if they are primiparous, are inhibited from mounting large, dominant cows. Clearly some cows are favoured by most cows for mounting, and rarely initiate mounting themselves. Social dominance can also influence the duration of oestrus, being prolonged when dominant cows are in oestrus.

Spatial distribution

Cattle are aggregated into non-random patterns, both when housed and at pasture. For economic reasons, stocking densities on farms are normally greater in housing than at pasture; however, milking cattle kept in sheltered woodland choose to live at greater interindividual distances than in the open range (Dudzinski *et al.*, 1982), suggesting that cattle under cover prefer a lower stocking rate than in the open. This dichotomy can lead to social tension in the cattle house as it has been seen that the maintenance of personal space is one of the main status symbols for cattle. The personal space is the envelope or 'bubble' around each individual that it attempts to keep free from interference by other animals. When this space is breached, the animal will attempt to flee from the intruder. Studies of both housed and grazing situations show that cattle expend a great deal of effort in maintaining the correct interindividual distances. Similarly, humans may feel uncomfortable when they move into a very different stocking density, e.g. when a person from the country enters a crowded environment, or a city dweller becomes agoraphobic in uninhabited countryside.

The distance from an animal's head to the edge of the 'bubble' is known as the flight distance (Fig. 9.20). Because the animal's senses are concentrated towards the reception of signals from the front, the flight distance is greater in front of than behind the animal (Fig. 9.21). The flight distance is determined by the environment, the type of cattle and their position in the dominance order. In intensive environments the flight distance is by necessity reduced, compared with, for example, an open range. Beef cattle have greater flight distance than dairy cattle, even in the same environment, demonstrating that short flight distance has been selected for during the domestic evolution of dairy cows. Cattle higher in the dominance order have greater flight distance and normally intersperse themselves throughout the herd to avoid contact with each other (Beilharz & Mylrea, 1963a,b). This means that less dominant cattle continually

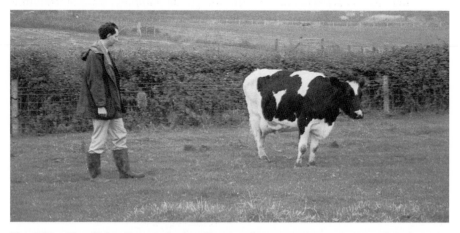

Fig. 9.20 The flight distance is the distance that someone can approach before the animal starts to move away. In dairy cows it is usually about 2 m.

have to move around to avoid contact with them. In a cubicle house they often seek respite in less preferred cubicles such as at the end of rows, but in an open yard or small paddock where there is no escape for subordinate cattle, the incidence of agonistic encounters is increased (Kondo *et al.*, 1989).

Forced movement of cattle initially creates an order unrelated to dominance, because the dominant cattle are interspersed throughout the herd. However, subordinate cattle gradually move to the front of the herd and the most dominant animals stay in the middle, leading the herd by 'pushing' rather than 'pulling'. They are reluctant to be right at the back of the herd because of their fear of humans driving them. Their attitude to humans is often more fearful than medium- and low-dominance cattle. Less dominant cattle have been found to be more likely to escape from the herd, as they are relatively less afraid of humans than the more dominant cattle.

In free movement of cattle at pasture, some benefit might be expected from leading the herd, because the leaders get first access to the pasture. This may not be very great, however, as Reinhardt (1983a) found that there was no relationship between dominance and position in the grazing herd. Not all cattle are closely associated with the herd. Some low-dominance cattle graze more independently, and presumably this demonstrates an antipathy to or a fear of agonistic interactions. Most cattle herds graze in a pear-shaped formation, which may be simplified into a parallel formation in small herds or where there is considerable benefit from having first access to the sward, e.g. in strip grazing. Normal interanimal distance under good grazing conditions when the size of the paddock is not limiting is about 10 m (Kondo *et al.*, 1989). The presence of flies, which are attracted to the secretions from the lacrimal and sebaceous glands (Fig. 9.22), causes the cattle to reduce the interanimal distance. With heavy fly infestation, cattle will rest from grazing by standing with their heads together or will seek elevated ground where wind may reduce the number of flies. Tail swishing and head movements, including ear flapping, reduce the infestation. Excessive heat may also disrupt the grazing process. Shade-seeking is not always

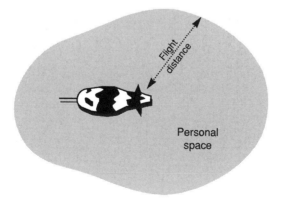

Fig. 9.21   Personal space and flight distance.

a synchronised behaviour, and may be performed in turn by members of the herd (Fig. 9.23).

Although the size of the enclosure for cattle is often dictated by economic considerations, the shape of the enclosure can be manipulated to allow for the social behaviour needs of the cattle. With housed cattle the perimeter:area ratio should be maximised because cattle use the perimeter ground more than any other. This ratio is greatest for a rectangle and increases as the length to breadth ratio increases; it is least for a circle. In the grazing context, overuse of pasture by the perimeter fence by some cattle, in particular bulls, suggests that this ratio should be minimised to graze the whole area of the field evenly. This will also minimise the contact area with wildlife or other cattle at the boundaries, which may reduce disease transmission, but will also reduce the area available for wildlife. Bulls develop individualistic behaviour as they mature, and will pace up and down perimeter fences. They will also overgraze corners of fields. On rangeland, these behaviours do not develop until the bulls are three to four years old, but in intensive grazing they occur much earlier. During the time when bulls develop their territoriality they show much agonistic activity, particularly head to head encounters. If space allows they create special areas, often choosing elevated ground, for display and threat behaviour, and subordinate bulls are often mounted or ridden to exhaustion after agonistic encounters. If space allows, the mature bulls will remain in their own territory to minimise agonistic encounters, and the most dominant bulls have the largest territories. In these circumstances grazing loses its synchronised character and bulls are not orientated in the same direction during grazing (Kilgour & Campin, 1973).

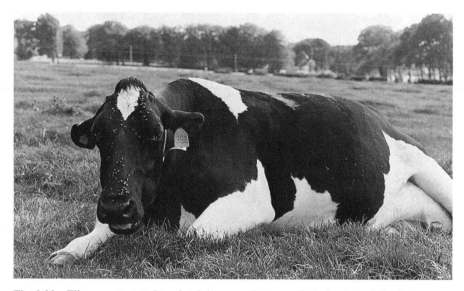

Fig. 9.22   Flies are attracted to glandular secretions, particularly around the face.

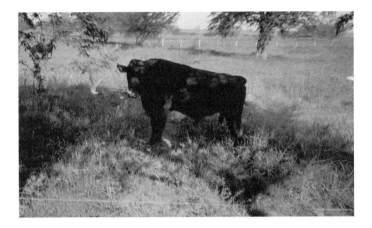

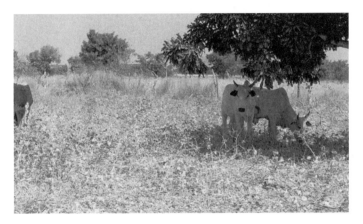

Fig. 9.23   Shade-seeking behaviour may be a solitary (above) or small group (below) behaviour.

Herd size and space allowance

Cattle are gregarious animals that have traditionally been kept in small herds (Reinhardt & Reinhardt, 1981). In developing countries most milking cows are kept in small groups of one to four animals (Nanging, 1989), but in most developed countries herd size is greater and is increasing. In England and Wales only 11% of dairy cows are kept in groups of fewer than 20 cows (Milk Marketing Board, 1991).

There are no wild cattle remaining to observe the natural group size, but a feral population of 140 cows has been observed to subdivide itself naturally into a number of distinct subgroups (Lazo, 1994). This accords with a model of forage utilisation by cattle in extensive grazing conditions, which has predicted that forage will be most efficiently utilised by groups of 10 to 40 animals (Wallis DeVries, 1996). Larger groups utilise forage less efficiently owing to overexploitation and exhaustion of forage resources, and smaller groups underexploit the forage resources and quality is reduced.

The excellent spatial memory of cattle (Bailey *et al.*, 1989) may assist in maintaining consistent spatial relationships between them during grazing. This could provide benefits of improved herbage utilisation or reduced agonistic interaction. Maintaining a required distance to the nearest neighbour is likely to be more difficult in large groups with a small area, but this may not be of significance in the grazing situation. In housed cattle, Kondo *et al.* (1989) reported that the frequency of agonistic interactions increased with group size, and the distance of each animal to its nearest neighbour decreased. As herd sizes increase, individual members have difficulty remembering the social status of other members. The frequency of agonistic encounters then increases, at least in cattle where a dominance order has been established. In young calves where no dominance order has been formed, group size has no effect on the frequency of agonistic encounter (Kondo *et al.*, 1989). The frequency of agonistic encounters decreases as space allowance increases. This may reduce stress but it does not always affect the growth rate of beef cattle or milk yield of dairy cattle or the time that the cattle spend grazing (Rind & Phillips, 1999).

Cattle decrease their interanimal distance in response to increased group size, especially calves, who have not learnt their position in the dominance order and the need to refrain from invading other animals' personal space (Fig. 9.24). The detrimental effects of a large group size can be overcome, where space allowance is adequate, by the formation of subherds or smaller groups within a population. This frequently occurs in beef cattle on rangeland, where herds typically break up into groups of 10 to 12 animals. Although subdivision of a smaller cattle population was not observed in the study of Hall and Moore (1986), Lazo (1992) reported that the extent of subdivision of a group of 130 cattle depended mainly on the abundance and distribution of food, the perceived predation risk and the reproductive state of the cows. The size of subgroups was greatest for cows, compared with bulls and growing cattle, and was also greater when the cows had calves with them and when the habitat was open.

When cattle are brought together for the first time there is initially aggression, to determine dominance, followed by aggregation. In the small groups agonistic encounters are initially more frequent but quickly these produce repeatable results and the encounters can then be ritualised and become less frequent (Kondo *et al.*, 1989). Small groups show more rapid aggregation, whereas large groups take longer to become stable.

The distance of dairy cows to their nearest neighbour was reported by Kondo *et al.* (1989) and Rind and Phillips (1999) to be approximately 5 to 15 m, but it was longer (25 m) for entire and castrated male cattle in the study of Hinch *et al.* (1982a). This difference is probably due to both gender and the extensive nature of the vegetation in the study of Hinch *et al.* (1982a). There are also genetic influences – cattle bred for fighting have greater distances between them at pasture than those not bred in this way (Plusquellec & Bouissou, 2001). Rind and

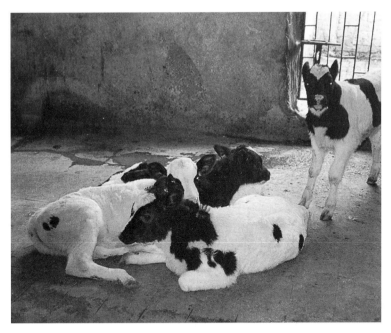

Fig. 9.24 Calves have not learnt the concept of personal space and do not refrain from close proximity of other calves.

Phillips (1999) found that the distance to the nearest neighbour increased with group size, which may demonstrate that cohesive behaviour is stronger in small groups because of fear of predation, or the effect may have been due to the increased aggression between cows in the large group. This is in contrast to the work of Kondo *et al.* (1989), where an increase in group size reduced the distance to nearest neighbour, but this may have been due to the reduction in space allowance per animal in the latter work. It is not clear to what extent fences, particularly electric ones that divide paddocks, represented boundaries to the cows' perceived space (Penning *et al.*, 1993).

An increase in space available to the herd results in an increase in the interanimal distance for both calves and adult cattle. Kondo *et al.* (1989) reported that the interanimal distance increases with space allowance, up to 10 to 12 m and reaches this maximum at a space allowance of 360 m^2 per animal. In adult cattle the need to retain cohesiveness of the group at high space allowances is evident, as they have this maximum interanimal distance of 12 m at large space allowances, e.g. on open range (Kondo *et al.*, 1989). The close proximity of cows in small groups may have an anti-predator function, as the cows could monitor the horizon more frequently and gain maximum benefit from aggregation from an attack by a predator (Rind & Phillips, 1999). Nevertheless, the opportunities for shared vigilance are reduced in small groups (Lazo, 1992), and Rind and Phillips (1999) also found an increased rate of lateral head movement in small groups (four cows) compared with groups of eight and 16 cows, which again may indicate greater individual vigilance. There is other evidence for a vestigial fear of predation in cattle, since Lazo (1992) found that feral cows aggregated into larger groups when they had young calves with them and when they were in an open habitat, even though they had never been exposed to predators. Herbivores also benefit from grazing in aggregations by maintaining the grass in a short state (McNaughton, 1984; Fryxell, 1991), and small groups of cattle may have to aggregate to a greater degree to achieve this. However, if the herbage height is too short, intake will fall, and the model of Wallis DeVries (1996) predicts that, when the dynamics of forage quality are included, cattle in large groups will travel further and visit more patches, which was substantiated by Rind and Phillips (1999). The increased energy expenditure for travel between patches is offset by increased forage intake and quality.

Space perception

An animal's perception of space is undoubtedly influenced by many environmental and physiological factors, and it is much more complex than, for example, a simple volume measurement. The quality of space available, and therefore the space requirement, are affected by building factors such as lighting; the number, design and size of cubicles; flooring characteristics; the width of feeding and other passageways; the waste disposal system and the number and type of feeding and drinking stations (Potter & Broom, 1987).

Animal factors which influence space requirements include the physiological state of the animal, its gender, the presence of horns and the breed of cattle. Physiological state is important, for example, when periparturient cows distance themselves from the rest of the herd. Gender is more important in adult than juvenile cattle, and even the body form (male or female type conformation) influences the behaviour and social space requirements. Bulls with more masculine body characteristics are more aggressive and more dominant, but surprisingly they initiate fewer and receive more mountings (Jezierski *et al.*, 1989). This may occur because bulls of the more dominant masculine type pose a threat to subordinate, more feminine type bulls, who attempt to meet this challenge by mounting their rivals.

Breed effects are clearly discernible in the social behaviour of cattle and probably relate to the length and type of domestication influences as well as the physical environment. Hill breeds normally dominate lowland breeds, even if they are smaller, e.g. Aberdeen Angus dominate (but are smaller than) Herefords (Stricklin, 1983). They also tend to have a greater flight distance and less readily accept artificial management practices, such as bucket rearing (Le Neindre & Sourd, 1984). Crossbred cattle dominate and are more aggressive than purebred cattle, which may be one reason for the popularity of purebred cattle for dairy herds, despite the production advantages for the crossbred.

Animal and environmental effects on space perception such as these must be included in the design of accommodation for any cattle farming system. Ideally the needs of all the cattle should be accounted for, but frequently, extremes of body size, temperament, age, etc., as, for example, in regard to cubicle size, do not receive special allowances.

Isolation

Isolation is generally not a natural state for such gregarious animals as cattle, but there *are* occasions when they prefer to be solitary. A cow that is about to calve normally seeks an isolated place so that she can give birth undisturbed and, more importantly, the calf will be drawn to the correct dam without the risk of mis-mothering (Edwards, 1983). Mature bulls also seek territorial isolation from other bulls, although they may remain within sight of one another. Subordinate and sick cows often graze away from the rest of the herd, presumably to avoid agonistic encounters with more dominant cows. Sexually active cows, either with a bull or other cows, usually isolate themselves from the rest of the herd. These are the situations in which cattle seek at least partial isolation from the rest of the herd, but modern husbandry methods often impose isolation at quite different times.

The most contentious period of isolation in modern cattle farming is that of the newborn calf. Calves are usually separated from their dam at about 24 hours post partum and offered artificial milk replacer for five to seven weeks in individual pens. This is done to prevent cross-infection at a time when the calves' natural immunity is not well developed. The imprinting or primary socialisation drive appears not to be fully satiated by the initial 24 hour contact between cow and calf, since longer contact increases the bond between the two, and hence the stress of separation. This isolation delays or eliminates the normal refractory period after primary socialisation and the calves attempt to create substitute bonding partners to replace the severed imprinting bond. Group-reared calves quickly form associations amongst themselves but delay the formation of a dominance order unless resources are restricted.

Individually reared calves have at most visual contact with a small number of calves and perhaps tactile contact with nearest neighbours. Stronger bonds may be created with stockmen and therefore, particularly if the same stockmen are responsible for the adult cattle, this will strengthen the relationship to the stockman in adult life. Signs of behavioural deprivation, however, are common and the calves' behaviour is affected for life. In their pens they often display redirected behaviours, particularly those related to the absence of suckling contact with the dam such as sucking the pen or buckets, or 'kissing' the nearest neighbour. That this is not solely caused by the deprivation of suckling is demonstrated by the absence of these behaviours in group-reared calves fed artificial milk replacer. Locomotion is by necessity limited and individually reared calves vocalise more by higher frequency 'baaocks' (see *(m)enh* described above) than the normal 'moos', indicating greater stress. When they are eventually put into groups they are socially maladapted, and this loss of experience is never compensated for. These calves are denied a crucial period of play which restricts their social development. In comparison with calves that are given contact with cattle from birth, they are less skilled, particularly in social contact situations, and they tend to be less dominant. They are also less successful in agonistic and sexual interactions, with more disorientated mounting behaviour (Silver & Price, 1986). These differences are maintained into adulthood.

The experience of stress at an early age is probably of benefit to calves if the environment during adulthood is going to be stressful (Creel & Albright, 1988). There is an argument that juveniles should be conditioned to adult stresses, and there is good endocrinological evidence that this will facilitate stress habituation in adulthood (Creel & Albright, 1988).

Other instances of enforced isolation in modern cattle farming systems include the separation of sick dairy cows and dairy bulls from the rest of the herd. Individual tethering of dairy cows is also still common in many countries, particularly in hot countries where feed must be cut and fed to the animals under shade, and/or countries where labour is readily available for this purpose. In developed countries loose housing, where the cows are given the free range of the building, is practised increasingly because of high labour costs. Frequent human contact can at least partially substitute for the intraspecific bonds, and hence the traditional system of keeping dairy cows in individual stalls can function satisfactorily with adequate labour inputs.

The isolation of sick cattle and dairy bulls causes stress, as evidenced by the frequent vocalisations of such animals (an attempt to increase social contact by vocal means where visual contact is prevented), increased aggression to stockhandlers and stereotypic behaviour. It could be argued that in the wild these animals would have been at least partially isolated from the herd, but it is the completeness of the isolation that causes the stress in the case of the dairy bull housed in a bull pen, as well as the suddenness of it in the case of a sick cow that is withdrawn from the herd. In the prevailing atmosphere of increased awareness of animal rights, regular social contact is probably one such 'right' that this social species should be afforded.

Mixing groups

When cattle groups are mixed, a new dominance relationship is created, usually within 24 to 72 hours, depending on the degree of change in the group. Minor changes result in an approximate doubling in aggression activity for about 24 hours, longer if dominant cattle are introduced to a stable group when cattle may continue fighting for up to 30 to 45 days as they create a new social order (Schein & Fohrman, 1955; Sato *et al.*, 1990), but they usually end up in approximately the same relative position in the dominance hierarchy as previously, with no loss of position as a result of the move (Brakel & Leis, 1976). In bulls and to a lesser extent steers the increased aggression is accompanied by an increase in homosexual mounting and chin-resting. This has given rise to the suggestion that mounting behaviour is stimulated by aggressive motivation rather than sexual attraction, but it would also be expected that the novel partners presented in a new group would stimulate sexual motivation. After regrouping there is a gradual transition from physical encounters to psychological (threat/avoidance) ones (Kondo & Hurnick, 1987).

Regrouping commonly occurs towards the end of an animal's life when it is mixed with other cattle in a truck and perhaps again in a market and/or abattoir. Creation of a new dominance order may be prevented, either by spatial restriction in a truck or lack of time in the market or abattoir. An increase in stress is evident during this period and has an adverse effect on meat quality due to a lowering of glycogen levels in the muscle tissue. This occurs during fighting and mounting activity in bulls pre-slaughter, so it is probably best to slaughter as soon as possible after the animals arrive at the abattoir (see Chapter 5).

In dairy cows changes in group structure may sometimes cause sufficient disruption to reduce feed intake and hence milk production. Most previous research has considered the mixing of groups of similar cattle, for example, as they change between feeding groups. Multiparous cows have experience of being regularly moved between groups during the lactation period as their yield potential changes. The frequent mixing diminishes the impact on milk yield (Sowerby & Polan, 1978). Following the mixing there is sometimes a reduction in milk yield, but there is considerable variation between studies: reductions of 19% (Vajner, 1978), 8% for ten days (Kovalcik & Kovalcikova, 1974), 5% for 40 days (Krohn, 1978), 4% for five days (Jezierski & Podluzny, 1984) and 3% for one day (Brakel & Leis, 1976) are reported, and others (Clark *et al.*, 1977; Collis *et al.*, 1979; Konggaard *et al.*, 1982) found no change. One study demonstrated that the extent of milk yield reduction is not directly related to the extent of agonistic encounters, but is more likely to reflect reduced feeding (Brakel & Leis, 1976), particularly in situations where there is limited access to the food resource. Grazing behaviour may also be affected by the introduction of strange cows during the development of a new group order (Syme & Syme, 1979). However, Hasegawa *et al.* (1997) found that milk yield was reduced following mixing only in cows that ended up considerably lower in the dominance hierarchy, in which case the yield fell by about 5% in the first two weeks. The number of cows being introduced to a new group probably influences the effects on milk production. Kovalcik and Kovalcikova (1974) reported a greater reduction in milk yield when batches of 15 cows were moved to new groups than when individual cows were moved. However, Sowerby and Polan (1977) found that under commercial conditions the number of cows introduced to a new group, between three and 20, did not influence the scale of the milk yield reduction, but the level of replication was low.

The entrance of the new uniparous cows into the herd can create social tension, and may depress performance (Brakel & Leis, 1976), especially as they are usually introduced in only one or two large groups per year and are often not used to changes in social structure. The new entrants would mostly be at the bottom of the dominance hierarchy because of their young age (Beilharz & Zeeb, 1982), small size (Brantas, 1968) and inexperience (Schein & Fohrman, 1955). A reduction in milk yield of 3% for one week has been reported, following the introduction of eight uniparous cows into a stable group of eight multiparous cows (Phillips & Rind, 2002b). Both uni- and multiparous cows grazed for less time and they stood for longer, particularly in the first week post-mixing. The multiparous cows in the mixed group increased their pasture biting rate and became more dominant than the uniparous cows, who spent more time grooming other cows and in aggressive interactions compared to the unmixed group of uniparous cows.

Temperament

Temperament may be described as a major parameter in the personality or mood of cattle in relation to their reaction to man. It is genetically unrelated to position within the dominance orders, which primarily refer to priority of access to resources between members of the herd. The within-breed heritability of temperament is low, between 0 and 0.15 (see Chapter 7), and there are strong environmental (management) effects on temperament. These relate mainly to previous handling experience – its frequency, the animal's age when it was handled (temperament develops at an early age) and the degree of pain or unpleasant feeling associated with the handling. Extensively reared cattle are more difficult to handle than cattle that have been regularly handled during rearing (Boivin *et al.*, 1994). However, there are clear genetic differences between the temperament of different breeds, particularly between *Bos indicus and Bos taurus* cattle (Voisinet *et al.*, 1997b), but also between different *Bos taurus* breeds and sires within breeds (Boivin *et al.*, 1994). Lanier *et al.* (2000) found that Holstein cattle were more sensitive to sound and touch in auctions than beef cattle breeds.

An animal's temperament should be measured in relation to its 'fearfulness' or reaction to fearful stimuli (Lanier *et al.*, 2000), not its 'aggressiveness'. Fearfulness will more often be expressed in an attempt to flee, or in excessive kinetic activity, rather than aggression towards the handler, which is more likely to reflect position in the dominance order. Fearfulness is best recorded in the parlour for dairy cows or in the crush for beef cattle. To a certain extent this represents a reaction to confinement as well as to the presence of humans. The optimal situation in which to measure fearfulness is when cattle are accustomed to the confinement, and it is the response to the approach or tactile stimulus from the handler that is recorded. A number of scoring techniques have been devised, some of which include descriptions such as 'placid', 'docile', 'nervous' and 'lively' (Nayak & Mishra, 1984), and they correlate well with the more objective measures of heart rate and breathing rate.

Table 9.2 The behaviour of dairy cows in high- and low-yielding units

Behaviour	High yielding	Low yielding
Mean entry time to parlour (s/cow)	9.9	16.1
Field flight distance (m)	0.5	2.5
Approaches to observer (no./min)	10.2	3.0
Defecation in the parlour (no./h)	3.0	18.2

After Seabrook (1984).

Despite the apparently low heritability, many breeding indices now include an assessment of temperament. Docile dairy cows tend to give higher milk yields, as seen when comparing the behaviour of cows in high- and low-yielding units (Table 9.2). *Bos taurus* cattle tend to be more docile when being milked than *Bos indicus*, which is presumably a result of prolonged breeding for this characteristic. In both beef and dairy cattle, the animal's temperament is particularly important in minimising the stress reaction, and higher productivity in both beef and dairy systems has been found in placid cattle in stressful situations. Stress-susceptible or 'fearful' cattle find it difficult to relax in a large, highly stocked, loose housing environment and they actually milk better in tie stalls (Devyatkina, 1986). Repeated stress reactions elevate blood cortisol concentrations. Cattle that react strongly to such stresses have reduced growth rate (Voisinet *et al.*, 1997b), and those with a very excitable temperament produce carcases with tougher meat and are more likely to be classified as dark cutters than cattle with calm temperament ratings (Voisinet *et al.*, 1997a). Some cattle react strongly to human presence, and can remember aversive handlers in the parlour, leading to reduced milk production (Mulkens & Geers, 1995; Rushen *et al.*, 1999b) and reproductive rate (via gonadotrophin inhibition) (see Table 9.3). The temperament of a dairy bull is also important for the ease of handling and safety of the stockman.

Table 9.3 Factors associated with the development of good empathetic stockmanship and possible actions to promote them

Factor	Action
Operant conditioning	Reward good behaviour of animal
	Use of food and other positive stimuli as a distraction for negative interaction
Physical contact	Stroking and patting
	Scratching animal's head
Social identification	Use of voice and social gestures
Stable environment	Consistent and confident actions
Handling	Non-aggressive behaviour

After Seabrook (1984).

Work rates are also reduced if stockmen find themselves chasing cattle or having to give excessive encouragement to animals to move, which are common problems both in the farm and at the abattoir (Grandin, 1993). Cattle of an excitable temperament are particularly difficult to handle in novel situations, such as the abattoir (Grandin, 1996).

Cattle usually improve their temperament and become less fearful with age (Roy & Nagpaul, 1986; Lanier *et al.*, 2000), probably because they actually experience little unpleasantness with most handling experiences and habituate to them. It is likely that handling experiences during calf-hood to a large extent formulate the animal's personality, as bad handling during this critical period will render an animal nervous and hypersensitive to stress (Boivin *et al.*, 1992). Calves receiving just ten days of handling during the first three months of age, or after artificial weaning at eight months of age, are easier to handle than non-handled animals (Le Neindre *et al.*, 1996).

The benefits of conditioning calves to a certain amount of stress by isolation have already been discussed (see 'Isolation' above). To some extent mood is relative, and an idyllic calf-hood followed by transfer to stressful intensive husbandry conditions (as could be experienced by, for example, feedlot cattle in the USA) will be more detrimental to the animal's welfare than some stress conditioning during early life followed by more benign conditions in later life.

Chapter 10
Nutritional Behaviour

Introduction

Nutritional behaviour includes all the activities concerned with obtaining and processing nutrients for maintenance and production – feeding, drinking, rumination and elimination. Cattle evolved primarily as grazing and browsing animals, that is they harvest feeds, usually still growing, from the strata of plant life either near the soil or from bushes and trees. By definition 'grazing' refers to the harvesting of grasses, but it commonly applies to the harvesting of other plants or parts of plants, such as legumes or maize stover (Fig. 10.1). Cattle will also feed from shrubs and trees (browsing), although their mouthparts are not well designed for this. Grazing by cattle usually entails harvesting of relatively large quantities of ground level plant material with little selectivity compared, for example, with sheep. Cattle will consume grass heads on tall reproductive stems individually, but this is not their main method of feed harvesting; rather it is an energetically expensive way of obtaining some palatable feed items (Ginnett *et al.*, 1999).

Cattle forage in matriarchal groups on natural grassland, and large groups of cows (more than 100 cows) often subdivide, depending on the abundance and

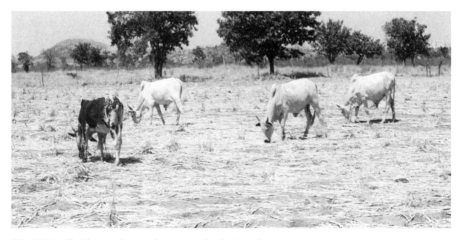

Fig. 10.1 Cattle grazing maize stover in the tropics.

distribution of food, the perceived predation risk and the reproductive state of the cows (Lazo, 1992). Large groups risk exhausting forage resources in a limited area, whereas small groups may underexploit the forage resources, with the result that quality declines.

Food procurement and ingestion

Foraging strategy

Cattle evolved, along with other ruminants, with a unique anti-predator foraging strategy. They consume primarily coarse grasses which need large amounts of chewing or mastication before they can be digested. To minimise the predation risk they consume the grasses as rapidly as possible, followed by mastication later in relative safety when they lie down, mostly at night. Boluses of feed are regurgitated during this mastication process (rumination) by reverse peristalsis. They are re-masticated and then swallowed.

The forage selection policies adopted by cattle must provide for the optimum nutrient intake. Nutrient requirements vary with the physiological state of the animal (e.g. pregnancy, body fatness), its genetic potential for production and the need to provide milk for offspring. Cattle are motivated to feed by hunger, which is alleviated by a feeling of satisfaction or satiation. Hunger is not, however, a broad-spectrum motivational force. Specific hungers (euphagias) exist to maintain the intake of the major nutrients (energy, protein and sodium at least), but the range is limited by the perceptive powers of the cattle (Fig. 10.2). For most cattle the major limiting nutrient is energy, even though they have a well-developed buffering system in the form of body fat stores. Energy intake is governed not just by feeding behaviour constraints, but also by gut and digestive capacities and the energy status of the animal.

Exactly how cattle acquire the necessary knowledge to achieve this nutrient selectivity remains unclear. Some believe they have acquired innate wisdom

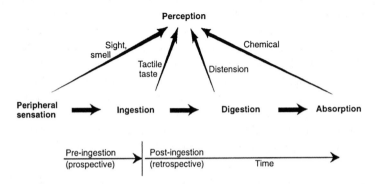

Fig. 10.2 Pre-ingestion and post-ingestion factors contributing to food perception.

(evidenced by euphagias) to select the optimum diet. However, they clearly learn some elements of selectivity, probably by operant conditioning and by allelomimicry. For example, avoidance of toxic plants such as ragwort is learnt not inherited. Cattle that have grown up with experience of ragwort in a field learn of its mild toxic effect when eaten in small amounts and subsequently avoid it. However, if cattle are suddenly introduced to a field with a lot of ragwort and little alternative forage, and they have not experienced it before, they will eat large quantities with often lethal consequences. Learning evidently has an important part to play in dietary selection, but there are inherited elements too. That the grazing process itself is learnt is not in doubt. At eight weeks of age calves graze at only 14 bites/minute but at 18 weeks this has increased to 50 bites/minute, a rate similar to that seen in adult cows (Hancock, 1953).

The manifestations of dietary selection are specific responses to feed characteristics – gustatory, olfactory and tactile. Some scientists believe that this is purely a hedonic response (hedyphagia) (see review by Provenza & Balph, 1990) but this ignores the fact that these hedonic responses almost certainly evolved in response to euphagias. However, although animals can be credited with a considerable degree of euphagia, this belief can be taken too far. There is, for example, the need for cattle to sample regularly the available forages to determine optimum intake (Illius & Gordon, 1990). Memory may therefore be limited. Even given a nutritionally optimum diet, it is likely that cattle would prefer variation in feed supply as an insurance against any one feed becoming scarce. One long-standing technique of achieving very high intakes, and consequently milk yields, is to offer a wide choice of feeds to cattle. This was ably demonstrated in the 1940s at the Royal Agricultural College when Professor R. Boutflour achieved yields that are high even by today's standards by offering a large range of feeds at regular intervals to cows. But for the difficulties of managing such a system, it would probably be popular today. This gives us evidence that some feed selection is hedyphagic rather than euphagic. Finally we must remember that we as humans do not always allow euphagia to influence our dietary selection, and hedonic responses often predominate. The food manufacturers utilise our hedonism by creating foods with unnaturally high sugar, fat and salt concentrations, which we find difficult to refuse. In the same way it is possible to exceed the euphagic capabilities of cattle and, for example, increase the intake of forage by increasing its sodium content over and above requirements (Chiy & Phillips, 1991). However, some euphagia definitely exists and feeds with excessive sweetness or salt content have a reduced palatability (Chiy & Phillips, 1999b). The appetite for salt is instinctive and is particularly strong in wild or feral cattle (Gupta *et al.*, 1999). It is also strong in lactating cows, owing to the loss of sodium in milk. However, experience plays an important part in controlling the salt appetite, and it is possible to increase the salt appetite of cattle by prior exposure. Increasing the sodium concentration of concentrate from 4 to 9 g Na/kg when feeding calves in the first six weeks of life increased the preferred feed sodium concentration of the calves at six months of age from 3 to 9 g/kg dry matter (DM) (Phillips *et al.*, 1999). There is also evidence that supplementing pregnant cows with sodium can increase the preferred salt content of the diet of their calves (Mohamed & Phillips, 2001). Research with other species, most notably the laboratory rat, suggests that depriving pregnant cows of sodium will also increase their calves' sodium appetite, manifested as excessive licking behaviour.

Another mechanism that controls foraging strategy, apart from nutrient (primarily energy) intake optimisation, is foraging cost minimisation. In the short term, the processing cost (mastication) is the main regulator of food intake rate (Gross *et al.*, 1993). In the long term, up to a certain point (probably about 50 000 grazing bites/day), there is only a small benefit in minimising foraging time, as the energy costs of grazing are low in relation to total energy intake. However, as intake increases or availability of feed decreases, the opportunity costs of grazing become relatively high. Foraging begins to infringe on other highly desirable activities, e.g. resting. Cattle prefer to maintain their lying time rather than feeding time, when they do not have sufficient time for both activities (Metz, 1984).

An overriding concern of all grazing cattle is to satisfy their motivation for gregariousness, i.e. to stay close together, whilst feeding. Small numbers of cattle in a group stay closer together while grazing than a large group of cattle (Rind & Phillips, 1999). Cattle also stay close together when they are in a small enclosure – Kondo *et al.* (1989) found that interindividual distance increases up to a space allowance of 360 m^2 per animal.

Other behaviours, such as parturition, can be accomplished alone, but grazing is a very social activity. Cattle develop preferred grazing partners (Reinhardt & Reinhardt, 1981) and adopt a common direction and interanimal distance during grazing. The influence of this social facilitation process is clearly demonstrated when cattle are offered supplementary feed (Table 10.1). Cattle offered supplements reduce their grazing time, and when they are grazed with unsupplemented cattle the grazing times of the latter are reduced as well.

Feeding mechanisms

Cattle feed and drink using their lips, teeth and tongue. During grazing all three are used to secure the feed in the mouth before ripping it from the sward. When cattle eat loose feed, i.e. not connected to the soil, the tongue is used to a greater

Table 10.1   The effects of social facilitation on the grazing response of cattle to a supplement of 3.6 kg oats per day (Bailey *et al.* 1974)

	Grazing separately		Grazing together	
	Unsupplemented	Supplemented	Unsupplemented	Supplemented
Grazing time (h/day)	8.4	6.5	7.7	6.4

extent to manipulate particles into the buccal cavity. More free-flowing materials like liquids or powders are sucked into the open mouth by expanding the lungs.

Feeds are masticated or chewed by compression and severance between the upper and lower molars. This alternates on either side of the jaw, because the upper jaw is considerably narrower than the lower one. The lower jaw is therefore moved upwards and inwards to contact the upper jaw on one side, followed by a similar action to achieve contact on the other side. Through this process and with the addition of saliva, which lubricates the food as well as having digestive functions, a bolus of the more fibrous material is prepared, with most of the cell solutes released.

Following chewing, this food bolus is manipulated into the pharynx by the tongue and contact with the pharynx triggers peristalsis, or contraction of the oesophagus behind the bolus, to deliver it into the rumen. After this swallowing process a new portion of food is obtained and the cycle recommences.

The grazing process

Cattle graze herbage by collecting it into the mouth and compressing it against the upper palate with the tongue and lower incisors. The herbage is then severed from the plants by jerking the head upwards. This is repeated several times a minute, typically 30 to 70, and the animal moves its head from side to side as it walks. Associated with the grazing bites are occasional chewing bites or manipulative movements of the tongue or lips to manoeuvre the herbage in the mouth. These are more common when the herbage is long and fibrous. They are much less common in grazing cattle than in cattle eating conserved food, or in grazing sheep.

Cattle generally prefer to graze tall, dense, dark-green pastures. Some selectivity occurs even in the most uniform pastures. Herbage height largely determines the bite size and mass. A tall sward gives the greatest ease of prehension and therefore minimum foraging time. However, cattle do not exclusively graze tall swards and leave short areas untouched. When offering cattle a choice of 3 or 6 cm grass swards, Phillips and James (1998) found that cattle only spent just over one-half of their grazing time on the tall sward, probably because they were balancing the need for high-quality herbage consumed slowly from the short sward with large quantities of low-quality herbage consumed rapidly from the tall sward.

Within any pasture there are tall areas of herbage close to faecal deposits that are not grazed. The rejection around each faecal deposit is greater in undergrazed swards because the cattle have the choice of other, clean areas to graze. Herbage around dung deposits is rejected initially because of the smell of the faeces and later because of its maturity. Typically it is lighter and browner than 'grazed' green herbage, and this indicates to the cattle that it has a low nutritive value. Darker green pastures are also usually preferred because this indicates a higher nitrogen content, and dense pastures because they give a greater bite weight.

Cattle extract a cylinder from the sward during a bite, and if the herbage is dense this cylinder has a greater weight of herbage in it because of the large herbage weight per unit volume. Researchers have studied this process using microswards, hand-constructed small swards which present uniform herbage for the animal to bite (Ungar *et al.*, 2001). Defoliation imprints can also be measured in a heterogeneous field sward (Cid & Brizuela, 1998). When cattle graze, their head subtends an arc as they move it to the right of their body and then to the left and back again, approximately every 10 to 20 seconds (Rind & Phillips, 1999). This movement is faster for cattle in small groups (less than eight animals), probably because of the perceived need for greater vigilance (Rind & Phillips, 1999). During this period they take several bites over an arc that is approximately 160 cm wide, at the same time as moving forward at about 2 m/min (Phillips *et al.*, 1999). They move more quickly on swards that are more suitable for grazing (e.g. high sodium swards; Phillips *et al.*, 1999), probably because of reduced time spent in selection.

Although cattle are not as selective as sheep, their grazing action usually allows them to select a greater proportion of leaf material than the sward contains as a whole, thereby increasing the digestibility of their diet (Fig. 10.3). This is primarily because of vertical selectivity: they graze the upper strata of the sward (i.e. above the pseudostems, normally about 2 cm above the soil surface), and this layer contains more leaf material. A greater proportion of young, expanding leaves is consumed, approximately 70% of the length, than older leaves, where only 35 to 50% of the leaf is consumed (Chiy & Phillips, 1999a). This is probably because the young leaves are more erect. Male cattle, with their faster growth rates and higher requirements, are less selective than female cattle of the same age (Phillips *et al.*, 1999).

Little is yet known about how cattle determine the height above ground level at which to defoliate the sward. They may balance a high leaf:pseudostem ratio (which would maximise nutrient content of the herbage) with achieving an adequate total intake. The extent to which they do this to optimise nutrient intake is as yet uncertain. Optimal foraging theory predicts that the mass and composi-

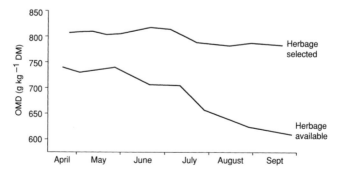

Fig. 10.3   The organic matter digestibility (OMD) of the herbage selected and of the available herbage.

tion of the plant eaten will be balanced against the energetic cost of grazing and possibly digestion in order to supply nutrient requirements at least cost in grazing time. The ease of severance of the bites is another factor which may influence grazing height (Phillips *et al.*, 1999).

Cattle also exhibit horizontal selectivity when grazing, for example when avoiding herbage around dung deposits or herbage with hairy or waxy leaves. The opportunity for horizontal selectivity is limited by their mouthparts. Possessing uncleft upper lips and a broad dental arcade, cattle cannot manipulate individual plant items to the same degree as sheep and goats.

The sweeping side-to-side grazing action of each individual animal as it walks forwards combines with the cohesive grazing action of a herd of cattle to result in a sward that is all, or nearly all, defoliated to a common height, with the exception of areas around dung deposits. In contrast, sheep select individual tillers and sever them much closer to the ground, resulting in an infrequent but more severe defoliation. Because of the reduced frequency of defoliation, more tillers escape grazing altogether and become rejected due to their maturity, especially if the stocking rate of the sheep is too low. With cattle this only usually occurs in herbage around dung deposits, and even this is limited if the stocking rate is high. This ability of cattle to keep a pasture relatively free from mature herbage has led to their commonly being kept to 'clean up old pasture' on sheep farms. There are even greater advantages if cattle and sheep graze together, as they accept herbage close to each others' faeces, but not from a member of their own species. This is because most parasites are specific to either cattle or sheep and there is little risk of cross-contamination by grazing close to faeces of another species grazing in the same field.

In a conceptual mechanistic model of the cattle grazing process, feed intake can be determined from the grazing time multiplied by the rate of intake (Fig.

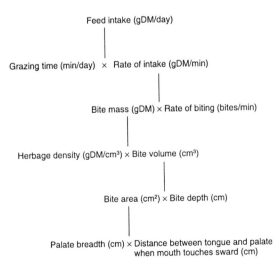

Fig. 10.4 Mechanistic model of the grazing intake of cattle.

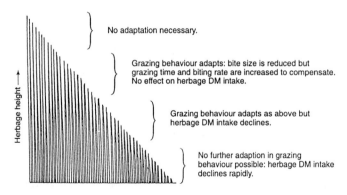

Fig. 10.5 Effect of declining herbage height on grazing behaviour and herbage DM intake.

10.4). The latter can be predicted from bite mass multiplied by the rate of biting, and the bite mass determined from the herbage density multiplied by bite size or volume. Bite volume is the product of bite area and bite depth. Bite area is a function of palate breadth and the distance between the palate and the tongue when the mouth touches the sward. Bite depth is the main factor regulating the other components of behaviour, and it is largely determined by sward height. Hence when cattle graze a 10 cm lush spring pasture, intake rate is about 25 to 30 g DM/min, whereas when they graze a 5 cm autumn pasture it will only be eaten at 15 to 20 g DM/min.

Cattle compensate for reduced bite depth by modifying other behavioural factors, principally grazing time and biting rate, which may enable herbage intake to be maintained when they graze short swards. The ability of cattle to compensate for inadequate herbage depends on the severity of the bite depth reduction and the animal's intake requirements (Fig. 10.5). If the intake requirements are high, the ability of the cattle to compensate is limited.

Maximum grazing times and biting rates normally occur at about 10 to 12 hours/day and 65 to 70 bites/minute, respectively (Fig. 10.6), although longer

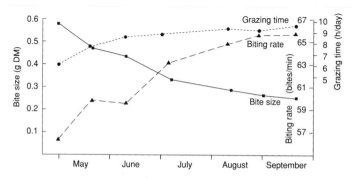

Fig. 10.6 Changes in grazing behaviour over a typical five-month grazing season in the UK, during which time herbage height declined from 10 cm at turnout to 5 cm at housing (Phillips & Leaver, 1985c).

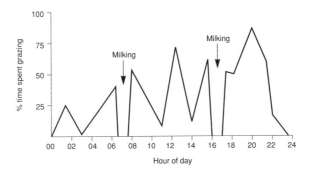

Fig. 10.7 Change in grazing intensity over the day for a lactating cow.

grazing times (13 hours/day) have been recorded on sparsely vegetated range-land (Smith, 1955). This gives a maximum of 50 000 bites/day on temperate swards, although individual cattle achieve more. High-yielding cows can only achieve long grazing times at the expense of lying and ruminating times (Cooper *et al.*, 2002). There is little else that they can sacrifice, and this emphasises the need to minimise the time that high-yielding cows are kept off the pasture for milking and other routine procedures.

Grazing lactating dairy cows typically have about five meals per day, each last-ing on average 110 minutes (Fig. 10.7). Cattle with lower intake requirements in relation to their weight (e.g. dry cows, mature bullocks) have fewer, shorter meals. Normally the first meal begins soon after dawn, followed by two or three meals between morning and afternoon milking, and the longest, most intensive meal in the evening ending shortly after dusk. This is to provide sufficient food to digest during the night period. High-yielding cows often have a short meal for approximately 30 minutes at about 1 AM, after which the rest of the night is spent ruminating and resting (Phillips & Denne, 1988).

Biting rate is usually constant for most of a meal except for a reduction at the beginning and end as time spent in other activities increases (Fig. 10.8). As the

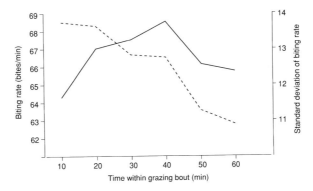

Fig. 10.8 Variation in biting rate (———) and the standard deviation of biting rate (- - -) during a one hour grazing bout (Phillips, unpublished data).

grazing bout progresses there is less difference between cows in biting rate. Grazing is an energetically expensive process usually followed by periods of just lying and then lying and ruminating. If cattle are starved for a period, they increase their rate of consumption mainly by increasing their bite size and pasture biting rate and decreasing the time spent masticating the food.

Grazing systems

Most cattle are either grazed on the entire available area (set-stocking) or rotated around sections of it. In intensive grassland conditions there is little evidence of major differences in behaviour and performance between the two systems. Rotationally grazed cattle, which are held on a smaller area at any one time, have less interanimal space and increased social interaction, but this does not appear to affect production. In rangeland grazing, where the areas covered by the cattle are much larger, the greater density of rotationally grazed range can reduce searching time and increase productivity (Olson & Malechek, 1988).

Topography

The ability of cattle to graze steep slopes is limited, and they also find it difficult to get adequate rest under such circumstances, as they cannot lie down. In a heterogeneous environment, they prefer to graze on level, lowland ground and only graze steep slopes if there is insufficient forage elsewhere (Hart *et al.*, 1991).

Breed/environment interaction

The main cattle genotypes – *Bos indicus* and *Bos taurus* – show marked differences in heat tolerance that interact with feeding behaviour. *Bos taurus* cattle spend less time grazing and more time in the shade in hot conditions. Perhaps because of this, and the greater nutritional requirements necessary to support their higher productivity, they are less selective than *Bos indicus* cattle and have a broader dietary spectrum. Criollo cattle (*Bos taurus* cattle that were taken to South America by early Spanish emigrants) also have a greater dietary selectivity than improved British cattle (Minon *et al.*, 1984). This suggests that the period of improvement of British cattle since the Agricultural Revolution may have resulted in these cattle developing a broader dietary niche as a result of being offered a wide variety of feeds.

External parasites

Many external parasites disturb the grazing behaviour of cattle. Biting parasites such as ticks have a greater effect than flies (e.g. *Hydrotea irritans*), which merely create a nuisance. The warble fly is particularly feared by cattle and a tape-recording of the flight sound alone causes evasive action (Nogge & Staack, 1969). Cattle affected by flies will change position frequently from grazing to standing, rather than lying down, and will stand with their heads facing each other. Regular tail swishing gives some protection against flies; consequently cows in susceptible areas should not have their tails trimmed. Skin rippling is also an effective method of removing flies in areas that cannot be reached by their tail, and in extreme circumstances leg kicks may occur (Baylis, 1996). Cows also seek areas of high ground and windy places where fly concentrations will be reduced and they avoid shade, thus making themselves more exposed to heat stress. Grazing is conducted in lines, with the cattle in close proximity. Stampedes occur only in exceptional circumstances (Ralley *et al.*, 1993).

Recently insecticide-impregnated eartags have been developed which reduce the facial concentrations of flies for several months. The normal activity of the cattle, e.g. ear flapping and grooming, causes the active ingredient, cypermethrin, to be transferred from the tag to the animal's body. Fly numbers are reduced substantially. Dipping or spraying may eliminate other parasites such as ticks.

Browsing

Browsing is feeding on plant material in the secondary storey in forests, i.e. shrubs and trees. In a forest environment, cattle do not consume woody parts of the plant but selectively eat the leaves and young shoots of accessible shrubs (Fig. 10.9), sometimes in preference to grasses, which are likely to be more lignified. Cattle have long tongues which are a valuable asset in selecting browse material, but they have a broad, flattened lower incisor arcade which is valuable for grazing. Selective browsers, such as giraffes, have narrow, pointed incisor arcades with which to sever leaves and young shoots from woody perennials (Gordon & Illius, 1988). Cattle are more adapted in both grazing and browsing to bulk harvesting, because they have a well-developed capacity for fermentation of coarse fodder by micro-organisms in their rumen.

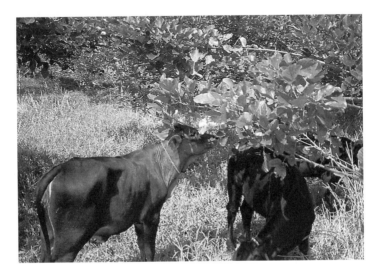

Fig. 10.9 Young cattle in the tropics browsing on leguminous trees.

Evidence that cattle are equally well adapted to both grazing and browsing comes from feral cattle in south-east Asia, which show considerable variation in their diet. They are least selective in the early morning and late afternoon, when their priority is to consume large quantities of food to maintain rumen fill before and after their quiescent period during darkness (Gupta *et al.*, 1999). At this time, they frequently consume grasses on the forest fringes. During mid-day they are more selective, often venturing into the forest to consume shrubs, that are less fibrous and contain more protein. Their foraging behaviour is also governed by the availability of water, particularly if the herbage consumed has a low moisture content, and salt, which is important for digestion of fibrous material.

Browsed plants do not normally make up a significant part of the diet of intensively managed cattle in temperate regions, because grasses are easier for farmers to maintain in a vegetative state. However, where suitable browse species grow and can be consumed without much selectivity, e.g. bamboo (Fig. 10.10), cattle exist on large quantities of leaves and young shoots. Browse is more important in tropical countries because:

(a) it survives the dry season better than shallow-rooted grasses
(b) the shortage of fodder during dry periods is not so easily buffered by conserved feed as it is in temperate countries
(c) the requirements of the cattle are not as high as in temperate regions.

In the diverse forest habitats remaining in tropical and subtropical regions, there is considerable overlap in the plant species selected by domestic cattle and wild ungulates (Fritz *et al.*, 1996). Competition therefore exists between domestic cattle and some herbivores, such as impala. Deer are particularly well adapted to selective browsing, and cattle may rely mainly on grazing if the deer are

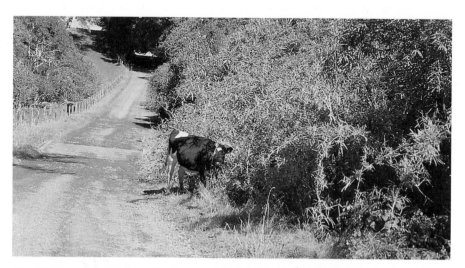

Fig. 10.10 A young steer feeding on bamboo on the edge of indigenous forest in southern Chile.

present in sufficient numbers (Pordomingo & Rucci, 2000). In most circumstances, cattle can be part of a heterogeneous landscape provided for a variety of ungulates with complementary feeding habits.

In some tropical regions, tree leaves are collected manually for cattle feeding, which prevents damage to the trees by the cattle and provides an income for those collecting the cattle food. Similarly tropical shrubs such as leucaena leucocephala and glyricidium sepium are often harvested manually for cattle. This browsing equivalent of zero-grazing can be a more efficient way to use the fodder provided by trees and shrubs.

Eating conserved feed

Both cereal grains and forages are harvested and preserved for use as cattle feed when grazing is scarce. As conserved feeds are usually presented in a readily prehensible form, suitable for large bites, the rate of consumption is high (Table 10.2). Conserved forages are often more fibrous than grazed herbage or concentrates, and need to be masticated for a longer period, during both eating and rumination. This helps to comminute the plant parts and expose more components of the cells to the slow process of fibre digestion.

Many factors influence the rate of an animal's intake of conserved feed. Lactating cows, for example, which have high intake requirements, eat particularly quickly, and dominant cows may eat more quickly than subordinates. Animal size has a major influence, hence small heifers take longer to eat their concentrate ration in the parlour than older cows.

Feed form and composition affect both acceptability of the food and the rate of prehension. Dusty pellets or meals are consumed slowly, because they have to be mixed with saliva before they can be swallowed. Acid feeds, such as silage, are eaten quite rapidly, but the meals are short, suggesting that there is negative inhibition of intake by rumen or buccal receptors. pH receptors in the tongue may control rumination by using information presented by the regurgitated boluses. Excessive saltiness or bitterness also reduces the rate of intake of concentrates, although a limited amount of salt mixed in with the feed increases palatability (Chiy & Phillips, 1999b). Indeed, it used to be a common practice to add salt to hay or silage to make it more palatable.

Table 10.2 Typical rates of eating conserved feed

	Rate of intake (g DM/min)
Oat straw	20
Hay	30
Grass silage	45
Ground and pelleted hay	80
Concentrate meal	250
Concentrate pellets	400

From Campling and Morgan (1981) and Phillips (1983).

Cattle are selective when consuming conserved feeds, although to a lesser degree than during grazing. When consuming silage and to some extent hay, they manipulate it with their nose to find herbage that tastes or smells best. While we cannot yet be sure exactly what they are searching for, it is likely that feed previously contaminated or 'marked' with another cow's saliva will be avoided since newly offered feeds are consumed at a rapid rate. Conceivably pheromones in the cow's saliva contaminate the feed, but no direct evidence is yet available to support this theory. Often when silage feeding, 'nosing' by the cattle turns into 'feed tossing' behaviour, which can result in a waste of feed (Fig. 10.11). First a mouthful of silage is taken; then by dipping the head and twisting the neck upwards the silage is thrown upwards into the air, sometimes landing on the back of the animal. Usually only a small proportion of the herd indulges in this wasteful behaviour, but it is particularly common if the feed is offered from a bunk or trough whose base is not at floor level (Fig. 10.12). Swallowing may be easier when the head is lowered, as it would be during grazing, but it is possible that the feed tossing behaviour is a redirected sward ripping action (which would normally be performed 30 000 to 40 000 times/day).

Whereas it is unlikely that space availability will limit the intake of grazing cattle, this is an important consideration with loose-housed cattle consuming conserved feed. A large area per animal is expensive to provide and can lead to abnormal behaviours such as lying on the floor instead of in cubicles. Too little space, however, increases competition between the cattle and reduces intake (Fig. 10.13). The inability of cattle to increase greatly their rate of consumption

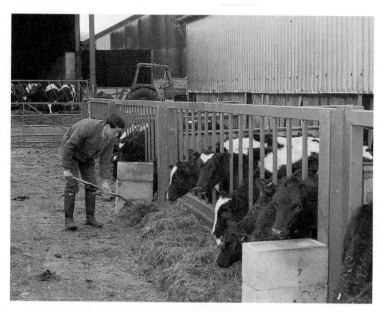

Fig. 10.11   Returning silage that has been manipulated and tossed forwards by cattle with their nose.

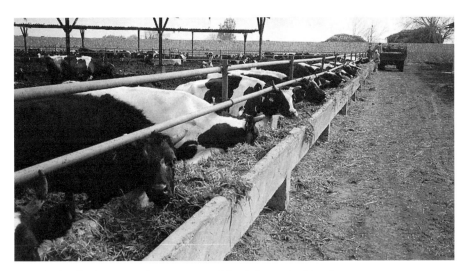

Fig. 10.12 Cattle consuming zero-grazed feeds in a raised bunk.

means that dominant cattle do not take all the feed when it is of restricted availability.

Housed cattle will typically eat silage or hay in 6 to 12 meals/day for a total of 4 to 7 hours/day. However, providing only this amount of time for the cows to eat will reduce intake by about 20% (Campling & Morgan, 1981), demonstrating the need for cattle to spread their feeds out over the day. Intake will also be

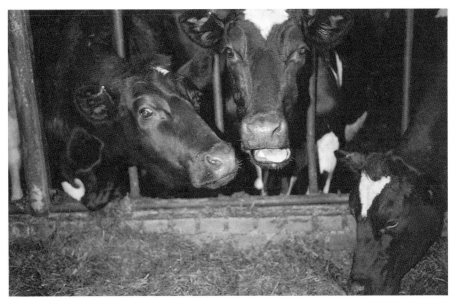

Fig. 10.13 The close proximity of cattle feeding at a barrier encourages competitive interaction.

restricted if less than 40 to 50 cm of feeding space is available per animal. Like grazing cattle, housed cattle prefer to take most feed during daylight hours, but there is often some feeding by subordinate cows overnight. Housed cattle exhibit less social facilitation when feeding than grazing cattle. This may weaken the social bonds and increase tension in the herd.

Self-feed silage

A common system of feeding silage that is popular in the UK and requires little mechanisation is for the cows to 'graze' vertically direct from a silage clamp. Feeding time and feed intake are usually similar to those of cattle consuming trough or floor-fed silage (Church *et al.*, 1999). However, the silage can be difficult to extract from the clamp, especially for young cattle losing their milk teeth and if the silage is not well chopped at harvesting. Heavily consolidated and finely chopped silage can also sometimes be difficult for cattle to extract from the clamp.

In the same way that an electrified wire can limit access to new grazing in the field, an electrified bar or a solid barrier about 0.9 m from the floor is needed to restrict consumption in the middle of the clamp, otherwise the top would fall down on top of the cattle. The stockperson must move the bar or barrier closer to the silage face at regular intervals, thereby allowing access to fresh silage.

Care must be taken if young heifers are required to feed with older cattle in this system, particularly if access to the feed face is limited. It will take some time for them to overcome their fear of an electrified wire, and they may also be bullied by older cows. In situations like this they inevitably resort to feeding at less favoured times, such as in the early morning. If the width of the feed face is limiting, a ring feeder holding cut silage may be used to provide a greater area of access.

Eating supplements

Most cattle in intensive farming are offered supplements to complement the nutritional value of the basal forage or grazed feed. Usually these supplements are of greater nutrient value than the forage and tend to be preferred to it. If supplied in small quantities, intake rate is increased and the greater the amount of supplement offered, the slower the intake rate will be. The rapid intake rate of supplements is of benefit to grazing cows, which are often short of time to harvest sufficient feed. There is no ideal time to offer the supplement because some substitution for the basal forage is inevitable, however undesirable it may be economically. Attempts to restrict its availability to non-preferred feeding times, e.g. at night, have not been successful in preventing the intakes of basal forage being reduced because the cow readily modifies its behaviour to cope with the new feeding times. In this respect, the preference for feeding mainly during daylight may arise not so much from the energetic benefits gained from adequate rest at night, as from a vestigial defence mechanism to restrict grazing when predators cannot be easily seen. There is, however, some evidence that morning supplementation is better than afternoon (Adams, 1985). Some cows prefer conserved supplements such as silage to grazed grass just because they can be eaten rapidly. This can even be to the detriment of their milk production; in this instance the cow is trading hunger satiation for more rest.

The rapid intake rate of conserved or zero-grazed feeds is primarily due to a large bite size (Fig. 10.12). Biting rate when prehending forage is low, for hay typically 15 bites/minute, but there are a large number of manipulative and chewing bites – about 60/minute – compared with cows at pasture where these rarely exceed 15/minute.

Environmental factors affecting feeding behaviour

Photoperiod and time of day

Cattle are mainly diurnal feeders, with concentrations in feeding activity at the twilight (crepuscular) times. When intake requirements are high or the day-length is short, nocturnal feeding will take place. Cattle attempt to spread out their meals over the daylight hours by manipulating meal number and length; hence in mid summer there are a large number of meals in the daylight but they are of short duration (Fig. 10.14). Nocturnal feeding is more likely to occur on a well-lit night, and in hot humid conditions night grazing is increased to limit exposure to the sun during the day (Coulon, 1984). Cattle may thus be regarded as facultative diurnal feeders.

The speed of grazing or biting the pasture also varies over the day. Speed is reduced at night, probably because the cattle do not have the necessary visual cues for fast herbage selection (Phillips & Hecheimi, 1989). Some experiments have found a marked increase in biting rate as the day progresses (Phillips &

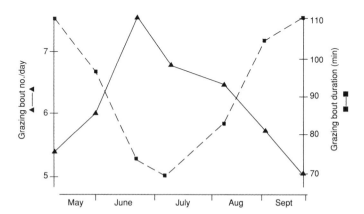

Fig. 10.14 Variation in grazing bout number and duration over the grazing season in the UK (Phillips & Hecheimi, 1989).

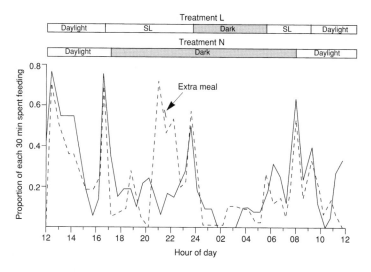

Fig. 10.15 Effect of supplementary light (SL) on feeding behaviour of housed dairy cattle: (– – –) treatment L with supplementary light; (——) treatment N with no supplementary light.

Leaver, 1985c). This is usually accompanied by an increase in grazing intensity – the proportion of time spent grazing. These two factors that increase the rate of herbage intake as the day progresses may be related to the increase in sugar content of the plant as photosynthesis proceeds (Orr *et al.*, 1997).

In rotationally grazed pastures, a fresh paddock is usually made available daily and there is an increase in grazing intensity when the fresh pasture is offered. Similarly the feeding intensity of cattle offered conserved feeds is greatest after a new feed has been provided.

Photoperiod manipulation in housed cattle can alter circadian patterns of feeding. Extending the daylength will increase the number of meals but will not increase the total daily feeding time (Fig. 10.15).

Feeding frequency

The offering of food to cattle is associated with increased activity and aggression between animals (Arnold & Grassia, 1983; Jezierski & Podluzny, 1984; Phillips & Rind, 2001), hence it may be advisable to limit the frequency of feeding. When they are fed once daily at the same time each day, the event is probably anticipated, as most mammals can anticipate up to two or three feeds per day (Mistleberger, 1994). However, mammals do not seem to be able to anticipate the offering of food at intervals greater than about 26 hours, and it is therefore likely that feeding cattle on alternate days eliminates anticipation of the event (Phillips & Rind, 2001). Varying the time of offering of milk to calves during the day, and thereby eliminating anticipation, can increase concentrate intake and feeding time, probably because it stimulates food searching behaviour (Johannesson & Ladewig, 2000).

Most research has shown no effect of the frequency of feeding total mixed rations (TMR) to stanchioned cows, between two and four times per day, on milk production or DM intake. In addition, feeding TMR between one and eight times per day to stanchioned cattle has little effect on rumen function (Nocek & Braund, 1985; Robinson & Sniffen, 1985), although there is evidence of reduced fluctuation in rumen ammonia and water-soluble carbohydrate concentrations (Burt & Dunton, 1967). Despite limited effects of frequent feeding on stanchioned cattle, it may disturb the social structure of loose-housed cattle because they are stimulated to feed when fresh food is offered. In primates, frequent feeding stimulates food searching behaviour, owing to an inability to anticipate the time of offering the food (Jordan *et al.*, 1984; Bloomsfield & Lambeth, 1995). There has been only one brief report on the effects of feeding loose-housed cows between once and three times daily on intake and performance (Goings *et al.*, 1975), which was not conclusive.

An early survey in the UK found that most farmers feed a complete diet once daily, but a small proportion feed every other day (Shingler *et al.*, 1979). Later, it was reported that feeding the complete diet occupied almost one minute/cow/day, or 16% of total labour requirements, making it the second most time consuming activity on dairy farms after milking (Agricultural Development and Advisory Service, 1980). Some saving in labour is possible by feeding every other day, because the time required for many components of the activity, such as opening silage clamps and preparing equipment for feeding, is a function of the number not the duration of feeds. The opportunity to reduce weekend work also exists, since a double ration can be prepared on Friday and offered on Saturday, with no further labour required for feeding until Monday.

Temperature and humidity

As inhabitants of nearly all parts of the global land mass, cattle may be considered thermolabile. However, they are prone to heat stress and unless some protection is provided their productivity declines. Both temperature and humidity increase the heat load and the necessity for cattle to seek shade during the day (thermoregulatory behaviour). Thus in hot dry conditions, particularly if there is a large circadian variation in temperature, cattle move their feeding to the night and reduce the heat load. In the humid tropics there is less circadian variation in temperature, and the high humidity reduces evaporative heat loss, making heat stress a common problem. This is particularly true for *Bos taurus* cattle, which need to spend much of the day in the shade, and feed intake is substantially reduced. Often about 60% of grazing is at night, but in many countries the cattle have to be housed at night to protect against predators (Ayantunde *et al.*, 2000). This can reduce grazing time to five hours a day or less, but pasture intake rate is usually increased to compensate for at least some of the reduction in grazing time.

High temperatures and humidity that cause heat stress will also alter feed preference. Concentrate feeds are preferred, and fibrous feeds should be avoided

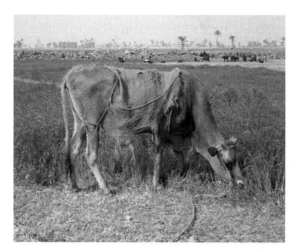

Fig. 10.16 Cattle that have evolved heat tolerance are more susceptible to cold stress. Baladi cattle in Egypt are provided with a hessian cover in winter, when temperatures rarely fall below 5°C.

because fibre produces a greater heat increment of digestion than other nutrients. In many tropical regions, however, only fibrous feeds are available for feeding to cattle, as concentrate feeds are required for human consumption.

The high heat of digestion of fibre enables cattle to survive remarkably low temperatures without loss of productivity, providing they have a functional rumen. Preruminant or sick cattle or those that are inadequately fed have reduced tolerance of cold stress. Feeding time for all cattle increases at low temperatures but healthy ruminant cattle can easily adjust to temperatures of −20°C or below. The major nutritional adjustment that they make is to speed up the rate of reticular contractions, increasing ruminating time and the heat increment of digestion (Gonyou *et al.*, 1979). Not suprisingly, cattle tolerant to heat stress tend to be more susceptible to cold stress. For example, Baladi cattle in Egypt, which are well adapted to the hot summer conditions, need protection from the cold in winter (Fig. 10.16).

Wind and rain

Wind and rain increase the feeling of cold in grazing cattle, forcing them to seek shelter in extreme conditions. However, wind also reduces heat stress, and forced air ventilation can be used for this purpose with housed cattle.

Cattle orientate their bodies to minimise adverse climatic effects. In cold temperatures they orientate themselves to be perpendicular to the sun's rays. In cold wind and rain they stand or graze with their hindquarters to the wind so that their faces, which are more thermally sensitive, are protected. Depending on their degree of hunger, heavy rain may stop them grazing altogether, particularly if shelter is available, but in most conditions they will graze with the wind, travelling faster and apparently grazing less intensively. Cattle are reluctant to lie on wet grass: if rain starts when they are already lying, they may not move, but if they are standing they will shelter rather than lie down. Sometimes a light shower can actually encourage lying cattle to get up and graze, which may be because they want to graze before heavy rain comes and the grass becomes too wet. A phenomenon which has puzzled farmers and scientists alike for many years is the low intake and productivity of cattle grazing lush temperate grasses during a prolonged period of wet weather. The rainfall has no effect on the rate of grass intake (in dry matter terms) but reduces the total amount of grass eaten daily, sometimes by 10 to 20%, and reduces grass digestibility (Phillips *et al.*, 1991). Addition of water to the rumen *per se* does not affect digestibility, so it is likely that the water in the buccal cavity reduces the efficiency of mastication and hence digestion – much as a lawnmower struggles to cut wet grass. The phenomenon occurs only with grass that already has a high water content. With grasses or other feeds of low water content (< 20%), intake may be increased if water is added. Cattle therefore have the highest intakes of feed dry matter between about 20 and 80% water content.

Feeding apparatus

The introduction of high-moisture bulky feeds such as silage and zero-grazed herbage has necessitated changes in the feeding apparatus for housed cattle from the conventional hayrack. The traditional feeding barrier was shaped like a row of tombstones, designed so that each animal had to lift its head to the top of the barrier before it could pull it back (Fig. 10.17). This deterred cattle from

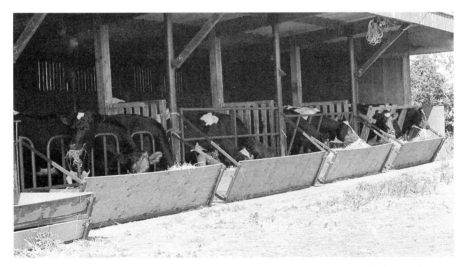

Fig. 10.17 Feeding barriers on trial at an experimental station. Left to right: tombstone, rectangular, diagonal and angled diagonal barriers.

pulling feed out of a trough and eating it in the feeding passage where it could be dropped and wasted. The tombstone and other similar barriers ensured that the animal's head remained over the feed trough whilst it ate. A diagonal feeding barrier, which is simpler to construct, achieves the same objective, as the animal must twist its head sideways to move backwards. An angled feeding barrier will more effectively contain the animal's forward thrust from the shoulders as it feeds and provide a more comfortable feeding position. Whereas cattle are content to consume feed from floor level, they prefer to masticate it with their head horizontal or slightly lowered.

Rumination

Rumination or 'chewing the cud' is the characteristic 'repeat consumption' process that enables cattle to digest coarse grasses. The principal function is to comminute further the plant cell walls so that cell solutes are released and the walls are exposed to microbial digestion in the rumen. An aid to this process is the mixing of the feed with saliva, which lubricates the chewing process, and adds chemical buffers and predigestive enzymes to aid digestion.

Rumination accounts for a substantial part of a cow's day, altogether about six to eight hours, usually interspersed between grazing bouts and with the most intensive period being several hours after dusk (Fig. 10.18). It is not a continuous process but it is performed in about eight bouts of 45 minutes each day. It is often associated with reduced alertness and its rhythmic action may induce a soporific or even hypnotic effect in the animal. It is characterised by a regular pattern of mastication, normally at about 60 to 70 bites/minute for adult cattle and more for calves. It is under voluntary control, and cattle that are disturbed and taken for milking, for example, will cease rumination. Most herdspeople recognise that only healthy and unstressed cattle will ruminate normally, and thus they look for ruminating activity as a sign of contentment in their cattle. The time that cattle spend ruminating declines at stressful times, such as close to calving (Bao & Giller, 1991; Lidfors, 1996). In hot climates, cattle prefer to ruminate in the shade (Sanchez & Febles, 1999).

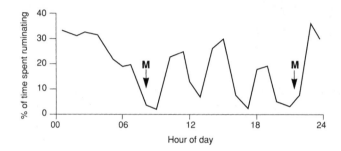

Fig. 10.18   Circadian variation in the ruminating behaviour of grazing dairy cows.

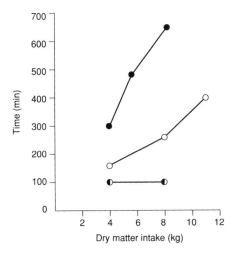

Fig. 10.19 Effect of dry matter intake of hay (●), dried grass (○) and concentrates (◑) on ruminating time of cows (Balch, 1971).

The extent of rumination required for a specific diet depends largely on its fibre content and also on the dry matter and surface water content (Fig. 10.19). Conserved forages that are normally harvested at a more mature stage than grazed grass are typically ruminated for longer, but total chewing time (eating and ruminating) is similar for different forages. This has led some researchers to propose that long rumination times constrain the intake of low-quality forages (Weigand *et al.*, 1993). With regard to surface water, wet grass is not ruminated efficiently and cattle increase rumination time to compensate.

Large ruminants generally have a more efficient fibre digestion process than small ruminants because of the size of their fermentation vat (the rumen) and the ease with which stable fermentation conditions can be created in the rumen. Older, larger cattle are therefore more efficient forage digesters than young cattle, which may be why they masticate more slowly. High-yielding cows seem prepared to forego some ruminating time to allow for other activities, such as grazing and resting. There is evidence that the best milking cattle have the fastest mastication rates (Deharang & Godeau, 1991), which enables them to utilise food more efficiently.

Drinking

Drinking is the consumption of liquids, usually water, by sucking it in through the mouth. The neonate also consumes milk by suckling, a specialist drinking action whereby milk is mainly squeezed out of the mother's teat rather than sucked. Water can also be lapped like a dog, particularly if there is any stray electrical current in the water.

Cattle need to drink at least every two to four days, depending on the temperature, the feed type and the drought resistance of the cattle. When they visit a watering place infrequently, as in rangeland grazing, they will usually spend a few hours there and drink three or four times. This sort of infrequent drinking is only found when the grazing is situated some distance (several hours' walking) from the available water.

When water is freely available, cattle drink more frequently, usually two to five times a day. There is considerable variation between individuals, with the range being two to ten times per day (Andersson, 1987). Cattle synchronise feeding and drinking, and for the ruminant there are digestive benefits in maintaining a constant rumen osmolality. Drinking is also synchronised with milking in lactating cattle, and as with feeding this is perhaps a learnt response to an impending osmotic demand. In fact voluntary water intake includes a 'luxury uptake', in much the same way that other nutrients (sodium, energy-rich feeds) are voluntarily consumed in greater quantities than required. This is despite the fact that some nutrients subject to 'luxury uptake', such as water and sodium, cannot be saved in any quantity in case of future deprivation.

Most of the drinking by grazing cattle, if water is provided at pasture, is either on being returned to the pasture just after milking or during a grazing bout, often in early evening. When cattle interrupt a grazing bout for water, they may speed up the rate of walking in the direction of the trough whilst they graze or they may break off from grazing altogether and walk to the trough. Grazing may be disrupted if the cattle have to wait too long for water or if they have to make many trips for a small amount of water each time, as happens if the refilling rate of the trough is slow because of low water pressure.

Sometimes, particularly in rotational grazing systems, grazing dairy cows are not provided with water at pasture and must obtain their water supply at milking. In this case a farmer must take into account the water requirements and the potential rate of water intake, which can be calculated from the weight of the cattle (Fitsimons, 1979). Water requirements vary with diet, temperature and physiological state of the cattle. Water intake is directly correlated with dry matter content of the diet, and cattle grazing very wet diets, e.g. lush spring grass, may drink little water. Normally even with wet diets some water is drunk out of habit or as 'luxury uptake' and the total water intake (free water plus feed water) varies inversely with feed dry matter content (Halley & Dougall, 1962). High protein feeds also usually require a high water intake, as do high sodium feeds. High water availabilities are very important in saline areas, where plants tend to have high sodium contents.

If water is in short supply, social factors can reduce the intake by subordinate cattle, as cattle often congregate around a water point and a dominance order develops for priority of access to the water, which does not necessarily accord with the social hierarchy (Andersson, 1987). Butting is common to prevent other cattle gaining access. Water intake is likely to be decreased if cows have to walk more than 250 m to the water. In this case they will reduce their luxury uptake, but not their water intake required for physiological purposes. Cattle can tolerate their water intake being reduced to 90% of *ad libitum* with little extra aggression, but if it is reduced to 50%, the consequences for some cattle will be severe (Little *et al.*, 1980).

Suckling

Both the calf's suckling drive and the cow's milk ejection reflex are innate but rapidly become habituated if not maintained. Some genotypes, especially *Bos indicus*, require the sight of a calf before the milk ejection reflex is initiated. Others, notably *Bos taurus* cattle, normally generalise the response from the sight of a calf to other premilking procedures such as washing and drying the udder or entry into the parlour or collecting yard. Within breeds there is variation in this response. It is possible that *Bos indicus* cattle could be selected for their willingness to release milk in the absence of the calf, which would facilitate machine milking. To establish a good conditioned reflex in *Bos taurus* cattle, the stimulus which acts as the signal for the conditioned reflex must precede the unconditioned stimulus, the cows must be healthy, unstressed and undisturbed, and the new stimulus must be benign and not upsetting to the cow in any way (Cowie, 1979).

The calf suckles mainly by squeezing the milk out of the teat cistern, but also by creating a vacuum around the teat. It squeezes the milk out by compressing the neck of the teat between its tongue and hard palate and squeezing the teat from the base to the tip with the tongue. A partial vacuum created by wrapping the tongue around the teat helps express the milk. After the milk is extracted, the bottom jaw is lowered and the pressure on the teat released so that the teat cistern can fill up again. This happens about 75 times a minute for the duration of the suckling bout. Newborn calves have five to eight suckling bouts each day. As the calf grows older this declines to three to five per day and the frequency with which the calf squeezes the teat declines. Cows suckling multiple calves permit a greater number of suckling bouts, up to 15 to 20 per day. In single-suckled cows each suckling bout lasts for 10 to 15 minutes, but it is shorter for multiple-suckled cows. Towards the end of each suckling bout the teat-squeezing frequency decreases as the calf bunts the udder to aid passage of the milk into the teat cistern.

During suckling, the calf moves rapidly from teat to teat, reaching under the udder to access those on the far side. A calf usually suckles between the back and front legs, normally with its body alongside that of the cow (Fig. 10.20). The cow often turns towards the calf to shield it. Sometimes, especially as the calf grows older, it will suckle at a right angle to the cow, or between the cow's hind legs. Younger calves often wag their tails whilst suckling, which may indicate satisfaction to the cow.

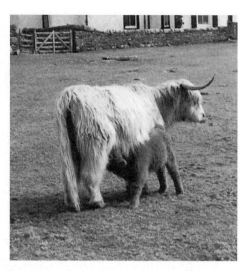

Fig. 10.20 Calves suckle between the front and rear legs, with their body alongside that of the cow.

Because the calf is taller than the cow's teats, suckling is usually performed with the calf's neck lowered and the head raised (Fig. 10.21). This position helps the oesophageal groove closure, where the milk bypasses the rumen to enter the abomasum directly. If calves are weaned from their mothers and given milk to drink from a bucket, the head-down position hinders the groove closure and makes the calf more likely to scour. Assistance in the form of two or three fingers placed in the bucket to simulate a teat may encourage the calf to drink in the head-down position (Fig. 10.22).

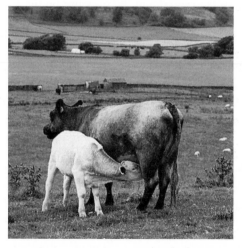

Fig. 10.21 Suckling in an older calf, showing lowering of the head to reach the cow's udder.

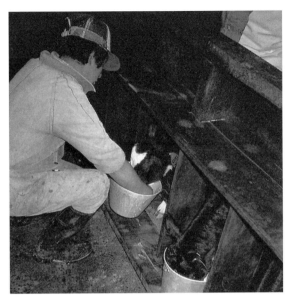

Fig. 10.22 Teaching calves to drink milk from a bucket involves encouraging them to suck two or three fingers covered in milk, simulating teat-sucking.

Elimination

Food and water that are not retained in the body for metabolic processes are eliminated either as solid material voided from the anus (faeces) or as a liquid from the penis in the male or vagina in the female (urine).

Defecation

When cattle defecate the tail is raised and there is light arching of the back to prevent the tail becoming contaminated with faeces. Defecation may be performed while the animal is walking, standing, grazing or getting up. Cattle normally defecate about 12 times a day, with surprisingly little variation (range 10 to 16). The pattern of defecation over the day is mainly determined by the grazing pattern, as most faeces are deposited during grazing. Cattle are likely to defecate when they stand up after a period of lying, and faeces therefore accumulates in an overnight camping area. This increases soil fertility and microbial activity (Haynes & Williams, 1999). If grazing cattle are more intensively stocked at night close to the parlour so that they can easily be brought in for milking, there may be a transfer in soil fertility due to more faeces being voided per unit area on the night pasture.

Some variation in faecal output occurs owing to intake and feed type. Highly digestible feeds such as spring grass produce more liquid faeces that will cover a greater area of grass. When the faeces are of low dry matter content, the projectile assumes a more horizontal trajectory and the tail may become soiled. Cattle that are nervous defecate more often and also produce more liquid faeces. An indication of a good stockperson is that the cows do not defecate excessively in the parlour (Seabrook, 1984).

In a grazing field, each faecal deposit occupies an area approximately of $0.07 \, m^2$, which means that at a normal stocking rate 6% of the pasture area will have received a deposit of faeces by the end of the grazing season. In practice there is some breakdown of faecal deposits so that by the end of a grazing season 2 to 4% of the pasture area is covered (Phillips, 1991). On average each faecal deposit causes an area of herbage six times its own area to be rejected. This is initially because of the odour and later because the herbage is more mature than the rest of the sward. Cattle will eat this 'rejected' herbage if there is little other feed available. Spreading slurry over a grazing pasture will also cause rejection by cattle, and if cattle *are* grazed on slurry contaminated pasture, walking time is increased because the cattle spend longer searching for uncontaminated pasture. Dry matter intake is likely to be reduced.

Several methods have been tested to overcome the reduction in herbage utilisation and intake due to faecal contamination. Conditioning cows to eat herbage near faecal deposits by feeding hay sprayed with dilute slurry or by grazing cattle on recently manured pastures has a very short-lived effect as the cattle habituate rapidly. Chain harrowing to disperse faeces and accelerate decomposition has met with little success, as it can damage the sward and does not disperse fresh deposits adequately. Covering the rejected herbage with molasses by spot spraying or a weed wipe attachment to a tractor has had some success, but the best method is to mix cattle with other grazing stock such as sheep or goats. Faecal rejection is largely species specific and is stronger in cattle than sheep, so complementary grazing of contaminated areas can readily be achieved. Zero-grazing (cutting fresh grass and feeding to the cattle indoors) is sometimes advocated to overcome the problem, as faeces and urine can be more evenly spread on the land at the most suitable times. The implications for pasture utilisation efficiency are small, but the potential increase in intake is considerable.

Indoors the constant proximity to faeces and urine in most loose housing systems may cause habituation to its offensiveness. As the ability to perceive odours is eliminated by constant exposure, this may not present as much of an offence to the welfare of cattle as is often perceived. However, several diseases are transmitted in slurry, including *E. coli* infection of the udder, tuberculosis, para-tuberculosis and brucellosis. Therefore, it is desirable to remove the faeces regulary with floor scrapers or to use slatted floors. Training cattle to defecate in one part of the building may be possible.

Urination

Urination in the female involves raising the tail, ceasing any activities, arching the back and sometimes splaying the legs to avoid their becoming wet. In the male urination can be accomplished while walking. A secondary function of urination is to transmit pheromonal information, especially during periods of stress (Boissy *et al.*, 1998) and oestrus (Dehnhard & Claus, 1996).

Cattle urinate less frequently than they defecate, on average about ten times a day (Hancock, 1953). At pasture urine presents less of a problem than faeces, although herbage may be scorched at high stocking rates and during dry weather. Cattle prefer to graze pasture that has recently received a urination, perhaps because of the herbage's increased sodium content, and will graze it lower than uncontaminated herbage (Jaramillo, 1990). Most urination takes place while cattle are grazing, not while they are resting. Urination is more frequent when cattle have high liquid intakes, e.g. when sodium intakes are high.

Chapter 11
Reproductive Behaviour

Reproductive strategy

Like most other sexually reproducing animals, female cattle produce a small number of gametes supplied with nourishment in the form of an ovum, and males produce large numbers of gametes with only minimum survival capacity. Because of their greater investment in the gamete, the females are responsible for nurturing the developing embryo and providing the parental care, particularly through lactation. The only 'parental investment' provided by the bull is to guard the cow during oestrus and prevent her from being inseminated by rival bulls. The minimal investment by the male encourages polygyny (individual males mating with many females), which in turn causes competition for females and sexual dimorphism. Therefore, bulls have increased size and strength compared to cows, especially in the parts necessary for effective combat – the shoulders, neck muscle and horns. Despite intense competition between males for access to females, coitus only occurs during the cows' oestrus. During guarding, a bull may attempt to mount and show other appetitive behaviour such as partial erection and dribbling of accessory fluid, but he will not force copulation.

Although most aspects of the reproductive strategy of cattle are typical for mammals, they differ by being essentially bisexual, with both sexes frequently exhibiting hetero- and homosexual behaviour. Homosexual cow behaviour (Fig. 11.1) was used in feral herds as a visual signal that the herd contained receptive cows. There has also probably been human selection for this trait for as long as the sexes were kept apart, to indicate when a cow was ready to be inseminated (naturally or artificially). What remains unclear is the apparent altruism in cow mounting behaviour. Why is a non-receptive cow mounting a receptive cow and not vice versa? It may be a form of reciprocal altruism, so the non-receptive cow will expect the same attention when she is receptive and *the population* therefore achieves greater reproductive potential. The mounting cow is usually close to oestrus herself and by drawing attention to the receptive cow, she is also drawing attention to herself and the sexually active group as a whole. Thus the mounting cow is signalling to the bull that she also expects his attention shortly, and given the bull's phenomenal serving capacity (77 ejaculations in

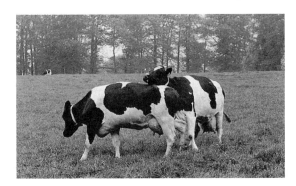

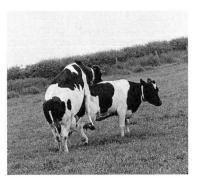 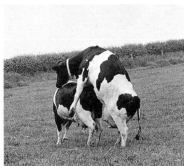

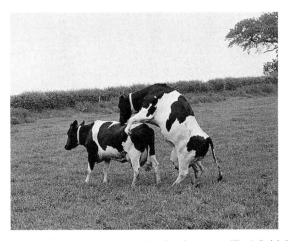

Fig. 11.1 Sequence of homosexual mounting in the cow. *(Top)* Initially the mounter orientates herself to the other cow, sometimes testing for the rigid back response by pressing her chin on the other cow's back. *(Middle)* The mounter raises her brisket onto the rear end of the other cow and clasps her with her front legs just in front of the pelvic bone. As the mounting proceeds the mounter may engage in rhythmic pelvic thrusting. *(Bottom)* As the mounter dismounts she drags her front legs over the flanks of the mounted cow, often leaving tell-tale muddy marks which indicate to the herdsperson that the cow has been mounted.

six hours have been recorded) and the libido boost that occurs when he changes his attention to a new cow in oestrus, this should not present difficulties for the male.

The stimulus for one cow to mount another is an inverted ∪, which is provided by the rump of the oestrous cow. Female–female mounting also involves pelvic thrusts in approximately 50% of cases. It is not clear what the immediate physical reward for the mounter is. Does she feel any satiation of libido during this potentially dangerous behaviour? The benefits for the mounted cow are more easily explained. Cows mounted by a bull experience a lowering of the electrical resistance of the skin immediately after the bull's ejaculation, suggesting an orgasm-like response (Hafez *et al.*, 1969). Probably a similar though weaker sensation is achieved by the rump pressure of a mounting cow, particularly during pelvic thrusting. This may be caused by pressure on the clitoris and vagina and is likely to be confined to the receptive period. Indeed genital stimulation helps to induce and synchronise oestrus via the hypothalamus. During oestrus the electrical resistance of the vaginal epithelium (Feldman *et al.*, 1978) and mucus (Schofield *et al.*, 1991) decreases markedly, allowing small pressure changes to trigger large electrical responses. The importance attached to homosexual mounting is demonstrated by the fact that cows even perform it in the presence of a bull.

Homosexual mounting in the male is most prevalent in a single sex group kept in stressful conditions, particularly from an early age. In such cases subordinate males may be excessively ridden by dominant males. This suggests that the motivation for the behaviour is less related to sexuality than to dominance. Homosexual behaviour in single sex male groups has also been explained, for other species including humans, as the maintenance of reproductive fitness in the absence of partners of the opposite sex. If this were the case, one would expect homosexual behaviour to occur more in the non-functional bulls in a mixed herd, which is not the case. Nor is it common in many other polygynous species, so it seems unlikely that this is the reason. Further evidence for the link to aggression comes from the fact that penile intromission does not normally take place during male homosexual behaviour. Since the behaviour is incomplete, play might be considered as a motive, but as about 50% of buller steers are forced into being mounted, rather than engaging in the behaviour voluntarily (Edwards, 1995), play is probably not the goal. The mounting can be considered an appeasement ceremony if the buller accepts the rider voluntarily, but if the buller is forced to accept the rider, the motivation of the latter is probably to show domination. In the case of forced mounting, the welfare of the buller is more seriously compromised. It is logical that bulls should associate mounting with an attainment of dominant status, as to achieve heterosexual mounting a dominance over most other males is required. Unlike homosexual behaviour in the female, which is comparatively rare in other mammals, homosexual behaviour does occur in other mammalian males and is likely to be explained by redirected aggression rather than the maintenance of reproductive fitness.

The ontogeny of reproductive behaviour

Mounting behaviour commences in calves as early as one week of age but develops mainly between the fourth and tenth month, especially between male calves (Fig. 11.2) (Reinhardt, 1983a,b). Males are more often mounted than females during the prepubertal period, which may reflect their tolerance of this behaviour rather than any sexual preference. Female calves often reject mounting attempts (Reinhardt, 1983a,b), perhaps to prevent any unwanted pregnancy before they are mature. Males gradually learn to target their advances to receptive females, but in feral herds they are inhibited from most mounting with females by the dominant male at ten months of age. By 16 to 18 months they have learnt to distinguish the finer points of oestrous exhibition.

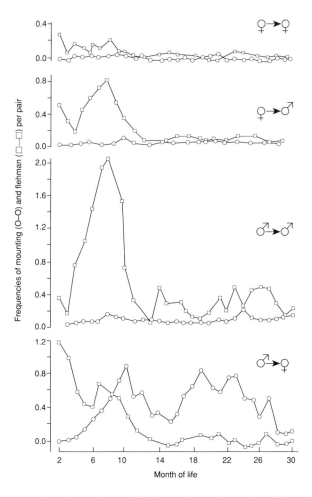

Fig. 11.2 Frequencies of mounting and flehman shown by male and female non-oestrous cattle during the first 30 months of life (Reinhardt, 1983b).

Homosexual mounting in immature feral bulls is a necessary mechanism to develop orientation ability, since only dominant bulls will have access to cows. In intensive housing situations, however, mounting can develop into redirected aggression between bulls, with the consequent exhaustion of subordinate animals that are excessively ridden. This behaviour can be prevented by hanging electrified chains just above the bulls, but it would be better to reduce the intensity of the housing system or more equally match the groups of bulls. Flehman develops mainly in male calves in response to males (Fig. 11.2), and is common between four and ten months of age during sexual behaviour development. It then goes through a quiescent period up to 16 months, after which it increases again as males take an interest in oestrous females.

Puberty represents a series of changes that commence in both male and female cattle at about six months of age and culminate in the attainment of full reproductive fitness when both the physiological and behavioural aspects of reproduction are functional. There is a strong positive correlation between growth rate and time to puberty in heifers (Mialon *et al.*, 1999). Whilst the development of the reproductive physiology, particularly in the female, occurs quite suddenly, the behavioural development takes place over a period of up to six months in both males and females. During this period males show increased mounting activity but without penile erection or ejaculation, and the proportion of head-to-side mounts gradually declines, demonstrating that correct orientation is learnt. Masturbatory activities may commence towards the end of puberty. Mixed rearing does not facilitate the development of reproductive behaviour, except that the first contacts between bulls and cows reared in sexual isolation are more hesitant, with delayed first mounting and less aggression between bulls to decide sexual priority. This does not imply that reproductive fitness is innate in either sex but rather that the development of the behavioural characteristics of mounting is achieved just as well in single sex as in mixed groups (Price & Wallach, 1990). The physiological development of reproductive fitness is, however, stimulated by mixed groups. In particular the presence of a bull will advance the age of first oestrus in heifers, probably through olfactory stimuli, but does not influence the intensity of oestrus. Biostimulation may be exploited commercially by using a teaser bull and may be of particular value for *Bos indicus* cows, which take longer to reach puberty than *Bos taurus* cattle (Chenoweth, 1994).

The female oestrus

Definition and description

Oestrus is the behavioural manifestation of sexual receptivity in the cow. The term derives from the similarity to the behaviour cattle show when attacked by the gadfly (spp. *Oestrus*). Oestrous behaviour is exhibited just before ovulation and is relatively short, lasting for only about 2.3% of the cycle. It is preceded by some signals that are detected by the bull, enabling him to guard a cow until full oestrus.

A method of describing oestrous activity by scoring the cow's receptivity (adapted from Lee, 1953) has been devised for farm and research recording purposes:

Score 1. Does not attract attention of other cattle for sexual purposes
Score 2. Attracts, but does not accept attention
Score 3. Attracts, and accepts attention under protest
Score 4. Attracts and accepts attention without protest or enthusiasm
Score 5. Attracts and accepts attention with enthusiasm

The mean oestrous cycle length is 21 days, with 60% of cows having cycles of 18 to 25 days. Oestrus is usually first observed about 50 days post-partum in weaned cows (Fig. 11.3) and about six months post-partum in cows that are suckling calves. There is usually at least one ovulation before this that is not accompanied by oestrous behaviour. The presence of the bull will accelerate the return to first oestrus (biostimulation), as will shortening daylength.

The oestrous cycle can be divided into the following stages: pro-oestrus, the preparatory period just before oestrus; oestrus; metoestrus, the refractory period; and dioestrus, when the cow's reproductive hormone output is dominated by the corpus luteum and she is said to be in the luteal stage. Of the 21-day cycle, mean duration of oestrus is 14 hours, with pro- and metoestrus approximately 10 hours each.

Variation in oestrous length is considerable: in one study over 33% of oestruses were less than six hours (O'Farrell, 1978), whereas another reported oestruses lasting for 30 hours (Hammond, 1927). Multiparous cows usually have

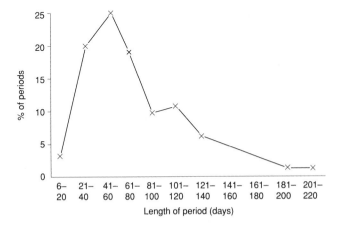

Fig. 11.3 Variation in the length of the period from parturition to first succeeding oestrus (Chapman & Casida, 1937).

cycles of approximately half a day longer than primiparous cows, and well-nourished cows tend to have shorter cycles than cows under nutritional stress (Schofield, 1988). There is also variation in oestrous behaviour due to genotype (the length of oestrus in *Bos indicus* cattle is only about 65% of that in *Bos taurus* cattle; Anderson, 1944; Mattoni *et al.*, 1988), gender (cows stand to be mounted longer for a bull than for each other; Marian *et al.*, 1950), temperature (cows at an environmental temperature of 27°C have been recorded as having 17% longer cycles than cows at 10°C; Pennington *et al.*, 1985), and season (length of oestrus has been reported as 15 hours in spring and 20 hours in autumn; Fraser & Broom, 1990).

Behavioural characteristics of oestrus

True oestrus is characterised by the cow being willing for other cattle, male or female, to mount her (Fig. 11.4). She indicates this by immobility when approached and a slight arching of the back. However, before mounting can be achieved the normal reluctance by cattle to breach each other's personal space must be overcome, and the cow's receptivity tested by the potential mounter. Hence oestrus is accompanied by extensive signalling and communication.

Visual signals include cows adopting the standing-to-be-mounted position (STBM), a generally increased activity level and tail raising and switching. Activity increases slowly during pro-oestrus, and then suddenly during oestrus, followed by an exponential decline during metoestrus (Arney *et al.*, 1994). In addition there is swelling and reddening of the vulva and production of cervical mucus, which is less viscous than usual (LopezGatius *et al.*, 1996) and may be

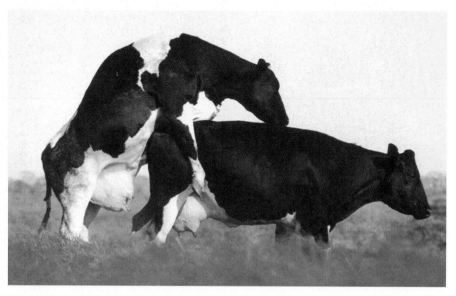

Fig. 11.4 During oestrus the receptive cow allows herself to be mounted by another cow.

seen hanging from the vulva. Additional visual signals to the herdsperson include cervical mucus on the end of a cubicle where an oestrous cow has been lying; dirty, steaming flanks from mounters with dirty hooves, which rub on the flanks as they dismount; and ruffling and abrasion of the rump hair over the sacral vertebrae.

Olfactory signals are provided in the form of pheromones released in the body fluids, especially sweat from glands in the flank and urine. During oestrus cows exhibit prolonged anovaginal sniffing and licking of the flank area. Flehman will also be exhibited to aid reception by the vomeronasal organ. The bull performs these behaviours too (Fig. 11.5) but finds it easier to test for pheromones by sampling the cow's urine. Olfactory signals from the cow enable the bull to detect a cow up to two days before oestrus, during which period he may guard her from the attentions of rival suitors. To increase the spread of pheromones the frequency of urination is increased.

Gustatory signals are provided by the oestrous cow being licked around the vulva, which either provides direct gustatory signals or aids olfactory pheromone reception. It is often followed by the flehman expression. Licking of the vulva may be naturally performed between cows, each head to tail.

Tactile signals are sometimes provided by an oestrous cow when she seeks out a bull and nudges and cajoles him into giving her his attention. She may sniff or lick his genitalia and mount him or other cows to attract him. She will also stand to receive chin pressing or rubbing behaviour by a cow or bull just behind the tailhead. This activity often precedes mounting and tests whether the cow has a

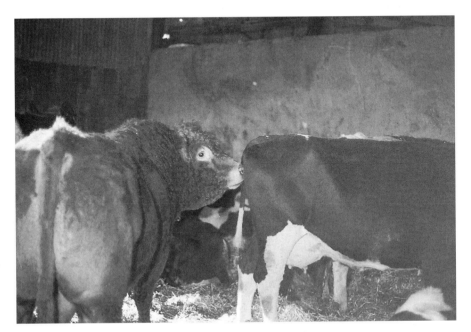

Fig. 11.5 Anovaginal sniffing of an oestrous cow by a bull.

rigid back or lordosis. Vocal signals in the form of repeated bellowing are also common.

Increased aggression occurs between sexually active cows. Cows higher in the dominance order are more likely to mount other cows (Reinhardt, 1983a,b; Schofield, 1988). Although some believe that oestrous behaviour is not related to the dominance hierarchy, the novel associations that cows make during oestrus would be expected to increase aggression. The sexual hierarchy and the space priority dominance hierarchy are not always related, as sexual hierarchy may be determined not so much by agonistic drive as by sexual preferences. Like other mammals, cattle have preferred partners, and the preferences may derive in part from personality and physical complementarity rather than superiority. Some preferences are evident when the bull selects cows; he is not likely to copulate with his family members, particularly his mother (Reinhardt, 1983a,b).

The external symptoms of aggression during oestrus may occur during circling behaviour when the cows engage in sniffing and licking each other's vaginal area, but more often takes the form of head-to-head tussles and butting the flanks. If we assume that the increased aggression arises from internal motivational forces rather than difficulties encountered in forming novel associations, it may enable an oestrus cow to fight for the attention of her intended partner, male or female. It may also serve to dissipate the increased motivation for activity that oestrous cows possess. Activity increases occur for virtually all oestrous cows (Fig. 11.6), with the mean walking rate being increased by a factor of 3.4 (Phillips, 1990a,b). This factor is inversely related to the normal distance that the cow walks, so that

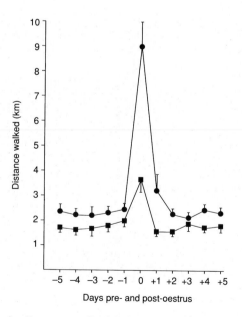

Fig. 11.6   Variation in distances walked before and after oestrus (●, night, ■, day) (Schofield *et al.*, 1991).

if, for genetic or environmental reasons, a cow only walks a short distance each day, her proportional increase in distance walked during oestrus will be large, and vice versa. Thus cows at pasture do not proportionately increase their activity at oestrus as much as cows in a cubicle shed.

Mounting behaviour

Cow receptivity to mounting is the best indicator of the oestrus state, with pelvic thrusting indicating that both partners are willing and confirming that the mounted cow is definitely in oestrus (Fig. 11.7). Pregnant cows occasionally stand to be mounted by cows or immature bulls, but never by an adult bull (Reinhardt, 1983a,b; Dijkhuizen & van Eerdenburg, 1997). This is most likely to

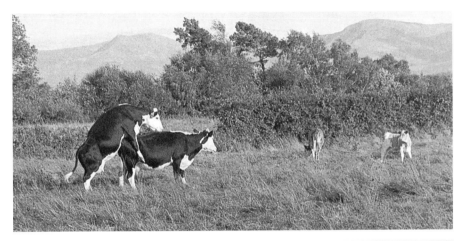

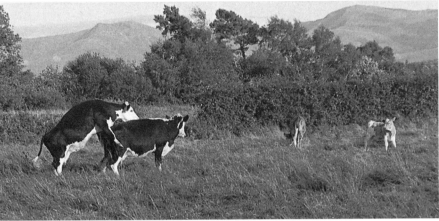

Fig. 11.7 Cow mounting with pelvic thrusting (above) and dismounting (below). As she dismounts she exerts pressure with her front legs and drags her chin over the mounted cow's back, whose legs bend with the pressure. On the right-hand side, a calf can be seen learning about the behaviour.

occur in mid gestation. They also perform other oestrous behaviour such as flehman and investigating other cows. Under normal criteria up to 10% of these cows would be predicted to be in oestrus, so checks must be made before inseminating any cows that might be pregnant.

When an oestrous cow is ridden by a dioestrous cow, it may reciprocate by trying to mount that cow and is most likely to be successful if the escape routes are blocked. Unsuccessful mounting attempts are frequent where escape routes cannot be blocked (Fig. 11.8). Given these exceptions, approximately 90% of all mounted cows are in oestrus, but only about 70% of mounting cows (Hurnik *et al.*, 1975). Cows are usually mounted 50 to 60 times during oestrus by other cows, but one-quarter of cows are mounted fewer than 30 times (Esslemont & Bryant, 1976). *Bos indicus* cows are mounted much less, typically only eight times during the entire oestrus (Mattoni *et al.*, 1988). Mounting activity in *Bos taurus* cattle increases from a negligible incidence in dioestrus to about six mounts/hour during peak oestrus (Fig. 11.9). More mounts are likely to be initiated in pro-oestrus than metoestrus, during which time cows are usually recovering from the excessive activity during oestrus.

Although the number of cows physiologically entering oestrus appears uniform throughout the day, there is a marked peak of oestrous behaviour in the early evening and a secondary peak in the early morning (Schofield, 1988). Probably oestrus expression is accentuated at times when cows are not preoccupied with other high-priority activities, such as feeding and milking, but are still normally active. Management details such as times of feeding and milking and degree of competition for feed will determine the most likely times for oestrus to be expressed.

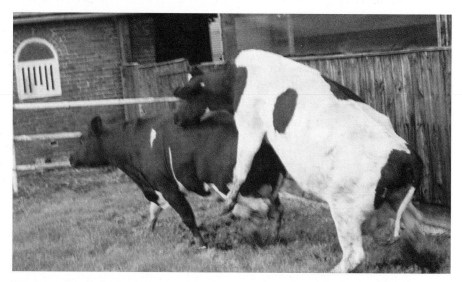

Fig. 11.8 Unsuccessful mounting attempt, with the mounted cow escaping and the mounting cow having to dismount rapidly.

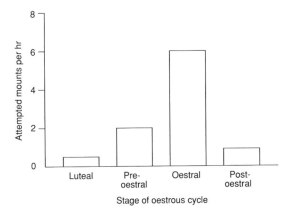

Fig. 11.9   Mean number of attempted mounts per hour by primiparous cows at different stages of an oestrous cycle as defined by levels of progesterone in blood (Helmer & Britt, 1985).

Both environmental and animal factors influence the frequency of homosexual mounting behaviour, and therefore are of importance for detection of oestrus by the herdsperson. Mounting by the bull is less frequent than by cows and will depend on the bull's libido and the bull-to-cow ratio.

Environmental influences on oestrous expression

Cold temperatures reduce mounting activity and alter the diurnal distribution of mounting to concentrate it into the middle of the day when it is warmest. In hot weather cows do most mounting in the early morning and late evening when it is cooler. Heavy rain suppresses mounting behaviour (Kilgour *et al.*, 1977).

Photoperiod also affects mounting behaviour, since artificially extending the daylength in winter can reduce mounting behaviour and activity in general (Phillips & Schofield, 1989). As this is often accompanied by a reduction in aggression, it may be due to the improvement of the environment and resulting pacifying effect on the animals.

The physical environment influences mounting. In a crowded building where the floor is slippery and space is limited, cows are reluctant to mount each other (Vailes & Britt, 1990) (Fig. 11.10). In such an environment cows reserve most mounting behaviour for late at night when the passageways are empty, which may make it difficult for the herdsperson to detect oestrus. Other oestrous behaviours such as chin rubbing are not reduced on slippery floors.

Close confinement can itself be a stimulus to mounting activity as more cows come into contact with each other. However, mounting can be thwarted in close confinement due to difficulties in obtaining all the necessary prerequisites: other cows in or close to oestrus, a floor with good slip resistance and adequate space for mounting and dismounting with safety. Highly stocked, straw-bedded yards may have inadequate space for oestrous behaviour to be fully expressed. Cows

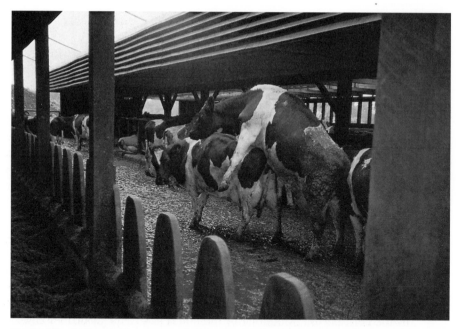

Fig. 11.10 A slippery floor covered with excreta often hinders cows from mounting each other. Dirty flanks that result from a mounting are a useful sign to a herdsperson that a cow is in or close to oestrus, but may also result from cows lying in passages.

usually lie down for longer in straw yards than in cubicles, presenting more of a hazard to mounting cows than in a cubicle house where lying areas are clearly defined and the passageways are free for mounting. In strawed yards teats may be trodden on by mounting cows. More mounting behaviour usually takes place in an open yard than in a building with cubicles. Where space permits mounting cattle usually move to the periphery of the herd, so disturbance to other cows is minimised. Routine, unstressful movement of cows often stimulates mounting, as cows are brought into contact with each other, for example during movement to a milking parlour.

Animal influences on oestrous expression

Genotypic differences are present in mounting behaviour (Rottensten & Touchberry, 1957) and there are probably breed differences (Boyd, 1977), but there has been little attempt to quantify these. The heritability of oestrous intensity estimated by Rottensten and Touchberry was low (0.21), as was the repeatability. It is probable that oestrus is stronger in pure dairy breeds such as the Friesian than in dual purpose and beef cows.

High-yielding dairy cows have reduced oestrous intensity (Michalkiewicsz *et al.*, 1984). Given the extensive selection for oestrous expression in the past, it seems unlikely that major increases could be achieved by selection, and even if they could, there would possibly be undesirable genetically correlated effects, such as a general increase in activity.

Older and heavier cows tend to show a stronger oestrus than small, light heifers, probably because the latter are inexperienced and more likely to be damaged, especially on slippery surfaces. It has been reported that maiden heifers showed 5.5 mounts/hour, first calvers 11.3 mounts/hour and older cows 7.9 mounts/hour (Gwazdauskas *et al.*, 1983), and that oestrous behaviour is reduced in senility (Boyd, 1977), which cows rarely reach. Within this age influence, there are preferences for individual cows and bulls as homosexual and heterosexual partners, respectively, which can influence oestrus. Nutrition does not greatly affect oestrous intensity but low-energy intakes can slightly restrict the increase in activity at oestrus (Arney *et al.*, 1994).

The most significant animal factor affecting oestrous expression is the number of cows at a similar stage in the cycle. A single oestrous cow in a group of dioestrus cows shows very little oestrous behaviour other than increased activity to search for potential partners. Mounting behaviour increases in proportion to the number of cows in oestrus up to four and then may decline (Esslemont *et al.*, 1980; Cortes *et al.*, 1999). When several cows are in oestrus, pro-oestrus or metoestrus, they form themselves into a sexually active group (Williamson *et al.*, 1972). Usually three to four in number, these interact together, with cows not fully in oestrus joining just for brief periods. Multiparous cows form more consistent groups than primiparous cows (Castellanos *et al.*, 1997). New partners stimulate sexual activity, whereas just two cows together lose interest in each other (Alexander *et al.*, 1984). The presence of people can also stimulate mounting activity (Williamson *et al.*, 1972), which may derive from imprinted sexual preferences or a general stimulation of activity.

Refractory behaviour

The oestrous behaviours described so far have all increased in time, so inevitably other behaviours must decline in priority, and these are usually resting and feeding. These are normally high priority behaviours in dairy cows, but during oestrus the motivation for activity, especially locomotion, is increased. It is not clear to what extent cows increase their *rate* of feeding during oestrus to compensate for reduced feeding time. The potential for this is probably greater for housed cattle than for grazing cattle, where the rate of intake is determined largely by sward height. In housed cattle receiving conserved forage, the number of manipulative and chewing bites can be reduced, as well as the length of the rumination period. This will increase intake rate and hence maintain short-term satiation but it will reduce digestibility. In the long term, feeding behaviour will be restored to its normal dioestrous level, and nutrient supply restored. The difficulties of increasing intake rate in grazed cattle are probably greater. Bite depth could be increased by biting closer to the sward but biting rate would decline and the digestibility of ingested material would fall. Mastication and manipulative bites are few in number and so cannot be reduced, but rumination time could be reduced. The difficulty in maintaining the intake of grazing oestrous cows may explain their smaller proportional increase in oestrous activity.

Metoestrus encompasses a sudden reduction in oestrous behaviour and a refractory period when the cow recovers from her exertions of the previous 10 to 20 hours. This usually takes the form of more time spent lying and less standing, walking and feeding. These differences are most evident in straw yards, rather than in cubicle housing, because the latter is not sufficiently comfortable for long periods of rest (Phillips & Schofield, 1990) (Table 11.1, Fig. 11.11). As with oestrus, the extent to which a reduction in feeding time during metoestrus can be compensated for by an increase in feeding rate is unclear. In any event ruminant animals are better able to withstand a reduction in feed intake than monogastric animals because of feed reserves in the rumen.

Oestrous detection

Most dairy cows are kept in single sex groups, and the herdsperson needs to know when individual cows are in oestrus to arrange for them to be inseminated, either naturally or artificially. Beef cows are more often run with a bull, because of the difficulty of detecting the oestrus, which is less intensive, and the irregular contact with humans. Many dairy cows are kept unrestrained in a building yard or at pasture, and the behavioural changes associated with homosexual oestrous interactions can be detected by the herdsperson. Observation is, however, often restricted to milking times and collection for milking (Williamson *et al.*, 1972), which gives detection rates of only 50 to 60% of oestruses. Detection rates for two, three, four and five observations/day of 20 minutes each have been recorded as 62, 78, 80 and 91%, respectively, with the best results being achieved during early morning and late evening observations (Esslemont *et al.*, 1985). As well as the proportion of oestruses missed, it is important to consider the proportion of cows detected 'in oestrus' that were actually in dioestrus (false positives). Depending on the experience of the observer and the time spent in observation, this is likely to be at least 5% (Williamson *et al.*, 1972).

Table 11.1   Time spent by cows in a straw yard and cubicles in different behaviours on the day of oestrus (0), day before oestrus (−1), day after oestrus (+1) and mean of other non-oestrous days (Rest)

Time spent (min per 100 min)	Straw yard				Cubicles			
	−1	0	+1	Rest	−1	0	+1	Rest
Lying	46	36	72	52	37	29	39	34
Standing	17	43	10	18	43	43	35	44
Feeding	37	17	18	29	18	22	24	20
Walking	0.3	3.1	0.3	0.8	1.9	5.5	1.3	1.7

From Phillips and Schofield (1990).

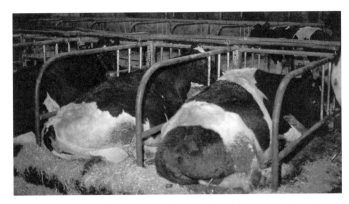

Fig. 11.11 Low levels of comfort of cows in cubicles discourage them from resting after oestrus.

Apart from behavioural changes, the herdsperson can look at changes in milk yield to assist in decisions about whether a cow is in oestrus (Horrell *et al.*, 1984). At the first milking after the onset of oestrus about 80% of dairy cows withhold some of their milk, and yield and fat content are reduced. In these cows there is a compensatory increase in yield at the second milking after the onset of oestrus (Schofield *et al.*, 1991). However, despite new parlour technology enabling milk yield to be automatically recorded and computed at each milking, the effect is not of sufficient magnitude or reliability to be used as the sole determinant of oestrus.

Tethered cows cannot exhibit interactive oestrous behaviours (such as mounting and investigation), although they may do so if they are taken in a group for milking. They exhibit a general restlessness, vulva swelling and mucus production, and increased vocalisation. The degree of personal attention required by tethered cows for such activities as feeding and milking means that oestrous detection rates are frequently as high as or higher than for loose-housed cows (Hackett & McAllister, 1984).

Aids to detecting oestrous behaviour

Although the best attributes for oestrous detection are diligence and patience in quantifying the intensity of oestrus, the herdsperson may be aided by a variety of instruments.

Pedometers can be used to indicate the extent to which walking activity is increased. Given accurate information on the number of steps taken by each cow during the previous two to three days, a mathematical formula or algorithm can be used to detect reliably all cows in oestrus with no false positives (Schofield *et al.*, 1991). The high success rate of this method is due to the large and predictable increase in walking rate at oestrus and the limited variation in dioestrous walking rate (Fig. 11.6). An important feature of this and other characteristic behaviour changes during oestrus is that each cow has a characteristic rate of locomotion and a separate threshold must be established for each cow.

Thus each cow must wear the pedometer for four to five half-day periods to establish a threshold. Pedometers are basically of two types. The simplest devices record stepping rate and telemetrically send the information for each cow to an in-parlour recorder, which is linked to an automatic identification device at each stall. In this case the pedometer can be small and unsophisticated, but considerable investment is required in parlour recording and data-processing facilities. The second type of pedometer is fully self-contained, and not only records step number and time, but also processes the data and indicates when the cow is in oestrus. This may be done visually by coloured lights or audibly by a repeated tone. Inevitably such a device is more expensive than a telemetric recorder for in-parlour processing, and a high degree of loss or breakage may occur. It has the advantage, however, of not requiring automatic cow identification and would therefore probably appeal to the smaller farmer.

The increase in activity and other oestrous behaviour can be monitored remotely using closed-circuit television. The benefits of this are limited unless the oestrous behaviour can be automatically detected. Possibilities for this include pixel monitoring to detect activity increases or infra-red sensors just above the level of the cows' backs to detect mounting behaviour. Neither has yet been exploited commercially.

Oestrous pheromone detection is not solely intraspecific. Interspecific tests have shown that dogs and rats can accurately detect the oestrous odours of cows, albeit not quite as successfully as the bull, who can olfactorily detect the onset of pro-oestrus. Direct chemical detection would avoid the need for expensive animal training, but oestrous odours are unfortunately a complex array of volatile compounds which cannot yet be automatically detected.

The most commonly used aids for detection of oestrous behaviour are those that are fixed to the tailhead of cows and respond to the pressure of the mounting cows. One device incorporates a small phial of red dye inside a larger plastic container. On pressure from the mounting cow the inner phial breaks to release dye into the larger container, a change which can be detected visually by the herdsperson. Alternatives include pressure-sensitive pads that record the time of mounting (Dohi *et al.*, 1993), and a small paint strip placed on the tail-head, which becomes abraded by the rubbing of the mounting cow. Both methods are subject to a high degree of false positives as cows may rub against cubicles or other inanimate objects or be subject to mounting attempts when in dioestrus. The former device also may be subject to a high loss rate, especially in spring when the cows moult. Such methods are only useful therefore as a complement to the herdsperson's observation.

Teaser cattle can also be used to detect oestrus, and they can be raddled with a pigmented marker on the brisket or chin. Teasers are usually either castrated or vasectomised bulls or testosterone-treated females. Nymphomaniac cows can also be used but they are unreliable and may become exhausted. False positives are common as cows may not be exhibiting the immobilisation response when they are mounted. Teaser bulls have the advantage that they will accelerate and synchronise the post-partum return to oestrus, but they are expensive to prepare and maintain, and they also present a danger on the farm. They may suffer reduced libido or develop a 'harem' of favourite cows (Schofield, 1988). Teasers are, however, useful if there is a problem in identifying oestrus, particularly in hot climates where it often occurs undetected at night.

Other methods of detecting oestrus automatically rely principally on the physiological changes accompanying oestrus. These include the progesterone concentration in milk (or blood in the case of nulliparous heifers), cervical mucus conductivity and body or milk temperature changes.

Anomalous oestrous behaviour

Ovarian malfunction may cause oestrous behaviour to be absent (anoestrus) or persistent (nymphomania). Ovarian cysts cause both, in the approximate ratio 75:25. Anoestrus, or the absence of oestrous behaviour, is usually anovulatory in the case of cysts, or ovulatory (silent heat), when it may be due to inadequate progesterone secretion. Silent heats mainly occur during the first ovulation post-partum, after which progesterone secretion by the corpus luteum allows the expression of oestrous behaviour. Silent heats are often confused with reduced oestrous intensity, which can be caused by high milk yield, inadequate nutrition, an adverse environment or most commonly inadequate observation by the herdsperson. Nymphomaniac cows generally adopt bull-like behaviour, with pawing of the ground, deep vocalisation at low frequency and excessive mounting. They rarely stand to be mounted themselves.

Sexuality in the male

The degree of motivation for sexual interaction is usually referred to as libido in the male, which together with courtship, copulatory ability and semen quality forms an important element in reproductive fitness. This is particularly true for cattle where the majority of cows are mated by just the dominant male, in which case the libido of the males may determine their motivation to achieve this dominant status.

Unlike female cattle, bulls do not exhibit cyclicity in reproductive fitness, and there is even little evidence of a relationship between libido and conception rate of different bulls. In high libido bulls the volume of each ejaculate is reduced owing to an increased mating frequency (Lang *et al.*, 1988), but conception rate is not affected (Makarechian & Berg, 1988).

Male libido can be classified according to the following categories (modified from Hafez *et al.*, 1969):

(1) Avoidance of or disinterest in an oestrous cow
(2) No apparent interest in an oestrous cow other than standing near her or following her

(3) Licking the vulval regions of an oestrous cow, but failure to mount her
(4) Attempted but unsuccessful mounting
(5) Successful mounting but without ejaculation
(6) Successful mounting with ejaculation.

Tests based on serving capacity are usually preferred to subjective assessments of this type. Unfortunately, the procedures for testing serving capacity have not been standardised so that results are not directly comparable. Normally one or more tests are conducted that determine the bull's rate of successful mounting (with ejaculation) over a certain time period, often about ten minutes but sometimes up to 40 minutes. This test can be conducted in a pen using restrained cows that are not in oestrus or synchronised or unrestrained cows, which is more realistic but costly to run. The correlation between different types of tests is high (Crichton & Lishman, 1989), but in some tests, for example those conducted at pasture, the bull's mating activity is influenced by environmental factors as well as his libido.

Other less common measures of libido include the number of successful mountings until the bull becomes exhausted, the time taken to first ejaculation, the inter-ejaculation interval and the proportion of failures to mount or ejaculate. In all the tests the importance of bull stimulation is of paramount importance. Bulls work better in pairs, since one stimulates the other. Bulls about to be tested may be brought within sight or sound of the activity in the testing pen, in which case the first animal to be tested that was not stimulated by another bull must be retested at a later date.

Male sexual behaviour

The bull initially exchanges signals with the cow to obtain confirmation that both animals intend to proceed to copulation. Since the cow is in oestrus only periodically but the bull is always prepared for copulation, it is he who shows the greater seeking and testing behaviour, with the cow delivering most of the responses.

In the first instance the bull may be attracted to an oestrous cow by the latter being ridden by another cow or calling in a loud, high-pitched manner. These 'broadcast' stimuli are produced by the cow in the absence of a mate and are largely visual or auditory. Confirmation occurs as the bull receives the olfactory, gustatory and tactile stimuli at close quarters. Olfactory signals are provided in the pheromones produced by the sweat glands in the flanks and also in the cow's urine. Flehman or lipcurl is a common response by the bull on receiving these odours. The importance of this is probably largely in sexual arousal, as well as detection of oestrous cows. Soon after flehman occurs, blood serum concentrations of testosterone and luteinising hormone increase, both of which are associated with the ejaculatory response in the male (Lunstra *et al.*, 1989). Flehman is exhibited primarily in response to urine sampling (Houpt *et al.*, 1989) and the secretions of the perineal skin glands (Blazquez *et al.*, 1988). It lasts for about five seconds and is performed perhaps two to three times a day by the bull. Occasionally a cow will exhibit flehman in response to a bull's urine.

A bull will also perform flehman in response to another bull, and it has been suggested that this constitutes part of an appeasement ceremony (Kilgour, 1985). The interaction between libido and social status in the bull has not been fully investigated, but it is possible that high-libido bulls are more dominant and produce more pheromones to stimulate a flehman response by a subordinate bull.

During oestrus cows increase their urination frequency so that the bull can sample both the odours and the taste (Fig. 11.12). The bull also sniffs and licks the anovaginal area frequently (Fig. 11.13). Visual signals are provided by the close alignment of the bull and cow, often with the bull just behind the cow in a position where he can control her movements. This positioning also precedes mounting, and during pro-oestrus several intention mounts (where the front legs are lifted off the ground) and half mounts may be attempted, although the cow will not stand to receive these, and will escape by moving forwards. The bull tests for a rigid back (lordosis) by resting his chin on the cow's back, just behind the tail-head, and rubbing it back and forth. These identification and synchronisation exchanges all take place during pro-oestrus. Once a bull has identified a cow in this stage he 'guards' her for up to two days, keeping close contact and reinforcing the stimuli exchange. Direct ovulatory stimuli may be provided by the bull nosing the cow's perineum.

Finally, as the cow enters true oestrus, coition occurs. This is usually immediately preceded by vulval stimulation. Alignment follows and the bull raises his fore legs off the ground and lifts his brisket onto the cow's tail-head. Clasping the cow just in front of the pelvis the bull contracts his abdomen, bringing the

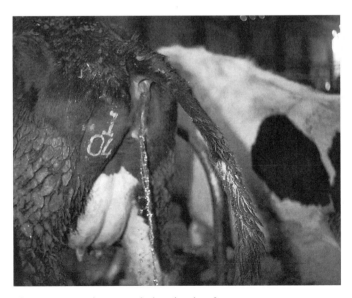

Fig. 11.12 Oestrous cows increase their urination frequency.

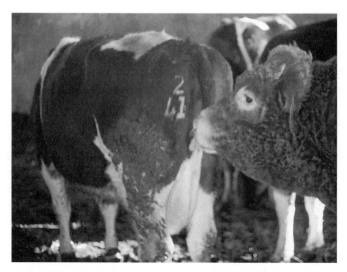

Fig. 11.13   The bull is attracted to the anovaginal area of an oestrous cow.

protruding penis near the vaginal orifice. Once penetration has been achieved, further abdominal contraction by the bull and vulval contraction by the cow achieve maximum penetration. Ejaculation of the semen follows quickly afterwards, accompanied by spinal rigidity in the bull and a strong abdominal contraction, the force of which may cause the bull's hind legs to leave the ground. Penile sensitivity is increased at this time, indicating that a hedonistic experience occurs.

Following ejaculation the bull quickly dismounts, drawing his chin over the cow's back as he does so. Attaching a crayon to the chin of a teaser bull (chinball marker) will thus mark a cow that has been mated. There follows a refractory period when the bull rests, until interest in the cow may be resumed. This refractory period varies from one to 20 minutes, depending largely on the bull himself. The coitus itself typically lasts for just two minutes, although some bulls will take longer. Most oestrous cows are served about five times by the bull, with a range of three to ten times (Chenoweth, 1983). Active breeding bulls can achieve an average of 20 services per day if stimulation is sufficient.

Animal factors affecting male sexual behaviour

Genotype strongly influences male libido, which has been reported as having a heritability of 0.6 (Blockey *et al.*, 1978). Bulls with low libido tend to have a reduced ratio of testosterone to oestradiol in the blood (Henney *et al.*, 1990). In general, dairy bulls have a greater libido than beef bulls, owing to greater selection by man. Older cattle have a higher libido than young cattle, provided that they are in good health and in particular that their feet are sound. They often develop arthritis, but this does not usually severely affect libido or mating performance (Fischerleitner & Stanek, 1987). Unlike many mammals, bulls are not inhibited from expressing their libido by the presence of humans or other animals. They do not prefer nocturnal mating (Crichton & Lishman, 1989), and this lack of inhibition may have been one factor favouring their domestication.

Bulls have a considerable serving capacity, which is immortalised in many legends, but it is usually assuaged by loss of interest in the cow. Their interest can, however, be maintained by the availability of new potential partners. Promiscuity of this type would clearly be well favoured by natural selection. Bulls used for artificial insemination are stimulated by minor changes in the environment. With relative ease bulls can be persuaded to mount dummy 'cows' that bear little relationship to the real thing. The sexual appetite of bulls was particularly revered by ancient civilisations, notably the Egyptians, for whom the bull was not just a domestic animal but a symbol of fertility. The high potential serving capacity of the bull is due to the seasonal breeding and polygynous mating patterns of cattle, both of which favour males with high serving capacity.

For the bull the key stimulus for mating activity is an inverted ∪, presented by the hindquarters of an oestrous female in a rigid stance when viewed from behind. A dummy 'cow' must be of the correct height (and strength) and must be immobile. Older bulls are more fastidious and prefer teaser cattle, ideally female, to dummies. Sexual preparation (prolonged stimulation) is important as it maximises the number of spermatozoa per ejaculate but is less effective in beef than dairy bulls. False mounts and delaying the ejaculation are methods of achieving this. Current recommendations for preparation of dairy bulls are one false mount, two minutes of restraint and two additional false mounts before ejaculation, and for beef bulls three false mounts before the first ejaculation and none before the second (Chenoweth, 1983). Beef bulls, therefore, not only have a lower libido than dairy bulls, but they also respond less to sexual preparation.

Masturbation occurs in both mixed and single sex groups of bulls and is more common in intensive rearing systems (MacFarlane, 1974). It is achieved by the bull repeatedly extending and retracting the penis through its preputial sheath and is more common when bulls are undisturbed, especially in early morning and late afternoon (Houpt & Wollney, 1989). It is stimulated by high protein diets. Only accessory gland fluids, not spermatozoa, are ejaculated, so that the concentration of spermatozoa in artificially collected ejaculates is increased. Masturbation does not confer any reproductive disadvantage on the bull and may serve to maintain reproductive fitness during periods when the male libido is not satiated by receptive females.

Parturient behaviour

Parturition and post-partum behaviour are critical stages in the bovine reproductive cycle (Fig. 11.14). It involves separation of the calf from its physical connection to the cow, and an increased risk of cow and calf mortality. In domestic cattle, there are risks of prepartum damage to the fetus, of difficulties in

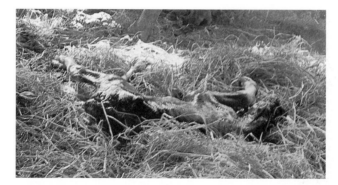

The expelled calf remains
recumbent for 15–30 minutes.

Vigorous nosing and licking by the cow encourages
activity by the calf.

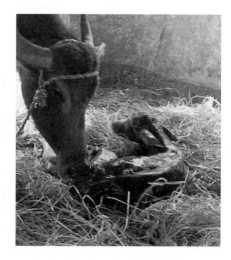

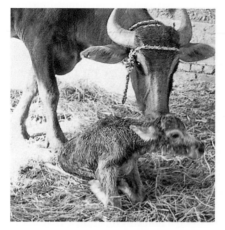

First attempts at standing
are aided by the cow.

Fig. 11.14   Post-partum behaviour in a buffalo calf (courtesy of M. Youssef).

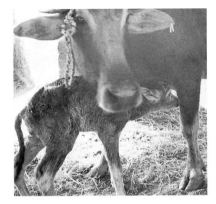

Teat-seeking behaviour. The calf is attracted to the junction of the legs and the body. This time the calf directs its search to the wrong end.

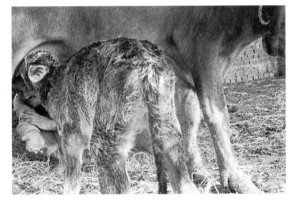

The herdsperson offers assistance by directing the calf's head to the teats.

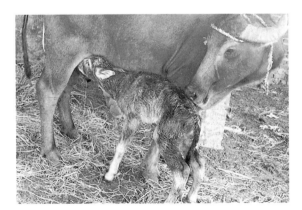

Further assistance is given by expressing milk from the teat. The cow sniffs the rear end of the calf.

Fig. 11.14 *Continued.* Post-partum behaviour in a buffalo calf.

expelling the fetus through the pelvic girdle, of failure of the calf to maintain its immune status by ingestion of colostrum post-partum, and of another cow stealing the calf. In feral cattle there is the added danger of predation of the neonate, which is highly vulnerable until it is mobile.

Early signs of impending parturition can be detected up to six weeks prepartum, when cows avoid aggressive interaction with other cattle to protect the fetus. This continues for a month or so and the cow is increasingly reluctant to engage in social encounters. She may even feed by herself or at the edge of a grazing herd. Then one to two weeks before parturition there is an increase in restlessness which intensifies in the last few days. This includes regular looking and turning around, calling, licking and pawing the bedding material, tail waving, frequent alternation of lying and standing, and interrupted eating patterns (Metz & Metz, 1987). At the same time there are morphological changes such as swelling of the udder and vulva and relaxation of the pelvic ligaments.

Finally the cow enters *stage one* of the parturition, which is characterised by cervical dilation and ends in the breaking of the waterbag and (in a normal presentation) the appearance of the calf's hooves. During this first stage tail raising and waving is common and usually occurs for at least two minutes each time (Schilling & Hartwig, 1984). The first stage normally extends to just over two hours (Table 11.2), but in primiparous cows needing help during calf expulsion it is considerably longer. This is probably because they are more likely to experience difficulties in expelling their calf through the pelvic girdle, whereas older cows are more likely to require help for other reasons, such as malpresentation or premature exhaustion.

Stage two of parturition – expulsion of the calf – normally takes about one hour. Initially the cow may be standing but she normally lies down to expel the head and shoulders. Usually she is laterally recumbent (on her side) and the two top legs are in the air. If the cow is frequently disturbed she often stands, and this can delay the labour. Uterine contractions during the second stage occur at regular intervals, usually every 15 to 20 minutes. Coinciding with these is a strong

Table 11.2   Duration of stages (minutes) of parturition in cows and heifers, with and without help. Obstetric help was provided from 70 minutes after rupture of the amnion

	Stage one (preparatory stage)	Stage two (calf expulsion)	Stage three (placental expulsion)
Multiparous cows			
Without help	146	64	270
With help	142	81	380
Primiparous cows			
Without help	131	61	324
With help	231	96	

From Schilling and Hartwig (1984).

abdominal straining to contract the diaphragm behind the calf and force it through the birth canal. The expulsion of the head is a critical point, and once this is accomplished the trunk follows quite quickly.

The timing of the second stage is important because the herdsperson usually prefers cows to calve during the day. The timing of parturition occurs naturally at random throughout the 24 hours of the day, however cows are able to avoid milking times (Edwards, 1979). Late evening feeding increases the number of night births (Yarney *et al.*, 1979), probably because the disturbance to the cows causes an increased risk of the waterbag breaking. At the end of stage two when the calf has been expelled, the cow usually stands up and licks her calf. Vocalisation by both cow and calf helps the two to bond. The cow may spend one and a half hours grooming the calf, and it is in the first few hours after birth that the calf is imprinted onto the cow. Normally the calf remains passive for the first half hour, but then attempts to stand, often aided by the vigorous nosing of the cow.

If the delivery has been difficult the calf may be anoxic and lethargic and may also suffer from neonatal acidosis. The cow attempts to overcome this by increased licking of the calf (Metz & Metz, 1987). If the cow herself is exhausted this will often by done in the lying position. In common with many prey animals, cattle are precocious so that they can reduce the predation of juveniles. Once the calf has stood, it starts to search for an inverted right angle. This it usually finds in the union of the cow's trunk and her leg, and this directs it to the udder. It is not necessarily the hind leg that the calf finds, but the cow positions her body alongside that of the calf and pointing in the opposite direction so that the calf is directed to the rear end. If the cow has a large, pendulous udder it may take the calf about 40 minutes to find the teat and obtain milk, i.e. about twice as long as normal. Also, if the delivery has been difficult, the time taken by the calf to stand and find the teat is considerably lengthened (Table 11.3). Assistance by the herdsperson has little detrimental effect. Some cows are not good mothers and may either show aggression to the calf or pay it little attention, which may be due to the effect of the cow's own rearing environment or her own maternal instinct (Donaldson, 1970).

Table 11.3 Duration of time intervals (minutes post-partum) between birth and the start of various activities in calves whose mothers received varying degrees of assistance during delivery

	Without help	With help from herdsperson	Difficult delivery
First attempt to stand up	13	16	29
First stood up	45	50	164
First looking for udder	65	62	>240
First suckling	116	131	>240

Supervision by a veterinarian required because either hooves did not appear at the end of stage one or traction by the herdsperson was not sufficient to allow the cow to expel the calf (Metz & Metz, 1987).

The final stage *(stage three)* of parturition is the passing of the placenta, generally four to six hours post-partum. The cow usually eats this, as well as the bedding contaminated with fetal and placental fluids. Calves in the wild are usually hidden, rather than following their dam as lambs do. In 'hider' species the dam eats the placenta to remove any traces of the birth that might attract predators, whereas in 'follower' species she usually does not.

Chapter 12
Locomotion and movement

Locomotion

Locomotion refers to a voluntary movement which displaces the whole body. This is usually confined to walking, trotting and galloping in cattle, but they can also jump, swim and canter. Other limb movements such as kicking or pawing are performed but do not involve whole body movement.

Locomotion in cattle and indeed all ungulates is primarily by forward motion. Sideways and backward motion *can* be performed but the muscles are designed for forward propulsion, and any other motion is much less efficient. During forward motion the centre of gravity is moved towards the front limb by the propulsive efforts of the hind limb, and the front limb is raised and repositioned to maintain the animal's balance. The positioning of the limbs may be in either a symmetrical or an asymmetrical pattern and the animal may be supported by three, two, one or no limbs at any particular time. The faster the gait, the fewer the supporting limbs (Alexander, 1987).

Cattle can only *walk* backwards, and they will do this when confronted with an obstacle in a narrow passageway, such as a race. The same stepping pattern is used as in forward motion and the head held high to place the centre of gravity as far back as possible.

Cattle change their gait according to their velocity requirements. There is a velocity above which it is energetically more efficient to trot than walk and another where galloping is preferable to trotting.

Walking

Walking is defined as a gait where each hoof is on the ground for at least 50% of the stride. The order of hoof movement is shown in Fig. 12.1. Each limb is lifted by shortening the leg through flexion of the joints, using especially the hip, knee, hock and digital flexor muscles. The limb then enters the swing phase (Fig. 12.2) and is placed on the ground through slow extension of the joint. Once the limb is on the ground, it checks and supports the load by tensing all the extensor muscles, particularly in the digital, hock and stifle regions (Nickel *et al.*, 1986). The sole is then pushed hard against the ground by contracting the digital flexors,

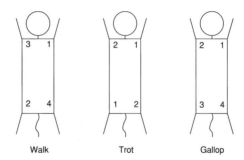

Walk   Trot   Gallop

Fig. 12.1 Sequence of limb movements in the walk, trot and gallop (Alexander, 1987).

thus enabling the pushing phase to begin, followed by the hanging limb and swing phases. The limb motion is therefore a cyclical, not an intermittent, process.

The walk in cattle can be considered as two people walking out of phase, one behind the other, so that four distinct sounds of the hooves contacting the floor are heard (Fig. 12.3). As the walking speed increases, efficiency decreases as the thrust phase (when the limb is supporting) is reduced at the expense of the hanging limb phase (Fig. 12.2). The major thrust is provided by the hind legs. The fore limbs, although supporting about 55 to 60% of the load of the animal, act mainly to position the limbs, enabling them to act as support agents and steer the load.

During turning the limbs on the outside of the turning circle are abducted or rotated outwards and those on the inside are adducted or rotated inwards (Fig. 12.4), resulting in a change in direction. The main pivots for the fore and hind limbs are the shoulder and hip, respectively. All limb movements contain an accelerative and a decelerative force. During turning the outer limbs increase their accelerative force while the inner limbs increase their decelerative force.

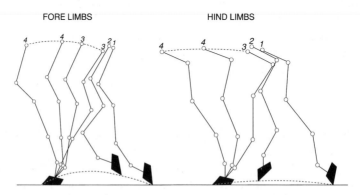

FORE LIMBS   HIND LIMBS

Fig. 12.2 Movements of the fore and hind limb during walking: 1, lifting, 2, swinging; 3, supporting; 4, thrusting. 1 and 2, Hanging limb period; 3 and 4, supporting limb period.

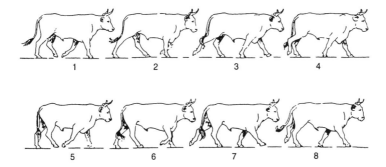

Fig. 12.3 Normal walk of cattle (Nickel *et al.*, 1986).

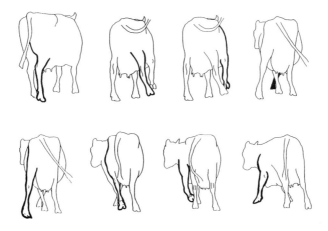

Fig. 12.4 Abduction of the outer limb (top) and adduction of the inner limb (bottom) during turning (Nickel *et al.*, 1986).

Some abduction and adduction occur during straight walking, but less in a young cow or a well-bred one than an old one (Fig. 12.5).

Walking behaviour changes with the degree of confidence that cattle have. If the floor is slippery or the building is poorly lit, cattle shorten their stride and slow down the rate of walking.

Trotting

The trot is used by many quadrupeds for long-distance motion where a faster gait than the walk is required. It is a symmetrical gait providing an even motion (Fig. 12.6). For this reason it is used frequently by cows with full udders, the pendulous nature of which makes the cow reluctant to increase her speed to that of a gallop. When stimulated to move quickly over long periods, as, for example, if a herdsman hurries a cow down a track for milking, she will trot, as this provides

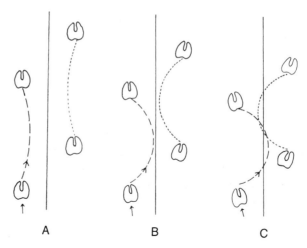

Fig. 12.5 Adduction path of the hindlimbs of: (A) a young non-lactating heifer; (B) a well-bred pedigree milking cow; (C) an old cow with poor breeding.

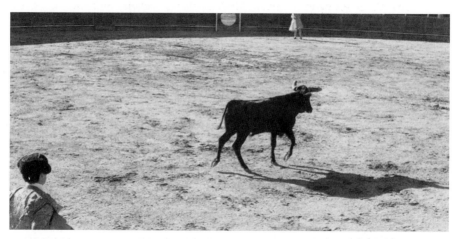

Fig. 12.6 The trot in a fighting bull. A symmetrical gait with diagonally opposite limbs used synchronously.

a fast, even motion so that the forces on the udder can be absorbed in a rhythmical swinging motion. In the trot, diagonally opposite limbs are used synchronously: left hind and right front are followed by right hind and left front. In a fast trot there is a period between limb changes when there are no limbs in contact with the ground.

Galloping

The gallop is the fastest gait and involves an asymmetrical step pattern and a lengthened free-gliding phase. Unlike in smaller mammals, the back in cattle does not contribute to the propulsive force, this being provided mainly by the hind limbs. In the gallop there is a leading front limb, followed by the other front limb, then a pause after which the two hind limbs are placed on the ground, one fractionally before the other.

Motivation for locomotion

Cattle are motivated to move in response to demand for food, water, companionship, shelter, grooming, a sexual partner, space and many other resources (Zeeb, 1983). This motivation increases with the duration and severity of resource restriction, especially of space (Dellmeier *et al.*, 1990), and is influenced by many factors, both genotypic and environmental (Fig. 12.7).

As animals whose progenitors roamed extensively in search of good grazing, today's cattle need exercise to keep healthy and productive. Regular exercise in the form supervised walking for tethered cattle will increase muscle and bone growth in growing animals (Melizi, 1985), prevent limb disorders, especially arthritis in bulls for semen collection, and also improve semen quality in bulls (Vetoshkira, 1985; Zaitser, 1985; Tizol *et al.*, 1987). Recommended allowances are for about one hour walking per day at about 3 to 4 km/hour. This recommendation, coupled with the observations that cows in a cubicle house walk for 2 to 4 km/day (Schofield *et al.*, 1991), suggests that cattle need to walk at least 3 km every day.

Range conditions in Africa may necessitate long-distance walks to water every two or three days. Such travel, which can be for up to 40 km, reduces feed intake and milk production (Homewood *et al.*, 1987; Nicholson, 1989).

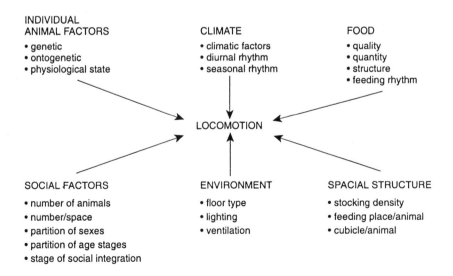

Fig. 12.7 Factors influencing cattle locomotion (Zeeb *et al.*, 1983).

Effects of the environment on locomotion

The environmental features with the greatest effect on cattle locomotion are the spatial structure and the type of accommodation, including lying and walking areas. These environmental effects undoubtedly interact with each other, and the animal's perception of the environment is modified by its experience.

Space availability

In both housed and grazing cattle the available space is one of the main determinants of locomotion. In the grazing situation an increase in area and reduction in food availability force cattle to walk further to search for food. Cattle on rangeland conditions in the Camargue have been recorded as walking three times as far as cattle on intensively managed pasture (Zeeb, 1983). In intensive grazing the cows only spend a small amount of time each day in between grazing bouts searching for new areas to graze, perhaps 10 to 20 minutes.

Increases in locomotion can be caused by external parasites such as flies (Hayakawa *et al.*, 1984) or bats (Delpietro, 1989), which interrupt grazing activity. This encourages cattle to move about and search for open, windy areas where they can lose the attention of the parasites, which normally attack when the cattle are stationary, especially lying down. An important consequence of excessive treading activity by cattle on poorly drained and clay soils is the loss of soil stability and eventual poaching damage (Schofield & Hall, 1986) (Fig. 12.8).

With housed cattle the provision of adequate space for locomotion is a complex issue. Although a considerable proportion of locomotion is still associated with feeding, and milking in the case of the dairy cow, a significant amount is

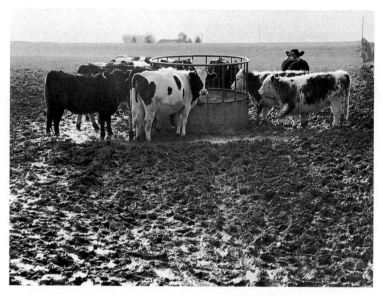

Fig. 12.8   Excessive locomotion can result in loss of soil stability and poaching.

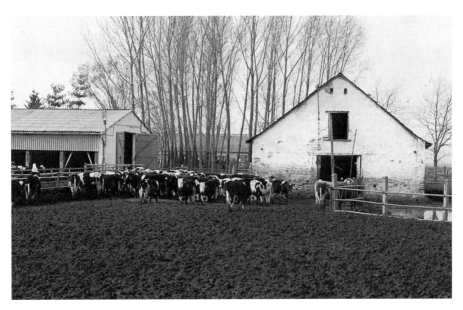

Fig. 12.9   Cow accommodation with exercise area.

associated with social and other activities. This is because cattle eating conserved food spend less time eating than grazing cattle, they are stationary while they eat, and the greater stocking density in a building than at pasture encourages more social interaction, especially grooming.

In a cubicle house for dairy cows the space for walking is provided in the passageways between cubicles, in the feeding passage and sometimes in a separate exercise area (Fig. 12.9). If the amount of space provided for locomotion is decreased below 4 to 5 m^2/cow, it is likely that locomotory activity will initially increase for a few days because of aggression caused by competition for space. In the long term, however, locomotion decreases owing to the restriction in space availability (Figs 12.10 and 12.11). If an insufficient number of cubicles are provided for lying, locomotion increases, particularly in subordinate cows.

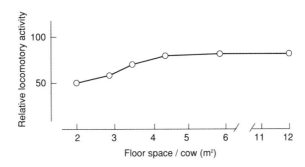

Fig. 12.10   Locomotion changes in relation to space availability (Zeeb, 1983).

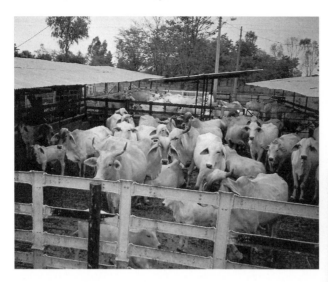

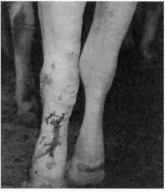

Fig. 12.11 Overcrowded cattle show reduced locomotion (above) and injuries to the limbs are common (below).

Floors

The floor is the most important part of the cattle house in its influence on cattle locomotion. Floor properties that influence locomotion include friction, which determines the slipperiness of the floor; hardness, which determines the loading on the limb; and the surface profile, which determines the stress loading on the hoof, as well as interacting with frictional properties of the floor.

Friction can be measured as the force required to start the motion of a cow's hoof across the floor (static friction) or that required to maintain this motion (sliding friction). There are both horizontal and vertical components to this force and the ratio is known as the coefficient of friction. The number of slip movements by the leg increases rapidly when the coefficient of static friction decreases below 0.4 (Fig. 12.12), but if the coefficient is above 0.5, cattle lying on the floor, as in tie stalls, may show injuries to the legs through hairless patches, swellings and wounds. There is probably therefore an optimum coefficient of friction of 0.4 to 0.5 (Phillips & Morris, 2001).

For loose housing systems where minimising slip is the main concern, the minimum coefficient of friction depends on the surface profile. For solid floors it should be at least 0.4, for slatted floors 0.35 and for perforated floors 0.25 (Irps, 1983). The frictional properties of a solid floor may be improved by cutting grooves in a squared pattern with 4 cm sides (Dumelow & Albutt, 1990). This

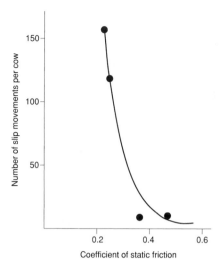

Fig. 12.12 Effect of coefficient of static friction on the number of slip movements of four cows during four eating periods (Webb & Nilsson, 1983).

disrupts the floor profile and gives the cow's hoof a greater vertical area against which it can apply pressure during the pushing phase of each stride. Also, the repeated passage of cows over a solid floor wears away the deformations in the floor profile created by initial tamping or grooving. Slips in excess of 500 mm are common on slurry-covered smooth concrete, especially during mounting behaviour (Mitchell, 1974). During the slip the hooves, especially in the front feet, turn outwards from the direction of travel.

Comparing different floor surfaces shows that soil is the most slip resistant, that a covering of slurry increases slip by 56% and that tamping increases slip resistance more than grooving (Table 12.1). On slippery floors cows modify their behaviour to reduce the incidence of slipping. They reduce their speed of

Table 12.1 Slip distances for back feet on different floor surfaces, either dry or covered with slurry

Surface	Slip (mm)
Dry	
Sandy soil	21
Tamped concrete	29
Steel float concrete	36
Steel flat concrete	41
Slurry covered	
Tamped concrete	40
Grooved concrete	54
Steel float concrete	81

From Albutt *et al.* (1990).

walking and reduce the angles of extension of the limbs to the floor (Phillips, 1990a, b), taking rapid, short steps (Phillips & Morris, 2001). Cattle can recognise differences in slipperiness in floors that humans have difficulty recognising (Phillips & Morris, 2002). Slip is most likely when the hoof first touches or leaves the floor and the vertical loading is least. The further the hoof is placed in front of or behind the centre of the stride, the less the vertical force and the greater the chance of slip. Hence stride length is reduced as the animal attempts to compensate for the floor conditions. The presence of slurry on the floor makes cows keep their legs more vertical at the end of the support phase to aid lifting the limb out of the slurry (Phillips & Morris, 2000). There is reduced risk of slip in deep slurry so cows place their fore limbs on the floor less vertically at the start of the support phase. Deep slurry reduces walking speed and may have adverse effects on the welfare of cattle. Cattle show strong avoidance of slurry in passageways when they spend most of the day at pasture, but if they are permanently in a building with slurry, they habituate to its presence (Phillips *et al.*, 2001; Phillips & Morris, 2002).

Slatted floors present a severe obstacle to normal cattle locomotion (Kirchner & Boxberger, 1987). Cattle cannot avoid the slots but their claws often slip into them, causing contusion of the sole and exungulation. To avoid excessive pressure on the sole, slot width should not exceed 25 to 30 mm and to prevent faeces building up on the slats each slat should not exceed 80 mm in width. Slats also cause cattle to slip more often and they alter their locomotion posture, orientating their heads more towards the floor (Sommer, 1985).

Light

Light is very important in determining the perception of the environment by cattle, which are by nature crepuscular. There is a pronounced diurnal rhythm of locomotion (Fig. 12.13), with greater activity during daylight hours, especially at sunrise and sunset if the cattle have peak grazing activity at this time or are mov-

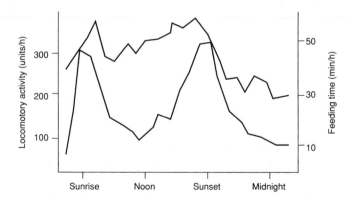

Fig. 12.13 Diurnal rhythm of locomotion (top line) and feeding time (bottom line) in Camargue cattle (Zeeb, 1983).

ing to or from their night resting area. Housed cattle show more activity at night than grazing cattle (Fig. 12.14), and reductions in locomotion have been recorded when a short winter daylength is supplemented with artificial light (Phillips & Schofield, 1989). This may be because aggression between cows is reduced, since unexpected encounters are rare when the house is lit, but common in the dark. Cattle show strong avoidance of dark passageways in cubicle houses (Phillips & Morris, 2001) and take short, rapid steps to maintain stability (Phillips *et al.*, 2000). The optimum light intensity is probably between 40 and 120 lux (Phillips *et al.*, 2000). In less hostile environments for cattle than a highly stocked cubicle house, for example at pasture or in a strawed yard, there is little effect of supplementary light on activity levels. Most cattle seem to prefer a daylength of about 16 hours and naturally have a quiescent period in the early hours of the morning.

Animal factors and locomotion

Younger cattle, particularly calves at play, are more likely to indulge in the faster forms of locomotion like gambolling and galloping than mature cows, who have little time for such activities and may be hindered from fast movement by the presence of a large udder. Bulls at pasture tend to be more active than cows, especially at night, perhaps because of reduced risk of predators. There is some evidence that hill breeds, such as French Salers cattle, are more active than

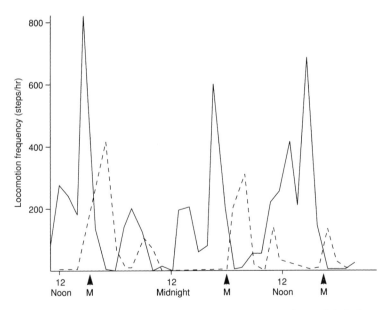

Fig. 12.14 Locomotion frequencies of two dairy cows, one active mainly before milking (——) and one active mainly after milking (– – –), measured with an electronic pedometer (Phillips & Owen, unpublished results).

lowland cattle like the Friesian (Veissier *et al.*, 1989). The introduction of new cattle into a stable group causes increases in activity connected with aggression as the dominance order is sorted out. For instance, the proportion of time spent walking increased from 4% to 6% for three days when ten cows were introduced to a stable group of 50 in a cubicle house (Botto & Zimmermann, 1986).

The oestrous state of cows has a major influence on locomotion, which is typically increased by a factor of three to four on the day of oestrus (see Chapter 11). Increased locomotion is also observed just before parturition, whereas it will often decrease after both oestrus and parturition.

Locomotion for draught power

A specialised requirement involving cattle locomotion is for draught power, where the cattle not only move not just themselves but also pull a trailed implement or wheeled vehicle (Fig. 12.15). Other common forms of work include carrying a load on their back or turning a turning a shaft connected to a power conversion unit, for example to raise water for irrigation (Fig. 12.16). The additional load created reduces the speed of locomotion, and cattle increase the thrusting period of the stride (Fig. 12.2) and reduce the hanging limb period. This also allows some of the energy normally used to decelerate the legs to be used for pulling the load. The load is transferred to the animal's shoulders by a collar or a yoke (Fig. 12.17), which may be for one or two animals. The energy cost of the work is related to the ground conditions, the gradient and the type of cattle used. A steady load is easier for cattle to manage than a varying one, and large cattle can counteract variation better than, for example, a donkey.

Cattle prefer to walk at between 0.6 and 1.0 m/s, and within this 'comfort zone' there is little change in the energetic efficiency of walking (Fig. 12.18). If the load

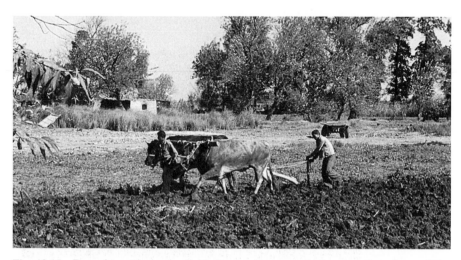

Fig. 12.15 Draught cattle in the field. During heavy work the thrusting phase of the stride is increased and the hanging limb period is reduced.

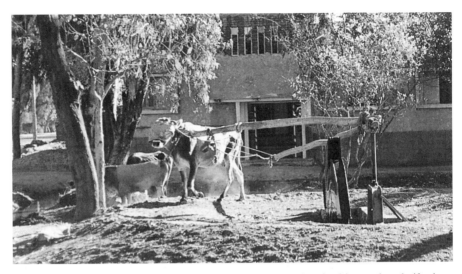

Fig. 12.16 Draught power is provided by regular locomotion, in this case by a heifer harnessed for raising irrigation water. Reducing sensory perception by applying blindfolds encourages compliance with the task.

is so heavy that the cattle have to pull it very slowly, they behave awkwardly. With heavy loads draught cattle have to use their back as well as their shoulders, and this reduces the energetic efficiency. Above 1 m/s the energetic efficiency of the work decreases (Lawrence & Stibbard, 1990). Saddles with loads are borne more efficiently if mounted on the animal's shoulders than its back, because the load is transferred directly to the ground through the front legs, rather than having to stress muscles to dissipate the load.

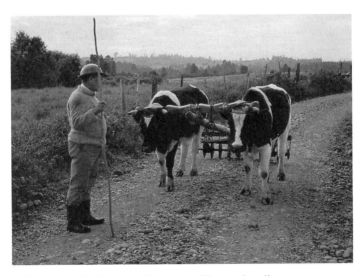

Fig. 12.17 Twin-yolked bullocks pulling a set of harrowing discs.

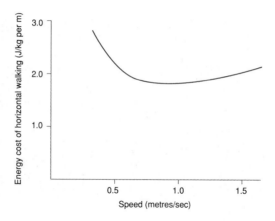

Fig. 12.18 Energy cost of horizontal walking at different speeds (Ribeiro *et al.*, 1977).

Lameness

Lameness is the clinical exhibition of an abnormality of the musculo-skeletal system in one or more limbs. This abnormality can arise from many different things: congenital defect, infectious or metabolic diseases, or trauma induced by environmental factors (Fig. 12.19). During lameness the supporting or swinging limb periods, or both, are shortened, so that the stride length is reduced. Reduction in the supporting limb period is most common with acutely painful lesions such as a sole abscess or chip fracture, as the pain is accentuated by pressure on the limb. Relief is gained also by reducing pressure on the diseased claw whilst standing (Fig. 12.20). When the swinging limb period is contracted this is often associated with increased abduction or adduction as the animals may attempt to decrease load bearing by a particular part of the hoof. Some unevenness of gait

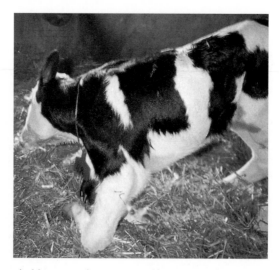

Fig. 12.19 Congenital lameness in a young calf.

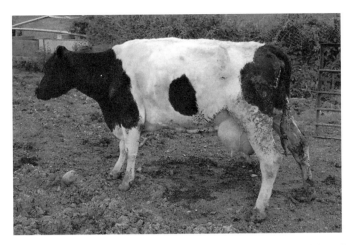

Fig. 12.20 Severe lameness in a dairy cow causes loss of body condition. In this case splaying the hind legs reduces pressure on the diseased outer claw.

is evident before and after each lameness incident, and in total the animal's gait may be affected for three months or more, with the animal being clinically lame on average for about eight weeks (Fig. 12.21) (Phillips, 1990a, b). A system of scoring cattle for the severity of lameness, based on the associated behavioural changes, has been devised by Manson and Leaver (Table 12.2). Alternatively, stride length may be measured in lameness research, but there are many sources of variation.

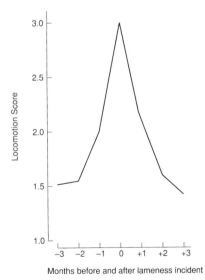

Months before and after lameness incident

Fig. 12.21 Change in locomotion score before and after a lameness incident. Locomotion score: 1, even gait with no observable adduction or abduction; 2, uneven gait but not lame; 3, lame (Phillips, 1990).

Table 12.2 Description of a locomotion scoring system

1.0	Minimal abduction/adduction, no unevenness of gait, no tenderness
1.5	Slight abduction/adduction, no unevenness or tenderness
2.0	Abduction/adduction present, uneven gait, perhaps tender
2.5	Abduction/adduction present, uneven gait, tenderness of feet
3.0	Slight lameness, not affecting behaviour
3.5	Obvious lameness, some difficulty in turning, not affecting behaviour pattern
4.0	Obvious lameness, difficulty in turning, behaviour pattern affected
4.5	Some difficulty in rising, difficulty in walking, behaviour pattern affected
5.0	Extreme difficulty in rising, difficulty in walking, adverse effects on behaviour pattern

From Manson and Leaver (1988).

Cattle are predisposed to lameness when walking and standing on wet concrete in cubicle houses (Mill & Ward, 1994). Concrete is a very hard surface that makes the hoof, and particularly the digital cushion, absorb much more force during walking than when the animal is on more natural, softer surfaces (Scott, 1989). It also becomes slippery when wet, and slipping is a regular cause of injury in cubicle-housed cows, as well as influencing the cows' behaviour (Mitchell, 1974).

The shape of the claw influences the lameness risk (Greenough, 1991), with steep claws and short toes conferring resistance. Most claw measurements have moderate to high heritabilities, but are not easily measured in the live animal (Hahn *et al.*, 1977; McDaniel *et al.*, 1984; Smit *et al.*, 1986, Andersen *et al.*, 1991). Visual scores of claw shape show little relationship with either actual measurements of claw shape or claw disorders and are also difficult to record repeatedly (Smit *et al.*, 1986; Murray *et al.*, 1994).

Large claw size could confer advantages of greater shock absorption. It has shown to be associated with a reduced risk of digital disorders in horses (Dyson, 1995) and it is highly heritable in cattle (Andersen *et al.*, 1991). It cannot be measured accurately on farms, but can be quite accurately predicted from hoof width at the top of the claw (Phillips *et al.*, 1996).

There are realistic possibilities of breeding animals that are more resistant to leg disorders, but measurement difficulties make this a distant goal.

Other forms of movement

Apart from locomotion, where the whole animal's body is moved, there are many other limb movements which have a variety of functions. Stretching is one such movement, which affects limb and other muscles. When cattle stretch they tense their muscles in the neck, back and limbs to maintain them in an active state and facilitate blood supply. Maintaining the muscle tone and exercising the joints is particularly necessary for the fetus since it cannot exercise its limbs by locomotion (Fraser, 1985).

Cattle also use their limbs, particularly the front ones, for manipulation in the same way that we use our hands. They will paw the ground to dig up earth and kick at objects. The limbs are also used to stand up and lie down and to change posture when standing or lying.

Behaviour during handling

Handling problems

Handling refers to the manipulation and movement of cattle by humans, which usually occurs for the purposes of slaughter, milking, restraint for veterinary work, movement to a different area of the farm on foot or movement in a vehicle to another farm, to market or to an abattoir. Because most cattle are not accustomed to being handled for these purposes, with the exception of milking, stress is likely to result unless the handling procedure is carried out with full regard for the animals' requirements for some continuity of nutritional, social and environmental resources. Their response to handling is highly likely to include abnormal behaviour, which can vary from the mild exhibition of stereotypies to acute distress and even death. Much can be done to improve the welfare of cattle during handling, both in refining the environmental and management practices during handling and in developing the handling skills of stock controllers, particularly those operating off the farm, who may have little relevant education or experience. This will have benefits of better labour efficiency and safety, better product quality (especially meat), and enhanced public perception of the cattle production industry.

Races, crowd pens and crushes

Cattle are put into a race either for one-by-one treatment such as drenching, or to move them single file into an area where they can be handled singly, as in a crush or dip. Although they move more easily in the race if it has solid sides, they will accustom to one with open sides, which should preferably be V-shaped to support the animal if they go down, and to discourage them from lying prostrate on the floor. Cattle prefer to move in a circular rather than a straight direction (Grandin, 1983), and if they are stressed, bunching may occur. Often an animal will then lie down, and it may be difficult to make it stand again.

In a crowd pen one side is angled at 30° to direct cattle to the entrance of a race. Crowd gates may be used behind the cattle to encourage them to move, but gates should not be electrified nor should electric goads be used or else bunching is likely to occur. Dogs are sometimes used in cattle handling and cause less stress than they do to sheep (Fig. 12.22). However, rushing cows down a lane with a dog is not a suitable preparation for milking.

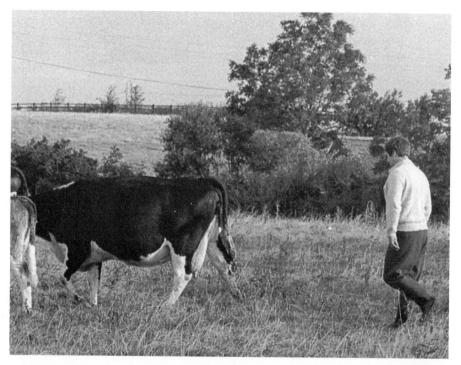

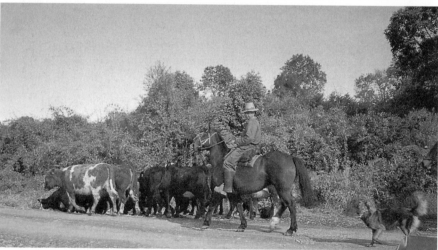

Fig. 12.22 Cattle movement on foot or with the aid of a horse and dog.

The ideal cattle crush has solid sides to make the animal feel secure, but frequently this is not possible as access is needed, for example to cows' hooves (Fig. 12.23). A winch or chain may be used to raise cows' hooves for trimming. A head restraint is useful and usually takes the form of two vertical bars which clamp around the animal's neck. For cattle that are not used to restraint this is not suf-

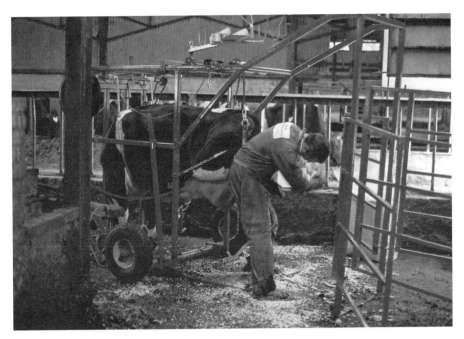

Fig. 12.23 An open crush with a winch to raise the hoof for trimming.

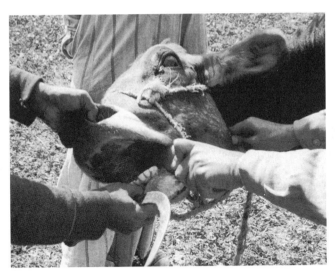

Fig. 12.24 Simple hand restraint by positioning the thumb and finger in the nasal orifices, in order to examine the teeth.

ficient, as vertical movement is still possible. Head restraint can also be achieved by holding the animal's nose with thumb and middle finger in the nostrils (Fig. 12.24). Bulls often have a permanent ring put in their nose so that they can be led. Other cattle may be led by training them to accept a halter.

Chapter 13
Resting Behaviour

Lying

Lying is important for recuperation and cattle demonstrate strong motivation for this behaviour (Metz, 1984). Symptoms of stress and physical exhaustion are evident when they are deprived of the ability to lie down (Munksgaard & Simonsen, 1996; Munksgaard et al., 1999). There is evidence of a link to production as cattle that lie down for longer grow faster (Mogensen et al., 1997a). Both the time spent lying (Haley et al., 2000) and the number of lying down attempts (Lidfors, 1989) could be included in a welfare index for cattle. Some practices, such as infrequent milking, reduce the comfort of cows while lying (Osterman & Redbo, 2001), and any welfare index should preferably be sufficiently sensitive to be able to detect small nuances in the behaviour, not just total lying time. Caution in the use of any index of lying should be exercised, since some factors contrary to welfare may increase lying time, e.g. diseases, in particular lameness (Singh et al., 1993), cold weather, owing to the need to minimise heat loss (Redbo et al., 1996), and possibly tethering (Munksgaard & Simonsen, 1995).

Lying is used for rest, predator avoidance and association. Predator avoidance is particularly evident in young calves, who like to hide in long grass (Langbein & Raasch, 2000). Some high-yielding dairy cows might need extra rest but actually spend less time lying because of the longer time required for feeding and ruminating (Venis et al., 1980; Fregonesi & Leaver, 2001). In these cows the amount of lying can increase as milk yield declines in mid to late lactation. The time spent lying is normally approximately 13 hours/day for calves (Weiguo & Phillips, 1991), 12 hours/day for bulls (Houpt & Wollney, 1989) and 7 to 10 hours/day for lactating dairy cows (in approximately five periods of 1.5 hours each) (Arave & Walters, 1980). However, lactating dairy cows may spend just five hours per day lying down if they are overcrowded (Leonard et al., 1996). It is difficult to determine the preferred lying time for cattle, since it is affected by many factors, but it is probably approximately ten hours per day.

Most adult cattle lie in the sternally recumbent position, that is, on the sternum or breast bone. Occasionally they will lie laterally recumbent (flat on their side), although this is not generally possible in cubicles because of restricted space. Prolonged lateral recumbency is prevented by the need to eructate gases

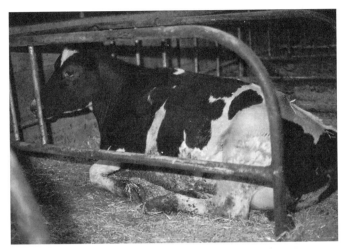

Fig. 13.1 The cubicle may prevent a cow from adopting a laterally recumbent position.

from the rumen at regular intervals (Fig. 13.1). Gravity plays an important part in reticulo-ruminal function and in releasing the gas bubble (normally present in the dorsal sac of the rumen) to the atmosphere via the oesophagus (Balch, 1955). Calves without a fully developed rumen often lie in the laterally recumbent position (Fig. 13.2). Mature beef cattle that are obese occasionally have difficulty in maintaining a sternally recumbent position and may roll over onto their side.

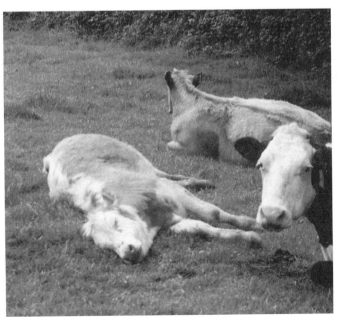

Fig. 13.2 The lateral recumbent position is most common in young, preruminant cattle.

Cubicles

A major change in the lying facilities offered to housed cows came with the introduction of the cubicle, or free stall. This is a solid bed raised off the floor, with partitions to create individual lying areas for the cows. If the cubicle bed is too small, which is common with the increasing size of the modern dairy cow, the cow will have difficulty lying down or getting up (Fig. 13.3). This leads to swellings on the carpal and tarsal joints and encourages cows to lie either half in the cubicle or in the passageway. Cows are more likely to accept cubicles if they have been trained as calves or heifers to accept small cubicles (Fig. 13.4).

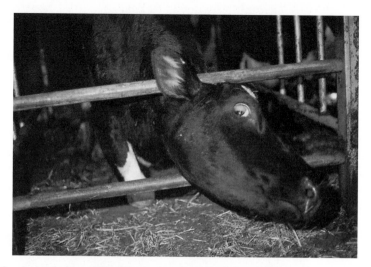

Fig. 13.3   A cow having difficulties in manoeuvring in a cubicle during rising, because of inadequate lunging space.

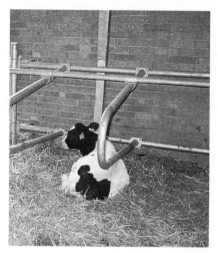

Fig. 13.4   A calf being trained to use small cubicles.

When a cow lies down in a cubicle she normally kneels down with one fore leg, then both, and then tucks one hind limb under her abdomen as she lowers her rear end (Fig. 13.5). The total process takes about 35 seconds, although it is twice as long in cows that are permanently tethered, owing to the poor condition of the limb joints (Gustafson & LundMagnussen, 1995). Thus when lying down, the cow eases her centre of gravity forwards along a longitudinal axis to minimise the stress on the limbs. Adequate space for forward motion is essential for cow comfort, both when lying down and when rising (Fig. 13.6). When rising, the cow first raises her forequarters slightly and then her hindquarters, using the outer hind leg primarily for vertical propulsion, then the inner hind leg that was tucked under, the fore leg on the same side and finally the outer front leg (Fig. 13.5).

Approximately one-third of cows show a clear preference for right- or left-side laterality, which is not shown by calves (Wilson *et al.*, 1999). Pregnant cows, especially those with twins, often prefer to lie on their left side, because the fetus

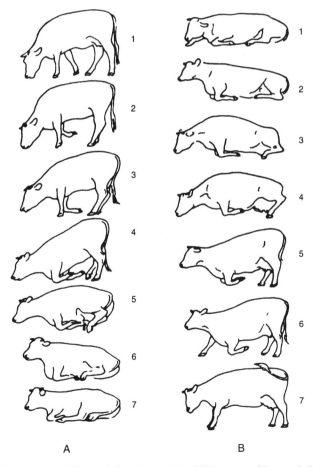

A   B

Fig. 13.5 The sequence of lying (A) and standing (B) in a cow (Fraser & Broom, 1990).

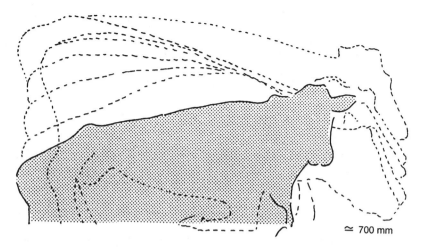

≃ 700 mm

Fig. 13.6 Forward space demand of the rising movement in a large Friesian cow (Cermak, 1987).

dwells in the right side of the abdominal cavity, at least in the latter stages of pregnancy (Bao & Giller, 1991). As cows get older they show less preference for left-side laterality, possibly because there is more room in the abdominal cavity and less chance of damage to the fetus by lying on the right side (Arave & Walters, 1980). If there is a sideways slope to the cubicle, cows prefer to lie with their dorsal side uphill. If a cubicle to one side is occupied, a cow prefers to lie with her back next to the back of the cow in the adjoining cubicle. If cubicles are positioned end to end with open fronts, as is sometimes advocated to allow adequate lunging space, cows may be reluctant to lie facing each other. Providing the cubicles are sufficiently large, cows prefer them to have a solid front, which may limit lunging space but gives greater comfort and a feeling of enclosed personal space.

There are many different types of cubicle divisions available (Fig. 13.7), all attempting effectively to separate the cows while minimising the hindrance to the cows' movements caused by the division (Fig. 13.8). A popular modern design that allows some space-sharing by virtue of the absence of a bottom rail at the back of the cubicle is the Dutch Comfort design. Cows prefer these cubicles to other designs, and this can even reduce lameness because they spend less time standing in slurry (Leonard *et al.*, 1994). If there is a bottom rail it should be about 50 cm from the cubicle base to avoid cows becoming trapped underneath. Front rails running perpendicular to the cubicle prevent the cow moving too far into it, preventing them from becoming trapped. They should be either near the floor (less than 25 cm from the floor) or fastened to the top rail, otherwise the rail will impede the cow from rising. In Dutch Comfort cubicles the front hoop should not be wider than 35 cm, otherwise small cows can get their shoulders stuck. There should always be some cubicles available that can accommodate the largest cows in the herd.

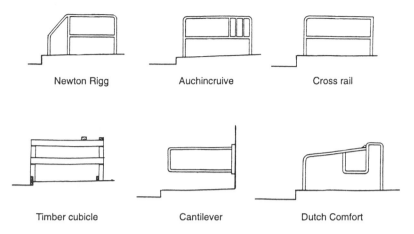

Newton Rigg   Auchincruive   Cross rail

Timber cubicle   Cantilever   Dutch Comfort

Fig. 13.7 Different designs of cubicle division for dairy cows (Loynes, 1985).

Optimum cubicle length in metres can be determined from the cow's weight as $1.75 + 0.00068 \times$ weight (kg) (Cermak, 1987), and the width is usually half the length. A variety of bedding materials can be used to increase cow comfort, especially when lying down, and also to absorb any urine deposited in the cubicle. A neck rail can be positioned perpendicular to the divisions, attached to the top rail 45 cm from the wall. This forces the cow to reverse out of the cubicle as she stands up and prevents the bedding being soiled. If cows are not able to stand fully in the cubicle, they will often stand half in and half out, which may increase stress to the hind feet. This is common in subordinate cows that use the cubicle as a place of escape.

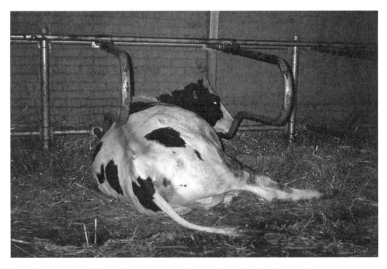

Fig. 13.8 Modern cubicles do not restrict the lying behaviour of cows – compare the more natural posture of this cow with that of the cow in Fig. 13.1.

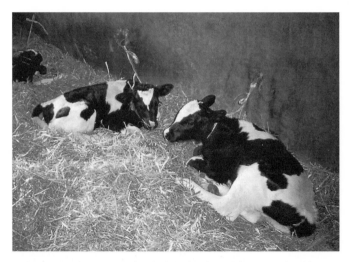

Fig. 13.9   Tethering cattle can restrict their behavioural freedom, in this case preventing lateral recumbency and posture changes.

Bedding material should be sufficient to cushion the shock to the cow's limbs as she lies down. It should also have insulatory properties for young calves kept at low temperatures. The lower critical temperature can increase from 8°C for a calf on dry straw to 17°C for the same calf on dry concrete. When the temperature falls outdoors, cattle lie down for longer so as to reduce heat loss from the underside of the body.

Tethering restricts the time cattle spend lying for the first few weeks, when they display more intention movements but few actual bouts of lying (Ladewig & Smidt, 1989; Haley *et al.*, 2000). In the long term the time spent lying may increase with tethering due to forced inactivity (Munksgaard & Simonsen, 1995). Stress levels are increased by tethering (Ladewig & Smidt, 1989) (Fig. 13.9). The act of lying is likely to stress the joints of tethered cattle, and a significant proportion show swollen joints (Krohn & Munksgaard, 1993). Cubicle systems for loose cows are less damaging to welfare than tethering systems, but the time that cows spend lying in cubicles is still less than in pens with deep straw bedding (Phillips & Schofield, 1994; Fregonesi & Leaver, 2001). High stocking rates of loose cows in straw yards or open yards should be avoided as they prevent cattle both sychronising their lying behaviour (Mogensen *et al.*, 1997b) and lying for their preferred time (Muller *et al.*, 1996).

Sleep

Sleep is characterised by a temporary period of inactivity and a raised response threshold. It is exhibited in a distinct diurnal rhythm and with a characteristic posture that allows the neck muscles to be relaxed. Cattle are usually sternally

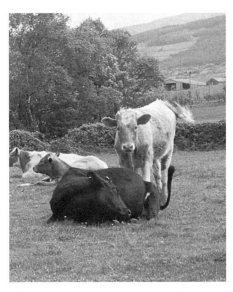

Fig. 13.10 Characteristic sleep position in cattle, with the head tucked round against the thorax to allow relaxation of the neck.

recumbent with the head either resting on the ground or tucked round and held against the thorax (Fig. 13.10).

Four levels of alertness can be distinguished in cattle (Ruckebush, 1972):

(1) *Alert wakefulness* (AW). Eyes fully open, characterised by a low-voltage, fast-activity electroencephalographic (EEG) brain output.
(2) *Drowsiness* (DR). Upper eyelid relaxed, increased arousal threshold and reduced alertness. Some high-voltage, slow-activity EEG output.
(3) *Quiet sleep* (QS). Eyes almost closed, increased arousal threshold and all EEG output of the high-voltage, slow-activity type.
(4) *Active sleep* (AS). Eyes fully closed, all EEG output of the low-voltage, fast-activity type, some rapid eye movement (REM), heightened arousal threshold. Otherwise known as paradoxical sleep.

The different proportions of the day that cattle spend in the different states of sleep are shown in Table 13.1. AW tends to predominate during the day and DR

Table 13.1 Proportions of the 24-hour day and of the night spent in alert wakefulness (AW), drowsiness (DR), quiet sleep (OS) and active sleep (AS)

	AW	DR	OS	AS
Percentage of 24 hours	52	31	13	3
Percentage of night	16	52	26	6

From Ruckebush (1972).

at night. AS only occurs at night and often after a bout of rumination. Rumination may accompany DR at night and also AW and occasionally QS. QS is often preceded by regular monotonous actions such as ruminating. Reticuloruminal motility is decreased at night, probably because of reduced basal metabolic rate during DR and QS.

The normal transition in the different types of sleep is from AW to DR to QS to AS. Periods of AS are short in cattle in comparison with other mammals, typically only five minutes long, but they are numerous, usually about ten occurring each night. Hence sleep in cattle can be considered as polyphasic, in contrast to that in humans. Sleep is also characterised by its consistency, as patterns vary little from day to day but are specific to individuals. Occasionally during AS, cattle demonstrate tachycardia (rapid breathing) and/or limb movements, both of which are indicative of dreaming. This phenomenon is not as common as in other ungulates and is most likely to occur in juveniles. The amount of both AS and QS declines with age, and the proportion of sleep that is AS declines from almost 100% at birth to 25% at maturity (Ellingson, 1972).

Functions of sleep

There are two probable functions of sleep in mammals: immobilisation and recuperation (Webb, 1979). In some animals regular, temporary immobilisation is beneficial in guarding against predation, providing that the sleeping site is secure. In large, herbivorous prey animals, such as wild cattle, the sleeping site is unlikely to be much safer than the area grazed during the day as they cannot hide or climb trees, and hence most grazing ungulates have evolved short sleep periods (Meddis, 1975, 1987). In contrast, for most forest-dwelling prey such as the dormouse, safe sleeping sites are available and sleeping times are long, even extending to hibernation in many species. Thus immobilisation offers two evolutionary advantages – energy conservation, which is of use to predator and prey alike, and security from predation.

Recuperation of brain function is likely to be of some benefit, since prolonged sleep deprivation leads to a state of exhaustion, the exhibition of abnormal behaviours and even hysterias. However, there is no evidence that longer sleep patterns occur more frequently in animals with a greater degree of cerebralisation, suggesting that recuperation is not very important. Indeed AS may specifically function to maintain the brain in a state of readiness during the subconscious state. Also animals that are more active physically do not have a greater reliance on sleep as a method of recuperation. On the contrary many inactive or sporadically active animals such as sloths, bears and lions sleep for long portions of the day. However, stressful and tiring procedures, such as transport, increase the time cattle spend resting and sleeping (Atkinson, 1992). It is not clear whether it is the stress or the physical effort needed to maintain balance that requires the cattle to increase sleeping. Sleep may also act as a redirected behaviour for cattle that are prevented from activity, for example, during transport and during the long, dark nights of winter (Phillips *et al.*, 1997). Individually penned cattle show no evidence of preferring to sleep in the dark (Phillips & Arab, 1998), but the opportunities for activity for individually penned cattle are similar in the dark and light. Cattle that are loose in a house or the field are invariably more active during the day, and sleep is therefore concentrated into the night.

In wild animals, the choice of whether to become an active feeder for most of the day and minimise sleep, or whether to save energy by maximising sleep, is determined by the security of the sleeping site and the rate at which the ingested food can be digested. Cattle developed the rumination process to be able to survive on low-quality food, but to achieve this they had to sacrifice many hours that could have been spent sleeping. Rumination only rarely accompanies QS and never AS. Hence the proportion of time spent in DR is much higher than in most other animals. Some reduction of basal metabolic rate is normal, but not as much as in QS.

Chapter 14
Behavioural Adaptation to Inadequate Environments

Behavioural needs

Keeping cattle in intensive environments inevitably leads to a modification of their behaviour compared with wild cattle. There are no wild cattle with which we can compare the behaviour of domesticated cattle, as the last members of the aurochs (*Bos primigenius*) were killed by poachers on a hunting reserve near Warsaw, Poland in 1627 (Felius, 1985). However, the behaviour of domestic cattle introduced into wild or semi-wild environments has been observed (e.g. Reinhardt & Reinhardt, 1981). This indicates the extent of 'normal' behaviour for the subspecies, although it can be argued that domestication has modified the behaviour sufficiently to make a consideration of behaviour in the wild irrelevant. Nevertheless it is accepted that farm animals have certain behavioural needs, if not rights, and one of these is to be able to express normal patterns of behaviour (Webster *et al.*, 1986). Other needs relate mainly to the avoidance of adverse conditions: freedom from thirst, hunger, malnutrition, prolonged discomfort, injury, disease, fear and stress (Webster, 1987).

Behavioural needs are best determined by first investigating which innate behaviours need to be performed, and secondly which behaviours are required to meet their physiological needs. The physiological needs include the absorption of adequate nutrient supply from the gastrointestinal tract, the perpetuation of the genotype by reproduction and the adequacy of the environment in terms of thermal and other sensory requirements. Taking these into account, the major behavioural needs can be summarised as follows:

- Reaction to danger (flight and escape)
- Ingestion
- Body care (including elimination)
- Motion
- Exploration/territorialism
- Rest
- Association (including social and reproductive behaviour).

Within this framework it must be recognised that most animals, and particularly domesticated animals, possess a degree of behavioural elasticity, i.e. they can modify their behaviour to meet their physiological needs. For instance, when a grass sward declines in height, cattle graze for longer and bite more frequently to maintain their intake. The extent of this behavioural elasticity is not yet known in sufficient detail, which is one reason why observation of wild cattle may not help much in analysing the behaviour of cattle in intensive husbandry systems. Behavioural elasticity can be estimated by depriving cattle of the opportunity to express two or more major behaviours. After the period of deprivation the cattle are observed to see which behaviour they perform. Alternatively, lever-pressing experiments are possible in which cattle are made to work in order to be allowed to perform a certain behaviour.

It seems likely that behavioural elasticity is limited with regard to innate behaviours in the neonate. In calves a particularly innate neonatal motivation is that of suckling. Preventing a calf from performing natural suckling behaviour is known to result in behavioural problems such as sucking the pen or nearest neighbour (kissing). These behavioural problems are relatively well studied in cattle. In the past many people referred to them as 'vices', but this implies that it is the cattle and not the system that are at fault. Such behaviours are also referred to as abnormal (Wiepkema *et al.*, 1983) but are difficult to define unless we know exactly what is meant by normal behaviour.

Behavioural problems are difficult to categorise, as each one has its own aetiology and function. However, we may discern the following major types, which are not mutually exclusive: stereotyped behaviours, injurious behaviours and redirected behaviours. These may create problems for either the animals, especially injurious behaviours, or the production system in which they are kept, e.g. feed tossing, where feed is wasted, or dark-cutting, which is common in bulls that have fought before slaughter. In addition there are numerous examples of behavioural elasticity or accommodation which are not necessarily deleterious to the animals or the farming system, e.g. abnormal styles of lying or standing, locomotion or nutritional modification, and are therefore not problems.

Behavioural problems

Stereotyped behaviours

In many situations cattle exhibit frequent repeated sequences of activity, which are stereotyped. These may be part of the normal behaviour, e.g. grazing or rumination, but in inadequate environments specific repeated sequences of movement may develop which appear to have no direct purpose in the context in they are performed. These are performed at more than the normal incidence and recur in nearly the same order in successive cycles. They may derive from conflict situations, where there was no solution to a behavioural problem. There is considerable variation between animals in the exhibition of stereotypies, but researchers believe that welfare of animals on a particular system is compromised when a significant proportion of a group of animals performs stereotypies, suggested to be more than 1 to 5% by Wiepkema (1983), and the welfare of an individual is compromised when it performs stereotypies for more than 10% of its waking life (Broom, 1983).

In cattle stereotypies are seen particularly in intensive housing situations and often relate to oral behaviours, such as bar-biting and tongue-rolling. Bar-biting is when a tethered cow clamps its jaws around a bar and moves its head back and forth while chewing on the bar (Redbo, 1992). In tongue-rolling (Fig. 14.1) the tongue is typically wrapped around an imaginary tuft of grass (with the head in the upright position) and rolled backwards towards the region of the pharynx inside the open mouth, and then protruded again (Redbo, 1990). Other forms, such as swinging the tongue from side to side outside the mouth or rolling the tongue inside the mouth, are also recognised (Sato *et al.*, 1994). Typically, in a high-risk population of artificially suckled calves fed inadequate roughage, tongue-rolling may be exhibited by 10 to 30% of cattle, and they will spend 2 to 5% of their time in this activity (Sato *et al.*, 1994). The behaviour may be a form of redirected sward grasping behaviour, as it is not observed in herbivores that bite rather than grasp and tear the sward as cattle do. As discussed with feed tossing behaviour (Chapter 10), which may conceivably be redirected sward tearing behaviour, grasps at the sward would normally be performed 30 000 to 40 000 times/day by grazing cattle. In addition, grazing cattle normally walk while graz-

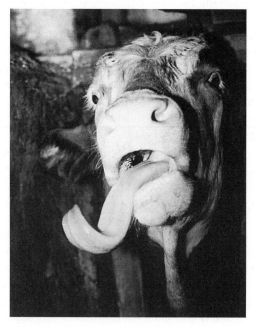

Fig. 14.1 Tongue-rolling in a bull (courtesy of H. Sambraus).

ing, whereas housed cattle are denied the opportunity to do this. Also, housed cattle do not spend a long time manipulating and processing feed, and cattle with restricted forage intakes show more oral sterotypies (Redbo *et al.*, 1996a; Redbo & Nordblad, 1997). Tongue playing is therefore believed to be the result of long-term frustration caused by suppressed suckling and feeding, and a boring environment (Seo *et al.*, 1998a,b).

Previous experience plays an important role in the extent of stereotypic behaviour, since it is more prevalent when cattle are tethered inside after a summer's grazing than just before being turned out to grazing (Redbo, 1990). Stereotypies are never performed when cattle are at pasture and have never been observed in animals in the wild. Much of the behaviour in intensive housing situations is related to feed searching behaviour, emphasising the relationship to inadequate feeding stimuli. One impact may be to lower the motivational hunger, and supporting evidence for this is provided by Redbo (1990), who observed that cattle spent more time in social behaviours immediately after performing stereotypies than before. In addition, high-yielding cows show more stereotypies than low-yielding cows, which may be because of greater energy deficit in the former (Redbo *et al.*, 1992). Usually stereotypic tongue-rolling and bar-biting are performed in the two to four hours after feeding (Redbo, 1990).

Non-nutritive sucking is common in calves where the sucking motivation is thwarted by supplying milk in a bucket rather than through a teat. Many modern systems now recognise this need and provide milk through a teat, even if it is only floating in the bucket. The satiation of the sucking motivation may otherwise be achieved by sucking the bars in the pen, the bucket handles or any other suitable protrusions. Sucking motivation also encourages calves to suck each other, either by oral 'kissing' or sucking ears and navels. This can lead to transfer of diseases and can be maintained into adulthood in the form of cows sucking each other's teats (and obtaining a further nutritive reward) or prepuce sucking (Fig. 14.2) and urine drinking in bulls. The importance of the sucking motivation has been demonstrated by Hammell *et al.* (1988), who showed that providing a dummy teat to bucket-fed calves partially satiates the motivation, which is particularly strong at feeding times.

One of the functions of stereotypies is to reduce the response threshold and pacify the animal to allow it to cope with a barren environment. Drowsiness is common in cattle during prolonged periods of rumination, and this may be one reason why stereotyped behaviours are less common in ruminant cattle in intensive environments than in other captive animals in intensive environments.

Stereotypies are most likely to occur where there is a specific releaser as well as a predisposing early experience of behavioural abnormalities. A common releaser is the lack of fibrous food, which has been linked to sham chewing in veal calves and tongue-rolling in bulls. Inadequacy of water supply may trigger prepuce sucking and urine drinking in bulls and milk drinking in cows (Sambraus & Gotthardt, 1985). In such cases these abnormal behaviours may develop in the majority of the animals and may occupy several hours each day.

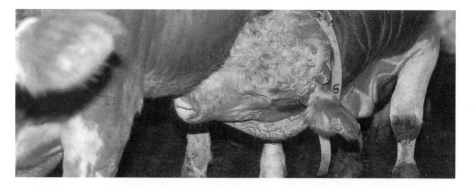

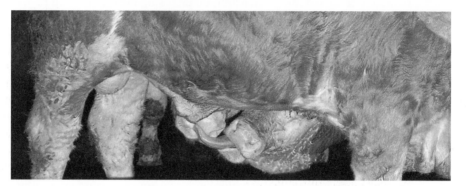

Fig. 14.2 Prepuce sucking in bulls. The sucker reaches under a bull (above) and stimulates it to urinate by licking the prepuce (below) (courtesy of H. Sambraus).

That these stereotypies perform a useful function in helping animals to cope with an inadequate environment is indisputable. Cattle performing stereotypies when they are tethered exhibit a lower cortisol response to an adrenocorticotropic challenge, compared to those that do not perform the stereotypies (Redbo, 1998). Also, they perform more exploratory behaviour in an open field test. Thus they appear to use stereotypies as a coping mechanism. Animals that do not learn to perform these behaviours frequently develop clinical disease problems, such as ulcers (Wiepkema *et al.*, 1987). In this respect stereotypies should be considered as indicators of an inadequate environment, not necessarily as behavioural problems in their own right. This does not necessarily mean that we should change all husbandry systems where stereotypies are displayed. Humans also exhibit a great deal of stereotyped behaviour in environments that do not cater for their needs, and they should perhaps have a higher priority for environmental modification. Nevertheless, where the incidence of stereotypies is widespread and lasts for a significant part of the day, this is an indication that the animal is having to devote considerable effort in coping with its environment. Modifying the environment could improve the productive efficiency as well as the welfare of the animal.

Stereotypies tend to increase with age, suggesting that they are learnt and not innate. This increase is probably associated with the positive feedback of sensory stimulation and possibly a progressive desensitisation of the repeatedly activated neural systems (Dantzer, 1986). The activation of neural systems has been demonstrated by administering psychostimulants, such as apomorphine (Sharman & Stephens, 1974). These block the neurotransmitters in the brain and cause stereotypies to be performed. In stressed cattle, particularly those suffering from inadequate space or nutrition, it is likely that the release of endogenous brain opioid peptides induces analgesia or a raised pain threshold. This compensates for the lack of arousal and helps the animal to cope with the environment (Dantzer, 1986).

Injurious behaviours

Behaviours that cause injury to other animals are most common where animals are group housed in a deficient environment. Bulls in a slatted floor building are one example of this, and deleterious behaviours such as excessive mounting and prepuce sucking will often develop. However, injurious behaviours are not normally as widespread in cattle as in pigs and poultry, where the degree of intraspecific aggression may even lead to widespread cannibalism. This species difference may be because of the more gregarious nature of ruminants, and a greater ability to tolerate close confinement, or it may be because of the natural pacifying effect of rumination.

The buller steer syndrome (Fig. 14.3), the welfare implications of which were discussed in Chapter 3 and the motivational aspects in Chapter 11, can be minimised by effective management, but the industry is not yet sufficiently motivated to act. Further pressure from the public and the multinational companies selling beef products may reduce this problem. The aetiology needs to be better

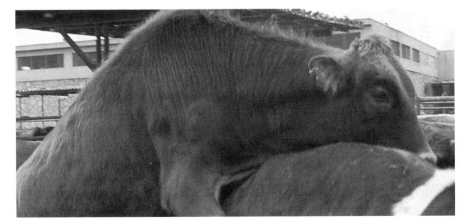

Fig. 14.3 The buller steer syndrome. Excessive mounting by steers can lead to exhaustion and slow growth.

understood, and particularly the role of stress. Maternal stress during pregnancy has been implicated in sexual deviance in human males (Dorner, 1989) and could be a factor in predisposing cattle to the buller steer syndrome, since nutritional stress in rangeland pregnant cows is common. Although the syndrome predominantly occurs in male cattle, in natural, heterogeneous groups of cattle the level of aggression in male and female animals is similar and mainly directed towards subordinate animals (Reinhardt *et al.*, 1987).

Another problem in groups of male cattle on slatted floors is tail tip necrosis, which has led some farms to dock the tails of cattle routinely (Busch & Kramer, 1995). The lesions are caused by damage to the tail following trampling by other cattle, and the incidence is closely linked to stocking density, with herds stocked at over 200 kg/m^2 being most at risk. A variety of micro-organisms infect the damaged tail and the ensuing pyrexia can result in death of the individual if not treated. Tail tip necrosis only occurs at warm temperatures, over 18°C. The reason for this is not clear. It may relate to the laterally recumbent position at high temperatures, exposing the tail to trampling. It is also not clear why only male cattle develop the problem, since it has never been observed in heifers.

Cattle may also unwittingly perform behaviours that are injurious to themselves, such as excessive self-grooming by individually penned calves, which can lead to the formation of hairballs in the stomach. Self-induced destruction of udder skin and teats by excessive licking at calving has been reported in primiparous cows in Israel (Yeruham & Markusfeld, 1996). The incidence of 0.4% of nearly 10 000 animals may have been genetically influenced by the widespread use of two bulls. Most of the cows had to be culled. Abnormal behaviours during stress often involve excessive toilet activity, particularly self-grooming if cattle are penned individually and allogrooming if they are in groups. The use of the tether, which prevents this important stress-dissipating behaviour from taking place, is now increasingly seen as unacceptable on welfare grounds. The process of adaptation to tethering includes initial escape attempts, followed by 'learned helplessness', accompanied by extreme passiveness, then the exhibition of stereotyped behaviours. These are initially directed to the environment but may increasingly involve self-attention as time progresses.

Redirected behaviours

Where the motivation for a behavioural need is particularly strong and is thwarted by environmental insufficiency, animals may attempt to redirect the motivation to the performance of a similar behaviour. This is especially common with ingestion.

An abnormal diet will often precipitate abnormal oral behaviours, and deficiencies of fibre, phosphorus and sodium will produce cravings for the nutrient, or pica. These may be satiated by unnatural food objects such as wood for fibre, bones for phosphorus and urine for sodium. Cattle that are deficient in sodium often induce urination by prepuce sucking (Stephens, 1974).

Although locomotion is common in free-ranging calves, including running, gambolling, cantering, and other movements like kicking and jumping, the use of redirected behaviours to overcome the restriction of activity in penned calves is limited (Fig. 14.4). In confined cattle, behaviours such as weaving, pacing and rocking from one leg to the other are used but in calves these are not commonly seen. Probably these behaviours do not have time to develop in the short period during which dairy calves are penned, and in veal calves other deficiencies, such as fibre – cause redirected oral behaviours to predominate, in particular self-grooming and licking objects in their pen (Dannenman *et al.*, 1985).

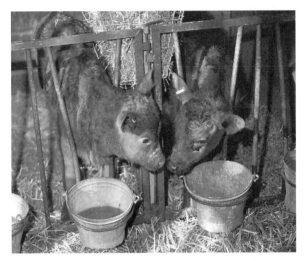

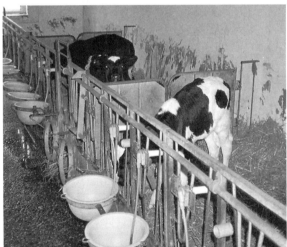

Fig. 14.4 Traditional calf-rearing systems limit contact with other calves and force calves to drink unnaturally from a bucket (above). Recently, systems have been developed where calves take the milk from a teat connected to the bucket by a pipe (below).

Conclusion

Cattle display a range of abnormal behaviours that are performed in inadequate environments, which help them to cope. Nevertheless, the performance of these behaviours is an indication that the environment is inadequate and that the welfare of the cattle is compromised. When these are performed in a significant proportion of cattle, perhaps 1 to 5%, the environment should be changed. In addition, if any individual performs abnormal behaviour for more than 10% of its waking life, then its welfare is likely to be reduced. Action should be taken to improve the environment for this individual, and consideration given as to whether the welfare of animals not performing the behaviour is also compromised.

Chapter 15
The Relationship Between Cattle and Man

Introduction – the domestic contract

By keeping domestic cattle in confined conditions, man reduces their freedom to perform certain desirable behaviours. It may not be essential that these behaviours are performed exactly as they would be in the wild, e.g. some reduction in locomotion can be accepted, and copulation can be replaced by artificial control by humans. However, if we are to demonstrate a healthy respect for the needs of other species with which we share the environment (which has been the hallmark of most successful and sustainable societies so far), we must recognise that the removal of the freedom to perform certain behaviours must be compensated by other provisions. Where we take away on the one hand freedom for locomotion, freedom to copulate and freedom to ingest feeds in a natural manner, we must compensate by, for example, providing adequate food of suitable composition, offering the freedom to develop bonds with similar livestock, and freedom from predation. This is the foundation for the formation of a domestic contract that demonstrates our respect for our husbanded livestock.

This respect was an essential feature of most primitive societies, and still is of many modern ones. In many ancient civilisations, this respect even went as far as the deification or sanctification of cattle, because of the dependence that man had on them as the major meat and milk producer (Fig. 15.1). However, in the western world many people are now far removed from the cattle that provide food for them and may through ignorance and/or greed encourage intensive production systems that provide cheap products at the expense of the welfare of the animals in these systems. A better knowledge of cattle behavioural requirements by stockmen, farmers and researchers should enable them to be kept in a manner in which we can truly say that they have enjoyed as good facilities and lifestyle as they would have had in the wild. Whether this happens or not will be for every civilised society to determine.

As this respect for the quality of life of cattle becomes integrated into our agricultural systems, it is imperative that we understand the relationship between man and cattle in more detail. Man could be regarded as a pseudopredator or a provider by cattle, and further information is urgently required so that the impact on the cattle of the human presence on farms can be accounted for in provision for their welfare.

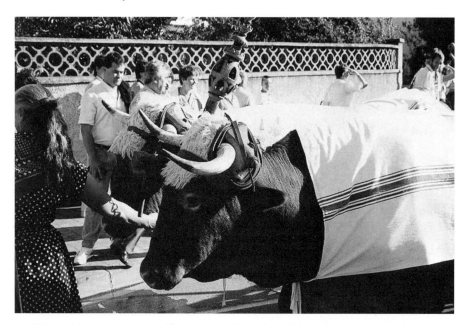

Fig. 15.1 The parading of decorated cattle in France during a local festival.

Recognition of people

Recognition of people by cattle has been demonstrated by both operant conditioning techniques and observational studies. Operant conditioning has shown that cattle can recognise people in most circumstances, with the person's face, height and type of clothing being the most important cues (Rybarczyk *et al.*, 2001). However, these cues have to be placed in their normal context to be effective – faces without bodies cannot readily be distinguished. The colour of clothing is likely to be important, with long wavelength colours being particularly easily distinguished. Little is known about the ability of cattle to recognise people by other cues, such as smell and voice, but their powers of perception are probably adequate for recognition at a distance. Observational studies have demonstrated that heart rates are elevated when cows are milked by a relief milker (Knierem & Warran, 1993) or when a person is present who previously mistreated them (Rushen *et al.*, 1999c). It is highly likely, therefore, that the person is recognised.

The bond between cattle and humans

Cattle, being social animals, seek alternative animals with which to bond if their matriarchal groups are disrupted. Man may assume the role of most dominant animal, mother, offspring substitute or leader. In the most extreme case, cattle managed by traditional herders, for example in sub-Saharan Africa, are tended by children during the day and by adults at night, both of which achieve a dominant role (Ayantunde *et al.*, 2000). The permanent contact with humans makes them easy to handle, since they learn to follow the human as their leader. Acting responsibly as the boss 'animal' brings stability to the herd, and there is evidence that cattle respond best to a person who is confident and consistent in handling them (Seabrook, 1984). The cattle also respond to regular communication with the stockperson, particularly during periods of stress such as calving. This communication may be in the form of touching the animals, petting, stroking or scratching, particularly around the head area. This mimics grooming by conspecifics and maintains the bond between man and cattle. Communication may also be verbal and visual, with good stockpeople regularly talking to and looking at the cattle in their charge. The importance of a stockperson's olfactory signals to cattle is not fully understood, but this could enable cattle to know a person's mood before any other communication has taken place.

Much of the effective communication between the stockperson and cattle should be to confirm the relationship between them. Firm handling to assume dominant status combined with the caring role of the matriarchal substitute is necessary if the cattle are to be contented. Modern production systems are designed for minimal labour input and the importance of the stockperson's role in the herd is not recognised. Abnormal behaviour problems in the presence of humans may increase as a result, and a farmer's time and money may be wasted devising physical methods to overcome these problems without recognising the psychological needs of the cattle for adequate social bonding.

Cattle and the human temperament

Cattle can recognise and respond to differences in human temperament and this will affect their response to handling. Seabrook and Bartle (1992) have identified three major types of interactions between animals and stockpeople: hand and arm (tactile) interaction, vocal interaction and holistic empathetic interaction (smell and other senses). Interactions may be either pleasant (patting the back, stroking, etc.) or aversive (hitting, etc.) and performed with a varying degree of confidence by the stockperson. However, even 'unpleasant' handling may be perceived as beneficial if it relieves the boredom of a sterile environment. Regular 'pleasurable' touching of cattle by the stockperson is desirable and can lead to reduced stress and paler meat in veal calves (Lensink *et al.*, 2001b), but some respect or fear of the stockperson is necessary to enable cattle to be moved with ease and to discourage the cattle from attempting to force interactions with the human. Reduced contact with humans makes group-reared calves more difficult to move than individually reared calves, but this can be overcome by increasing the degree of contact (Lensink *et al.*, 2001a). It is important for stockpeople to be able to assess an animal's temperament, so that they can predict its behavioural reactions to handling, milking, etc., and modify their own behaviour accordingly.

Human–cattle interactions and the productivity of dairy cows

Some studies have been briefly reported in which the authors claim that there is a relationship between the milk yield of dairy cows and their response to their handler (Seabrook, 1984; Hemsworth *et al.*, 1995). The same authors have made similar, brief reports of relationships between aversive handling and milk yield (see review by Rushen *et al.*, 1999b). Other authors (Dickson *et al.*, 1970; Purcell *et al.*, 1988) have failed to find any relationship between the personality of cows and their milk production. In the absence of more detailed reports, the results claimed by Hemsworth *et al.* and Seabrook must be viewed with caution, since the studies used only small numbers of herds, 12 to 14, and there was little evidence that other factors, such as environmental differences, had been adequately controlled for. Hemsworth *et al.* (1995) also reported that there is a strong relationship between the frequency of negative interactions between the stockperson and the cows, and the cows' proximity to a novel person, which is more plausible. Seabrook (1984) produced evidence from a study of 12 farms that a change in herdsperson is associated with a decline in production. However, if there is a relationship, it could be due to a change in management rather than the person themselves. As herds become larger, and there is less contact between the herdsperson and the cattle, there is less likelihood that there will be a major effect of the herdsperson's personality on milk production. However, the contacts between the herdsperson and the cattle are now more often ones from which the animal does not benefit, whereas previously tasks involving positive interaction, such as feeding, were largely accomplished manually (Rushen *et al.*, 1999b). Milking may represent a positive stimulus to high-yielding cows, but the reluctance of cows to enter an automatic milking plant suggests that the relief of udder pressure does not provide a major positive stimulus.

Fear of humans by cattle

Fear of humans is more likely to develop in cattle when they have unpleasant experiences as a result of contact with humans, however, there is also evidence that it is innate. Feral mithun cattle and wild gaur cattle in south-east Asia are fearful only of humans and tigers, even though they have little close contact with man (Gupta *et al.*, 1999). Regular positive contact leads to a respectful relationship between cattle and humans, as there is symbiosis between the needs of each species.

The herdsperson plays a major role in shaping the temperament of cattle in their care. Extra handling in the first nine months of life reduces the flight distance of heifers from humans (Boissy & Bouissou, 1988). This is not just a response to the person shaping the animal's behaviour, it is generalised to other animals. Receptiveness to the influences of shaping diminishes with age, so interactions with calves are particularly important in determining the behaviour of adult cattle. Regular contact between calves and humans reduces the strength of the adverse reaction to later handling and reduces the frequency of stress-related diseases, such as abomasal ulceration (Lensink *et al.*, 2000b). An important indicator of stress is the frequency of defecation and the faecal consistency, with cattle that are more stressed showing increased frequency of defecation and faeces of low dry matter content (Lensink *et al.*, 2000a).

The potential exists for a herdsperson to influence the behaviour of dairy cows by having positive contact with the cows before their first calving. Normally most contact with older cattle has neutral or negative associations, the latter being exemplified by procedures such as delivering injections, which has associated pain. Moving animals, inserting intrauterine devices and weighing, which all disrupt the normal social structure, bring the animals into abnormally close contact with each other and with humans and increase the risk of physical damage when the animals are in races, crushes, going through gates, etc. Young cattle may associate human presence with feeding, especially bucket-fed calves, but it is doubtful whether this extends to cattle fed from a tractor and feeding wagon. The adult cow requires a labour input of about 30 hours/year (Seufert, 1997), but much of this will involve only indirect contact providing neutral impact.

Primiparous dairy cows present particular difficulties to herdspeople when they join the rest of the herd, particularly as they often have problems adjusting to machine milking (Bertenshaw *et al.*, 2001). Farmers recognise that adverse handling may make cows difficult to milk. Positive interaction between pregnant primiparous cows and their herdsperson can reduce kicking behaviour in the parlour and increase milk flow rate in the subsequent lactation (Bertenshaw & Rowlinson, 2001). There is also less inhibition of milk let-down as a result of stress in the parlour, but no effects on milk yield have been demonstrated.

Cattle in sport

Throughout the period of domestication, cattle were not just kept for the production of milk, meat, faeces and traction, but also for sport and leisure. Cattle were so intrinsically part of primeval human society and were revered for their fertility and strength, that it was almost inevitable that they became part of our sporting activities.

Fighting bulls

The traditional fights between men and bulls may be one of the most obvious affronts to the welfare of cattle. However, there are people that believe that the sport is justified because of its cultural heritage or because it is no worse than other blood sports, such as fox hunting. The sport is legalised in the European Union by special exemption from slaughter regulations on the grounds of cultural heritage. It has its traditions in the time of the Roman empire and is now pursued in Spain, Portugal, parts of South America and, more recently, south-west France. It has its greatest following in Spain, where there are just over 1000 bull rings, which host about 1500 fights per year, killing approximately 4000 bulls. There are also many practice fights with animals that are not thought suitable for a major event. A big industry has developed to support the sport, with approximately 200 000 people employed in rearing bulls, maintaining the bull rings, etc. The fights are accompanied by much celebration and fiesta. Over the years they have developed into a more elaborate spectacle, with glittering costumes and large prizes for successful matedors, However, many young people have little interest in bullfighting (Llamas, 2001), and there is concern that the close-up pictures of the fight, and in particular the death of the bull, on television is bad for the moral upbringing of children and will desensitise them to violence. Children under 14 years of age are banned from attending fights in some regions of Spain, and other parts of Spain have banned bullfighting altogether.

Preparation of the bulls

The animals are bred to be brave and to respond rapidly and vehemently to the challenge by humans. Their courage is exemplified by a willingness to charge a man on horseback, a target which is far larger and heavier than itself. The animals must be so reactive to provocation that they charge up to the point of death, and they must not cry out or retreat when wounded. The breeding programme has led to the development of animals that are hypersensitive and nervous, quite different to cattle that are used for milk production, which have been bred for docility. Females are selected for breeding by testing the ferocity of their charge at horses, when provoked with lances jabbed into their back.

For the fight the bulls must be lean, strong and not too heavy, or their charge would be slow. To achieve this they mainly graze on natural pasture with little supplementation, which would make them deposit fat tissue. They are weaned at about eight months and branded. Their slow growth makes them late-maturing and typically they fight at four years of age, by which time they weigh about 600 kg. They have little contact with humans until the fight, and there are no practice fights for these animals before they enter the ring. Their welfare up to this point is therefore comparatively good, except that they are not allowed access to females, and therefore cannot fulfil their natural mating urge.

The fight

The bull must come to the fight well nourished, to give him enough energy to be able to charge with vigour to the last. He should be kept under as little stress as possible, otherwise his performance will suffer. A veterinarian is present at each fight and has to certify the animal's welfare before the fight.

There are regional variations in the bullfight, with a fight to the death normal in Spain and South America but not Portugal, where the bull is professionally slaughtered immediately after the event. After the extreme stress suffered by bulls during the fight, the best course of action for the bull on welfare grounds must be slaughter as soon as possible, regardless of whether it is in front of a crowd of spectators. However, if the slaughter encourages people to watch bullfights, and there are therefore more fights in total, then immediate slaughter could be opposed on utilitarian grounds.

Each fight lasts for about 20 minutes, with four to six bulls per event. There is considerable danger to the matedor, who normally fights two bulls at each event. He has assistance from two picadores, who carry long pikes with 10 cm steel tips, and three bandilleros, who are on horseback with decorated wooden sticks that end in a barbed harpoon. Initially the picadores thrust the pikes two or three times into the bull's shoulder muscle as he charges, to weaken his tossing ability. Next the bandilleros jab up to eight of their harpoons into the bull's back to weaken it further. A brave bull does not cry out when the harpoons are inserted and indeed shows no signs of pain throughout the event. Next the matedor taunts the bull by tempting it to charge a large piece of cloth, coloured fuchsia and yellow, held outside his body. The movement of the cloth take the bull's attention away from the matedor. This taunting continues until the matedor has complete control of the charging bull, which may take about 20 charges. During this period the bull may also charge the matedor, which challenges his speed and bravery. Then, with his sword in his right hand, the matedor attracts a final charge at a small bright red cape held directly in front of his body with his left hand. It seems likely that the bright red colour and the positioning of this cape are designed to extract the last vestiges of aggression in the bull (Phillips & Lomas, 2001). As it charges, the sword is plunged between the shoulder blades, which if correctly positioned causes instant collapse and death. If the bull fails to die, the matedor will lance the neck with a short sword, causing immediate death. A bull is considered to be more courageous and honourable if it dies with its mouth closed.

This description of bullfighting attempts to demonstrate the obvious cruelty involved in the procedures, but also to emphasise that there is considerable risk to the welfare of the matedors. The attraction of the sport, therefore, to the general public is probably not so much the cruelty to the bull, as the high risk to the matedor.

Bull-running and rodeos

A related practice in a small number of Hispanic communities is the running of bulls through a town, behind a group of young men who have to escape. Although the running through the town is less of a welfare problem to the bulls than bullfighting, the bulls are undoubtedly severely stressed and may suffer injury. Following the bull-running, bulls may be used in a traditional bullfight, as in the town of Pamplona in Spain.

Tribal slaughter

In the traditional societies of the Asian tribes, local cattle (of the mithun genotype) are still raised for ritual sacrifice. They are more highly prized for this purpose than any other domesticated animal and are reserved for religious, social and community feasts (Gupta *et al.*, 1999). The slaughter techniques are often barbaric and involve taunting the animal and torturing it before slaughter. In some cases, the animal is paralysed with a cut to the loins, after which tribesmen cut lumps of flesh from the live animal. Repeated spearing is another method practised in Bangladesh, but some tribes use methods that are less painful for the animal, such as cutting its throat and blows to the back of the head. The methods may have evolved partly because of their ability to cause major blood-letting, thereby helping to preserve the meat, but could now be considered as just as damaging to the animal's welfare as bullfighting.

Conclusion

The types of interaction between any domesticated animal and their human keepers are important for their welfare, but particularly in the case of cattle where human contact with individual animals is common. The behaviour of cattle is easily shaped by early contact with humans, which may have lasting effects on their temperament and reaction to humans. Effects on efficiency of milk or meat production have not yet been conclusively demonstrated. The use of cattle for sport has a very negative effect on their welfare, although usually only for a short period at the end of their life and this is only for a small proportion of the total cattle population. The widespread viewing of cruel treatment of cattle on the television may have adverse effects on human behaviour, and in particular people's tolerance of cruelty to animals.

References

Adams, D.C. (1985). Effect of time of supplementation on performance, forage intake and grazing behaviour of yearling beef steers grazing Russian wild ryegrass in the fall. *Journal of Animal Science*, **61**, 1037–1042.

Agricultural and Food Research Council. (1993). *Energy and Protein Requirements of Ruminants.* CAB International, Wallingford.

Agricultural Development and Advisory Service. (1980). Complete diet feeding of dairy cows. Supplementary report on investigations carried out during 1978–1979, 38 pp. Ministry of Agriculture, Fisheries and Food, London.

Agyemang, K., Clapp, E. & Van Vleck, L.D. (1982). Components of variance of dairymen's workability traits among Holstein cows. *Journal of Dairy Science*, **65**, 1334–1338.

Albright, J.L. & Arave, C.W. (1997). *The Behaviour of Cattle*. CAB International, Wallingford.

Albright, J.L. & Stricklin, W.R. (1989). Recent developments in the provision for cattle welfare. In *New Techniques in Cattle Production* (ed. C.J.C. Phillips), pp. 149–161. Butterworths, London.

Albright, J.L., Gordon, W.P., Black, W.C., Dietrich, J.P., Snyder, W.W. & Meadows, C.E. (1966). Behavioural responses of cows to auditory training. *Journal of Dairy Science*, **49**, 104–106.

Albutt, R.W., Dumelow, J., Cermak, J.P. & Owen, J.E. (1990). Slip-resistance of solid concrete floors in cattle buildings. *Journal of Agricultural Engineering Research*, **45**, 137–147.

Alexander, N. (1987). Locomotion. In *The Oxford Companion to Animal Behaviour* (ed. D. McFarland), pp. 347–356. Oxford University Press, Oxford.

Alexander, T.J., Senger, P.L., Rosenberger, J.L. & Hagen, D.R. (1984). The influence of the stage of the oestrous cycle and novel cows upon mounting activity of dairy cattle. *Journal of Animal Science*, **59**, 1430–1439.

Andersen, B.B., Madsen, P. & Smedgard, H.H. (1991). Genetic analysis of claw and leg traits in young bulls. *Beretning fra Statens Husdyrbrugsforsog*, **701**, 52.

Anderson, D.M., Hulet, C.V., Shupe, W., Smith, J.N. & Murray, L.W. (1988). Response of bonded and non-bonded sheep to the approach of a trained border collie. *Applied Animal Behaviour Science*, **21**, 251–257.

Anderson, J. (1944). The periodicity and duration of oestrus in Zebu and Grade cattle. *Journal of Agricultural Science*, **34**, 57–68.

Andersson, M. (1987). Effects of number and location of water bowls and social rank on drinking behaviour and performance of loose-housed dairy cows. *Applied Animal Behaviour Science*, **17**, 19–31.

Anil, M.H., McKinstry, J.L., Gregory, N.G., Wotton, S.B. & Symonds, H. (1995). Welfare of calves. 2. Increase in vertebral artery blood-flow following exsanguination by neck sticking and evaluation of chest sticking as an alternative slaughter method. *Meat Science*, **41**, 113–123.

Appleman, R.D. & Gustafson, R.J. (1985). Source of stray voltage and effect on cow health and performance. *Journal of Dairy Science*, **68**, 1554–1567.

Arave, C.W. & Walters, J.L. (1980). Factors affecting lying behaviour and stall utilisation of dairy cattle. *Applied Animal Ethology*, **6**, 369–376.

Arave, C.W., Albright, J.L. & Sinclair, C.L. (1974). Behavior, milk yield, and leucocytes of dairy cows in reduced space and isolation. *Journal of Dairy Science*, **57**, 1497–1501.

Arave, C.W., Albright, J.L., Armstrong, D.V., Foster, W.W. & Larson, L.L. (1992). Effects of isolation of calves on growth, behavior, and 1st lactation milk-yield of Holstein cows. *Journal of Dairy Science*, **75**, 3408–3415.

Arendzen, I. & Scheppingen, A.T.J. (2000). Economical sensitivity of four main parameters defining the room for investment of automatic milking systems on dairy farms. In *Robotic Milking* (eds H. Hogeveen and A. Meijering), pp. 201–211. Wageningen Pers, Wageningen.

Arney, D.R. Kitwood, S.E. & Phillips, C.J.C. (1994). The increase in activity during oestrus in dairy cows. *Applied Animal Behaviour Science*, **40**, 211–218.

Arnold, C.W. (1984). Spatial relationships between sheep, cattle and horse groups grazing together. *Applied Animal Behaviour Science*, **13**, 7–17.

Arnold, G.W. & Grassia, A. (1983). Social interactions amongst beef cows when competing for food. *Applied Animal Ethology*, **9**, 239–252.

Atkinson, P.J. (1992). Investigation of the effects of transport and lairage on hydration state and resting behaviour of calves for export. *Veterinary Record*, **130**, 413–416.

Axford, R.F.E., Bishop, S.C., Nicholas, F.W. & Owen, J.B. (1999). *Breeding for Disease Resistance*, 2nd edn. CABI Publishing, Wallingford.

Ayantunde, A.A., Williams, T.O., Udo, H.M.J., Fernandez-Rivera, S., Hiernaux, P. & van Keulen, H. (2000). Herders' perceptions, practice, and problems of night grazing in the Sahel: case studies from Niger. *Human Ecology*, **28**, 109–130.

Baehr, J., Schulte-Coerne, H., Pabst, K. & Gravert, H.O. (1984). (The behaviour of cows in cubicles.) *Zuchtungskunde,* **56**, 127–138.

Bailey, D.W., Rittenhouse, L.R., Hart, R.H. & Richards, R.W. (1989). Characteristics of spatial memory in cattle. *Applied Animal Behaviour Science*, **23**, 331–340.

Bailey, P.J., Bishop, A.H. & Boord, C. (1974). Grazing behaviour of steers. *Proceedings of the Australian Society of Animal Production*, **10**, 303–305.

Baker, A.E.M., & Seidel, G.E. (1975). Why do cows mount other cows? *Applied Animal Behaviour Science,* **13**, 237–241.

Balch, C.C. (1955). Sleep in ruminants. *Nature*, **175**, 940–941.

Balch, C.C. (1971). Proposal to use time spent chewing as an index of the extent to which diets for ruminants possess the physical property of fibrousness characteristic of roughages. *British Journal of Nutrition*, **26**, 383–391.

Baldwin, B.A. (1981). Shape discrimination in sheep and calves. *Animal Behaviour*, **29**, 830–834.

Baldwin, B.A. & Start, B. (1981). Sensory reinforcement and illumination preference in sheep and calves. *Proceedings of the Royal Society*, London, **B211**, 513–526.

Ballou, J.D. (1992). Potential contribution of cryopreserved germ plasm to the preservation of genetic diversity and conservation of endangered species in captivity. *Cryobiology,* **29**, 19–25.

Bao, J. & Giller, P.S. (1991). Observations on the changes in behavioral activities of dairy-cows prior to and after parturition. *Irish Veterinary Journal*, **44**, 43–47.

Barnard, C.J. & Hurst, J.L. (1996). Welfare by design: the natural selection of welfare criteria. *Animal Welfare,* **5**, 405–433.

Barrio, J.P., Zhang, S.Y., Zhu, Z.K., Wu, F.L., Mao, X.Z., Bermudez, F.F. & Forbes, J.M. (2000). The feeding behaviour of the water buffalo monitored by a semiautomatic feed intake recording system. *Journal of Animal and Feed Sciences*, **9**, 55–72.

Barroso, F.G., Alados, C.L. & Boza, J. (2000). Social hierarchy in the domestic goat, effect on food habits and production. *Applied Animal Behaviour Science*, **69**, 35–53.

Baylis, M. (1996). Effect of defensive behaviour by cattle on the feeding success and nutritional state of the tsetse fly, *Glossina pallidipes* (*Diptera: Glossinidae*). *Bulletin of Entomological Research*, **86**, 329–336.

Beaver, J.M. & Olson, B.E. (1997). Winter range use by cattle of different ages in southwestern Montana. *Applied Animal Behaviour Science*, **51**, 1–13.

Beaver, J.M., Olson, B.E. & Wraith, J.M. (1996). A simple index of standard operative temperature for mule deer and cattle in winter. *Journal of Thermal Biology*, **21**, 345–352.

Beilharz, R.G. & Mylrea, P.J. (1963a). Social position and behaviour of dairy heifers in yards. *Animal Behaviour*, **11**, 522–528.

Beilharz, R.G. & Mylrea, P.J. (1963b). Social position and movement orders of dairy heifers. *Animal Behaviour*, **11**, 529–533.

Beilharz, R.G. & Zeeb, K. (1982). Social dominance in dairy cattle. *Applied Animal Ethology*, **8**, 79–97.

Beilharz, R.G., Butcher, D.F. & Freeman, F.E. (1966). Social dominance and milk production in Holsteins. *Journal of Dairy Science,* **49**, 887–892.

Bell, F.R. & Sly, J. (1983). The olfactory detection of sodium and lithium salts by sodium deficient cattle. *Physiology and Behaviour*, **31**, 307–312.

Bennett, R. & Cooke, R. (2001). *Economic Assessment of TB and Alternative Control Strategies.* Proceedings of a Workshop, University of Reading, 4 July 2001. University of Reading, UK.

Berghash, S.R., Davidson, J.N., Armstrong, J.C. & Dunny, G.M. (1983). Effects of antibiotic treatment of nonlactating dairy cows on antibiotic resistance patterns of bovine mastitis pathogens. *Antimicrobial Agents in Chemotherapy,* **24**, 771–776.

Bertenshaw, C. & Rowlinson, P. (2001). The influence of positive human–animal interaction during rearing on the welfare and subsequent production of the dairy heifer. In *Proceedings of the British Society of Animal Science*, 17.

Bertenshaw, C., Rowlinson, P. & Ness, M. (2001). A survey to investigate the influence of commercial human–animal interactions during rearing on the welfare and subsequent production of the dairy heifer. In *Proceedings of the British Society of Animal Science*, 170.

Beverlin, S.K., Havstad, K.M., Ayers, E.L. & Petersen, M.K. (1989). Forage intake responses to winter cold exposure of free-ranging beef cows. *Applied Animal Behaviour Science*, **23**, 78–85.

Biozzi, G., Mouton, D., Stiffel, C. & Bouthillier, Y. (1984). A major role of the macrophages in quantitative genetics regulation of immunoresponsiveness and anti-infectious immunity. *Advances in Immunology,* **36**, 189–234.

Blackshaw, J.K., Balckshaw, A.W. & McGlone, J.J. (1997). Buller steer syndrome review. *Applied Animal Behaviour Science*, **54**, 97–108.

Blair West, J.R., Denton, D.A., Nelson, J.F., McKinley, M.J., Radden, B.G. & Ramshaw, E.H. (1989). Recent studies of bone appetite in cattle. *Acta Physiologica Scandinavia Supplement*, **583,** 53–58.

Blaschke, C.F., Thompson, D.L., Humes, P.E. & Godke, R.A. (1984). Olfaction, sight and auditory perception of mature bulls in detecting estrual responses in beef heifers. In *Proceedings of the 10th International Congress on Animal Reproduction and Artificial Insemination*, 10–14 June 1984. Paper 284. University of Illinois, Urbana, USA.

Blazquez, N.B., French, J.M., Lang, S.E. & Perry, G.C. (1988). A pheromenal function for the perineal skin glands in the cow. *Veterinary Record*, **123**, 49–50.

Blecha, F., Boyles, S.L. & Riley, J.G. (1984). Shipping suppresses lymphocyte blastogenic responses in Angus and Brahman × Angus feeder calves. *Journal of Animal Science*, **59**, 576–583.

Blockey, M.A. (1978). Serving capacity and social dominance of bulls in relation to fertility. In *Proceedings of the First World Congress of Ethology and Applied Zootechnology*, Madrid, pp. 523–530.

Blockey, M.A. de B., Straw, W.M. & Jones, L.P. (1978). Heritability of serving capacity and scrotal circumference in beef bulls. Abstract No. 92, 70th Annual Meeting of the American Society of Animal Science, East Lansing, Michigan.

Bloomsmith, A.M. & Lambeth, S.P. (1995). Effects of predictable versus unpredictable feeding schedules on chimpanzee behaviour. *Applied Animal Behavioural Science*, **44**, 65–74.

Boissy, A. & Bouissou, M.F. (1998). Effects of early handling on heifers' subsequent reactivity to humans and unfamiliar situations. *Applied Animal Behaviour Science*, **20**, 259–273.

Boissy, A., Terlouw, C. & Le Neindre, P. (1998). Presence of cues from stressed conspecifics increases reactivity to aversive events in cattle: evidence for the existence of alarm substances in urine. *Physiology and Behaviour*, **63**, 489–495.

Boivin, X., J.P. Garel *et al.* (1998). Is gentling by people rewarding for beef calves? *Applied Animal Behaviour Science*, **61**, 1–12.

Boivin, X. & Le Neindre, P. (1994). Influence of breed and rearing management on cattle reactions during human handling. *Applied Animal Behaviour Science*, **39**, 115–122.

Boivin, X., Le Neindre, P., Chupin, J.M., Garel, J.P. & Trillat, G. (1992). Influence of breed and early management on ease of handling and open-field behavior of cattle. *Applied Animal Behaviour Science*, **32**, 313–323.

Boivin, X., Le Neindre, P., Garel, J.P. & Chupin, J.M. (1994). Influence of breed and rearing management on cattle reactions during human handling. *Applied Animal Behaviour Science*, **39**, 115–122.

Botto, V. & Zimmermann, V. (1986). Effect of group formation on the ethological regime and milk efficiency of cows under conditions of large-scale production. *Zivocisna-Vyroba*, **31**, 983–988.

Botts, R.L., Hemken, R.W. & Bull, L.S. (1979). Protein reserves in the lactating dairy cow. *Journal of Dairy Science*, **62**, 433–440.

Bowman, J.G.P. & Sowell, B.F. (1997). Delivery method and supplement consumption by grazing ruminants, a review. *Journal of Animal Science*, **75**, 543–550.

Boyd, H. (1977). Anoestrus in cattle. *Veterinary Record*, **100**, 150–153.

Bradley, R. (1993). The research programme on transmissible spongiform encephalopathies in Britain with special reference to bovine spongiform encephalopathy. *Developments in Biological Standards*, **80**, 157–170.

Brakel, W.J. & Leis, R.A. (1976). Impact of social disorganization on behaviour, milk yield and body weight of dairy cows. *Journal of Dairy Science*, **59**, 716–721.

Bramely, A.J. (1978). The effect of subclinical *Staphylococcus epidermis* infection of the lactating bovine udder on its susceptibility to infection with *Streptococcus* or *Escherichia coli*. *British Veterinary Journal*, **134**, 136.

Brantas, G.C. (1968). On the dominance order of Friesian-Dutch dairy cows. *Zeitschrift Tierzuchtung Zuchtungsbiologie*, **84**, 127–151.

Breland, K. & Breland, M. (1966). *Animal Behaviour*. Macmillan, New York.

Breuer, K., Hemsworth, P.H., Barnett, J.L., Matthews, L.R. & Coleman, G.J. (2000). Behavioural response to humans and the productivity of commercial dairy cows. *Applied Animal Behaviour Science*, **66**, 273–288.

Broom, D.M. (1983). Stereotypies as animal welfare indicators. In *Indicators Relevant to Farm Animal Welfare* (ed. D. Smidt), pp. 81–87. Martinus Nijhoff, Boston.

Broom, D.M. (1986). Indicators of poor welfare. *British Veterinary Journal*, **142**, 524–526.

Broom, D.M. & Leaver, J.D. (1978). The effects of group-housing or partial isolation on later social behaviour of calves. *Animal Behaviour*, **26**, 1255– 1263.

Broom, D.M., Kirkden, R., Blokhuis, H.J., Canali, E., Dijkhuizen, A.A., Fallon, R., Le Neindre, P., Saloniemi, H., Webster, A.J.F. & Van Houwelingen, P. (1995). *Report on the Welfare of Calves*. Scientific Veterinary Committee Animal Welfare Section. EU Directorate-General for Agriculture VI/BII.2.

Brown, W.G. Jr. (1974). Some aspects of beef cattle behaviour as related to productivity. *Dissertation Abstracts International* B, **34**, 1805.

Brownlee, A. (1954). Play in domestic cattle in Britain: an analysis of its nature. *British Veterinary Journal*, **110**, 48–68.

Bryson, R.W. & Thomson, J.W. (1976). Laboratory and field control of clinical mastitis in dairy cows around Bulawayo. *Journal of the South African Veterinary Association*, **47**, 201–203.

Buddenberg, B.J., Brown, C.J., Johnson, Z.B. & Honea, R.S. (1986). Maternal behaviour of beef cows at parturition. *Journal of Animal Science*, **62**, 42–46.

Bumstead, N., Millard, B.M., Barrow, P. & Cook, J.K.A. (1991). Genetic basis of disease resistance in chickens. In *Breeding for Disease Resistance* (eds J.B. Owen and R.F.E. Axford), pp. 10–23. CABI, Slough.

Burrow, H.M. & Corbet, N.J. (1999). Genetic and environmental factors affecting temperament of zebu and zebu-derived beef cattle grazed at pasture in the tropics. *Australian Journal of Agricultural Research*, **51**, 155–162.

Burt, A.W.A. & Dunton, C.R. (1967). Effect of frequency of feeding upon food utilization by ruminants. *Proceedings of the Nutrition Society*, **26**, 181–190.

Busch, B. & Kramer, S. (1995). Prophylactical tail docking in fattening bulls. *Deutsche Tierarztliche Wochenschrift*, **102**, 127–129.

Campling, R.C. & Morgan, C.A. (1981). Eating behaviour of housed cows – a review. *Dairy Science Abstracts*, **43**, 57–63.

Castellanos, F., Galina, C.S., Orihuela, J.A., NavarroFierro, R. & Mondragon, R. (1997). Estrous expression in dairy cows and heifers (*Bos taurus*) following repeated PGF(2 alpha) injection and choice of selecting a mounting partner. *Applied Animal Behaviour Science*, **51**, 29–37.

Cermak, J. (1987). The design of cubicles for British Friesian dairy cows with reference to body weight and dimensions, spatial behaviour and upper leg lameness. In *Cattle Housing Systems, Lameness and Behaviour* (eds H.K. Wierenga and D.J. Peterse), pp. 119–128. Martinus Nijhoff, Dordrecht.

Chambers, J.D. & Mingay, G.E. (1966). *The Agricultural Revolution, 1750–1880*, pp. 30–33. Batsford, London.

Chapman, A.M. & Casida, L.E. (1937). Analysis of variation in the sexual cycle and some of its component phases with special reference to cattle. *Journal of Agricultural Research*, **54**, 417.

Charlier, C., Coppieters, W., Farnir, F., Grobet, L., Leroy, P.L., Michaux, C., Mni, M., Schwers, A., Vanmanshoven, P., Hanset, R. & Georges, M. (1995). The mh gene causing double muscling in cattle maps to bovine chromosome 2. *Mammalian Genome*, **6**, 788–792.

Chaves, A.H., da Silva, J.F., Pinheiro, A.J.R., Valadares, S.D. & de Campos, O.F. (1999). Selection of isolates of *Lactobacillus acidophilus* used as probiotic for calves. *Revista Brasileira De Zootecnia – Brazilian Journal of Animal Science*, **28**, 1093–1101.

Chenoweth, P.J. (1983). Sexual behaviour of the bull: a review. *Journal of Dairy Science*, **66**, 173–179.

Chenoweth, P.J. (1994). Aspects of reproduction in female *Bos indicus* cattle: a review. *Australian Veterinary Journal*, **71**, 422–426.

Chiy, P.C. & Phillips, C.J.C. (1991). The effects of sodium chloride application to pasture, or its direct supplementation, on dairy cow production and grazing preference. *Grass and Forage Science*, **46**, 325–331.

Chiy, P.C. & Phillips, C.J.C. (1999a). Sodium fertilizer application to pasture. 8. Turnover and defoliation of leaf tissue. *Grass and Forage Science*, **54**, 297–311.

Chiy, P.C. & Phillips, C.J.C. (1999b). The rate of intake of sweet, salty and bitter concentrates by dairy cows. *Animal Science*, **68**, 731–740.

Church, J.S., Hudson, R.J. & Rutley, B.D. (1999). Performance of American bison (*Bos bison*) in feedlots. *Journal of Animal and Feed Sciences*, **8**, 513–523.

Cid, M.S. and Brizuela, M.A. (1998). Heterogeneity in tall fescue pastures created and sustained by cattle grazing. *Journal of Range Management*, **51**, 644–649.

Clark, P.W., Ricketts, R.E. & Krause, G.F. (1977). Effect on milk yield of moving cows from group to group. *Journal of Dairy Science*, **60**, 716–721.

Clarkson, M.J., Downham, D.Y., Faull, W.B., Huughes, J.W., Manson, F.J., Merritt, J.B., Murray, R.D., Russell, W.B., Sucherst, J.E. & Ward, W.R. (1996). Incidence and prevalence of lameness in diary cattle. *Veterinary Record*, **138**, 563–567.

Clutton Brock, T.H., Greenwood, P.J. & Powell, R.P. (1976). Ranks and relationships in Highland ponies and Highland cows. *Zuchtungskunde Tierpsychologie*, **41**, 202–216.

Cockwill, C.L., T.A. McAllister *et al.* (2000). Individual intake of mineral and molasses supplements by cows, heifers and calves. *Canadian Journal of Animal Science*, **80**, 681–690.

Coffey, E.M., Vinson, W.E. & Pearson, R.E. (1986). Potential of somatic cell concentration in milk as a sire selection criterion to reduce mastitis in dairy cattle. *Journal of Dairy Science*, **69**, 2163–2172.

Collis, K.A. (1976). An investigation of factors related to the dominance order of a herd of dairy cows of similar age and breed. *Applied Animal Ethology*, **2**, 167–173.

Collis, P.W., Kay, S.J., Grant, A.J. & Quick, A.J. (1979). The effect on social organisation and milk production of minor group alterations in dairy cattle. *Applied Animal Ethology*, **4**, 61–70.

Connell, J. (1984). International transport of farm animals intended for slaughter. CEC report EUR 9556 EN. Commission of the European Community, Brussels.

Cooper, M.D., Arney, D.R. & Phillips, C.J.C. (2002). Differences in the behaviour of high and low yielding dairy cows selected by genetic merit. *Proceedings of the British Society of Animal Science*, p. 220.

Cortes, R., Orihuela, J.A. & Galina, C.S. (1999). Effect of sexual partners on the oestrous behaviour response in Zebu cattle (*Bos indicus*) following synchronisation with a progestagen (Synchro-mate B). *Asian-Australasian Journal of Animal Sciences*, **12**, 515–519.

Coulon, J.B. (1984). Feeding behaviour of crossbred Charolais cattle in a humid tropical environment. *Revue d'Elevage et de Medicine Veterinaire des Pays Tropicaux*, **37**, 185–190.

Cowie, A.T. (1979). Anatomy and physiology of the udder. In *Machine Milking* (eds C.C. Thiel and F.H. Dodd), pp. 156–178. National Institute for Research in Dairying/ Hannah Research Institute Technical Bulletin No. 1.

Craig, J.V. & Muir, W.M. (1996). Group selection for adaptation to multiple-hen cages: beak-related mortality, feathering, and body weight responses. *Poultry Science* **75**, 294–302.

Creel, S.R. & Albright, J.L. (1988). The effects of neonatal social isolation on the behaviour and endocrine function of Holstein calves. *Applied Animal Behaviour Science*, **21**, 293–306.

Crichton, J.S. & Lishman, A.W. (1989). Factors influencing sexual behaviour of young *Bos indicus* bulls under pen and pasture mating conditions. *Applied Animal Behaviour Science*, **21**, 281–292.

Dannenmann, K., Buchenauer, D. & Fliegener, H. (1985). The behaviour of calves under four levels of lighting. *Applied Animal Behaviour Science*, **13**, 243–258.

Dantzer, R. (1986). Behavioural, physiological and functional aspects of stereotyped behaviour: a review and a reinterpretation. *Journal of Animal Science,* **62**, 1776–1786.

Das, S.M., Redbo, I. & Wiktorsson, H. (2000). Effect of age of calf on suckling behaviour and other behavioural activities of Zebu and crossbred calves during restricted suckling periods. *Applied Animal Behaviour Science*, **67**, 47–57.

Dawkins, R. (1976). *The Selfish Gene*. Oxford University Press, Oxford.

Debreceni, O. & Juhas, P. (1999). Milk-sucking in dairy cattle in loose housing in Slovakia. *Livestock Production Science*, **61,** 1–6.

DeGrazia, D. (1996). *Taking Animals Seriously*, 312 pp. Cambridge University Press, Cambridge.

Deharang, D. & Godeau, J.M. (1991). The durations of masticating activities and the feed energetic utilization of Friesian lactating cows on maize silage-based rations. *Journal of Animal Physiology and Animal Nutrition*, **65**, 194–205.

Dehnhard, M. & Claus, R. (1996). Attempts to purify and characterize the estrus-signalling pheromone from cow urine. *Theriogenology*, **46**, 13–22.

Dellmeier, C., Friend, E. & Cbur, E. (1990). Effects of changing housing on open-field behaviour. *Applied Animal Behaviour Science*, **26**, 215–230.

Delpietro, H.A. (1989). Case reports on defensive behaviour in equine and bovine subjects in response to vocalisation of the common vampire bat (*Desmodus rotundus*). *Applied Animal Behaviour Science*, **22**, 377–380.

De Passille, A.M. (2001). Sucking motivation and related problems in calves. *Applied Animal Behaviour Science*, **72,** 175–187.

De Passille, A.M.B., Metz, J.H.M., Mekking, P. & Wiepkema, P.R. (1992). Does drinking milk stimulate sucking in young calves? *Applied Animal Behaviour Science*, **34,** 23–36.

De Passille, A.M.B., Christopherson, R. & Rushen, J. (1993). Nonnutritive sucking by the calf and postprandial secretion of insulin, CCK, and gastrin. *Physiology and Behavior*, **54**, 1069–1073.

Devyatkina, G.S. (1986). Selection of cows for stress resistance. *Zhivotnovodsto*, **9**, 40–42.

Dickson, D.P., Barr, G.R. & Wieckert, D.A. (1967). Social relationships of dairy cows in a feed lot. *Behaviour*, **29**, 196–203.

Dickson, D.P., Barr, G.R., Johnson, L.P. & Wieckert, D.A. (1970). Social dominance and temperament of dairy cows. *Journal of Dairy Science*, **53**, 904–907.

Dijkhuizen, T.J. & van Eerdenburg, F.J. (1997). Behavioural signs of oestrus during pregnancy in lactating dairy cows. *Veterinary Quarterly*, **19**, 194–196.

Doenhoff, M.J. & Davies, A.J.S. (1991). Genetic improvement of the immune system: possibilities for animals. In *Breeding for Disease Resistance* (eds. J.B. Owen and R.F.E. Axford), pp. 24–53. CABI, Slough.

Dohi, H., Yamada, A., Tsuda, S., Sumikawa, T. & Entsu, S. (1993). A pressure-sensitive sensor for measuring the characteristics of standing mounts of cattle. *Journal of Animal Science*, **71**, 369–372.

Donaldson, S.L. (1970). The effects of early feeding and rearing experience on social maternal and milking parlour behaviour in dairy cattle. PhD thesis, Purdue University, Indiana.

Dorner, G. (1989). Hormone-dependent brain development and neuroendocrine prophylactics. *Experimental Clinical Endocrinology,* **94**, 4–22.

Dougherty, C.T., Knapp, F.W., Burrus, P.B., Willis, D.C. and Bradley, N.W. (1993a). Face flies (*Musca autumnalis Degeer*) and the behaviour of grazing beef cattle. *Applied Animal Behaviour Science*, **35**, 313–326.

Dougherty, C.T., Knapp, F.W., Burns, P.B., Willis, D.C., Burg, J.G., Cornelius, P.L. & Bradley, N.W. (1993b). Stable flies (*Stomoxys calcitrans* L.) and the behaviour of grazing beef cattle. *Applied Animal Behaviour Science*, **35**, 215–233.

Dudzinski, M.L., Muller, W.J., Low, W.A. & Schuh, H.J. (1982). Relationship between dispersion behaviour of free-ranging cattle and forage conditions. *Applied Animal Ethology*, **8**, 225–241.

Dumelow, J. & Albutt, R. (1990). The effect of floor design on skid resistance in dairy cattle buildings. In *Update in Cattle Lameness* (ed. R. Murray), pp. 130–142. British Cattle Veterinary Association, University of Liverpool.

Dumont, B. & Boissy, A. (1999). Impact of social on grazing behaviour in herbivores. *Productions Animales*, **12**, 3–10.

Dyson, S.J. (1995). No foot, no horse. In *Welfare Problems of Food Animals and Horses 1. The Foot*, pp. 4–8. Symposium Proceedings. The Animal Health Trust, BVA Animal Welfare Foundation and RSPCA, Newmarket.

Edfors-Lilja, I. (1996). Genetic analysis of immune capacity in pigs. *Book of Abstracts of the 47th Meeting of the European Association for Animal Production*. Wageningen Pers, Wageningen.

Edmondson, A.J., Lean, I.J., Weaver, L.D., Farver, T. & Webster, G. (1989). A body condition scoring scoring chart for dairy cows. *Journal of Dairy Science*, **72**, 68–78.

Edwards, S.A. (1979). The timing of parturition in dairy cattle. *Journal of Agricultural Science, Cambridge*, **93**, 359–363.

Edwards, S.A. (1983). The behaviour of dairy cows and their newborn calves in individual or group housing. *Applied Animal Ethology*, **10**, 191–198.

Edwards, T.A. (1995). Buller syndrome: what's behind this abnormal sexual behavior? *Large Animal Veterinarian*, **50**, 6–8.

Edwards, S.A. & Broom, D.M. (1982). Behavioural interactions of dairy cows with their newborn calves and the effects of rarity. *Animal Behaviour*, **30**, 525–535.

Ekman, P. (1979). About brows, emotional and conversational signals. In *Human Ethology* (eds M. von Cranach, K. Foppa, W. Lepenies and D. Ploog), pp. 169–248. Cambridge University Press, Cambridge.

Elcher, S.D., Morrow-Tesch, J.L., Albright, J.L. & Williams, R.E. (2001). Tail docking alters fly numbers, fly-avoidance bahavior and cleanliness, but not physiological measures. *Journal of Dairy Science*, **84**, 1822–1828.

Ellingson, R.J. (1972). Development of wakefulness–sleep cycles and associated EEG patterns in mammals. In *Sleep and the Maturing Nervous System* (eds C.D. Clemente, D.P. Purpura and F.E. Mayer), pp. 165–174. Academic Press, New York.

Emanuelson, U., Danell, B. & Philipsson, J. (1988). General parameters for clinical mastitis, somatic cell counts and milk production estimated by multiple trait restricted maximum likelihood. *Journal of Dairy Science*, **71**, 467–476.

Eriksson, J.A. (1991). Mastitis in cattle. In *Breeding for Disease Resistance* (eds J.B. Owen and R.F.E. Axford), pp. 394–412. CABI, Slough.

Esslemont, R.J. & Bryant, M.J. (1976). Oestrous behaviour in a herd of dairy cows. *Veterinary Record*, **99**, 472–475.

Esslemont, R.J., Glencross, R.C., Bryant, M.J. & Pope, C.S. (1980). A quantitative study of pre-ovulatory behaviour in cattle. *Applied Animal Ethology*, **6**, 1–17.

Esslemont, R.J., Bailie, J.H. and Cooper, M.J. (1985). *Fertility Management in Dairy Cattle*. Collins Professional and Technical Books, London.

Esteban, E., Kass, P.H., Weaver, L.D., Rowe, J.D., Holmberg, C.A., Franti, C.E. & Troutt, H.F. (1994). Reproductive performance in high producing dairy cows treated with recombinant bovine somatotropin. *Journal of Dairy Science*, **77**, 3371–3381.

Evans, A. (1990). Moosic is for cows, too. *Hoard's Dairyman*, **135**, 721.

Fagen, R. (1981). *Animal Play Behaviour*. Oxford University Press, Oxford.

Fall, A., Pearson, R.A. & Lawrence, P.R. (1997). Nutrition of draught oxen in semi-arid west Africa. 1. Energy expenditure by oxen working on soils of different consistencies. *Animal Science*, **64**, 209–215.

Farm Animal Welfare Council. (1991). Report on the European Commission proposals on the Transport of Animals. Farm Animal Welfare Council, London.

Faye, B. & Lescourret, F. (1989). Environmental factors associated with lameness in dairy cattle. *Preventive Veterinary Medicine*, **7**, 267–287.

Feddersen-Petersen, D. (1991). (Behavior disorders in dogs – study of their classification). Verhaltensstorungen bei Hunden–Versuch ihrer Klassifizierung. *Deutsch Tierarztliche Wochenschreib*, **98**, 15–19.

Feldman, R., Aizinbud, E., Schindler, H. & Broda, H. (1978). The electrical conductivity inside the bovine vaginal wall. *Animal Production*, **26**, 61–65.

Felius, M. (1985). *Genus Bos: Cattle Breeds of the World*, p. ix. MSD Agvet, Rahway, New Jersey.

Fernandes, C.G., Schild, A.L., Riet Correa, F., Baialardi, C.E. & Stigger, A.L. (2000). Pituitary abscess in young calves associated with the use of a controlled suckling device. *Journal of Veterinary Diagnosis and Investigation*, **12,** 70–71.

Fernandez, G., Alvarez, P., San Primitivo, F. & de la Fuente, L.F. (1995). Factors affecting variation of udder traits of dairy ewes. *Journal of Dairy Science*, **78**, 842–849.

Fischerleitner, F. & Stanek, C. (1987). Arthritic lesions in the digital, carpal and tarsal joints of AI bulls and their influence on sexual behaviour and semen production. *Wiener Tierarztliche Monatsschrift*, **74**, 157–163.

Fisher, A.D., Crowe, M.A., de la Varga, M.E.A. & Enright, W.J. (1996). Effect of castration method and the provision of local anesthesia on plasma cortisol, scrotal circumference, growth, and feed intake of bull calves. *Journal of Animal Science*, **74,** 2336–2343.

Fisher, A.D., Crowe, M.A., O'Kiely, P. & Enright, W.J. (1997a). Growth, behaviour, adrenal and immune responses of finishing beef heifers housed on slatted floors at 1.5, 2.0, 2.5 or 3.0 m^2 space allowance. *Livestock Production Science*, **51**, 245–254.

Fisher, A.D., Crowe, M.A., Prendiville, D.J. & Enright, W.J. (1997b). Indoor space allowance: effects on growth, behaviour, adrenal and immune responses of finishing beef heifers. *Animal Science*, **64,** 53–62.

Fisher, A.D., Knight, T.W., Cosgrove, G.P., Death, A.F., Anderson, C.B., Duganzich, D.M. & Matthews, L.R. (2001). Effects of surgical or banding castration on stress responses and behaviour of bulls. *Australian Veterinary Journal*, **79,** 279–284.

Fitsimons, J.J. (1979). *The Physiology of Thirst and Sodium Appetite*, p. 121. Cambridge University Press, Cambridge.

Flower, F.C. & Weary, D.M. (2001). Effects of early separation on the dairy cow and calf: 2. Separation at 1 day and 2 weeks after birth. *Applied Animal Behaviour Science*, **70**, 275–284.

Fordyce, G. & Goddard, M.E. (1984). Maternal influence on the temperament of *Bos indicus* cross cows. *Proceedings of the Australian Society of Animal Production*, **15**, 345–348.

Fordyce, G., Goddard, M.E. & Seifert, G.W. (1982). The measurement of temperament in cattle and the effect of genotype and experience. *Proceedings of the Australian Society of Animal Production*, **14**, 329–332.

Fraser, A.F. (1985). Kinetic behaviour of the fetus and newborn. In *Ethology of Farm Animals* (ed. A.F. Fraser), pp. 111–125. Elsevier, Amsterdam.

Fraser, A.F. & Broom, D.M. (1990). *Farm Animal Behaviour and Welfare*. Baillière Tindall, London.

Fregonesi, J.A. & Leaver, J.D. (2001). Behaviour, performance and health indicators of welfare for dairy cows housed in strawyard or cubicle systems. *Livestock Production Science*, **68**, 205–216.

French, J.M., Moore, G.F., Perry, G.C. & Long, S.E. (1989). Behavioural predictors of oestrus in domestic cattle. *Animal Behaviour*, **38**, 913–919.

Friend, T.H., Lay, D.C., Bushong, D.M. & Pierce, D.W. (1994). Wisconsin's stale calf issue and a study designed to resolve some of the animal-welfare concerns. *Journal of Animal Science*, **72**, 2260–2263.

Fritz, H., de Garine Wichatitsky, M. & Letessier, G. (1996). Habitat use by sympatric wild and domestic herbivores in an African savanna woodland: the influence of cattle spatial behaviour. *Journal of Applied Ecology*, **33**, 589–598.

Fryxell, J.M. (1991). Forage quality and aggregation in herbivores. *American Naturalist*, **138**, 478–498.

Gadbury, J.C. (1975). Some preliminary field observations on the order of entry of cows into herringbone parlours. *Applied Animal Ethology*, **1**, 275–281.

Gardner, L.P. (1937). The response of cows in a discrimination problem. *Journal of Comparative Psychology*, **23**, 35–37.

Garner, F.H. (1989). *Farming in Our Lifetime*. Royal Agricultural Benevolent Institution, Oxford.

Gendin, S. (1989). What should a Jew do? *Between the Species*, **5**, 25–32

Gilbert, B.J. & Arave, C.W. (1986). Ability of cattle to distinguish among different wavelengths of light. *Journal of Dairy Science*, **69**, 825–832.

Ginnett, T.F., Dankosky, J.A., Deo, G., & Demment, M.W. (1999). Patch depression in grazers: the roles of biomass distribution and residual stems. *Functional Ecology*, **13**, 37–44.

Godfrey, R.W., Lunstra, D.D., French, J.A., Schwartz, J., Armstrong, D.L. & Simmons, L.G. (1991). Estrous synchronization in the Gaur (*Bos gaurus*) – behavior and fertility to artificial-insemination after prostaglandin treatment. *Zoo Biology*, **10**, 35–41.

Goings, R.L., Braund, D.G., Dodge, K.L. & Steele, R.L. (1975). Effect of TMR feeding frequency on performance of lactating cows. Cooperative Research Farms Trial, Charlotteville, New York (Agway Inc., Syracuse, NY). Cited in Nocek and Braund (1985),

Gonyou, H.W., Christopherson, R.J. & Young, B.A. (1979). Effects of cold temperature and winter conditions on some aspects of behaviour of feedlot cattle. *Applied Animal Ethology*, **5**, 113–124.

Gordon, I. & Illius, A.W. (1988). Incisor arcade structure and diet selection in ruminants. *Functional Ecology*, **2**, 15–22.

Graf, B. & Senn, M. (1999). Behavioural and physiological responses of calves to dehorning by heat cauterization with or without local anaesthesia. *Applied Animal Behaviour Science*, **62**, 153–171.

Grandin, T. (1983). Welfare requirements of handling facilities. In *Farm Animal Housing and Welfare* (eds S.H. Baxter, M.R. Baxter and J.A.C. McCormack), pp. 137–149. Martinus Nijhoff, The Hague.

Grandin, T. (1993). Behavioral agitation during handling of cattle is persistent over time. *Applied Animal Behaviour Science*, **36**, 1–9.

Grandin, T. (1996). Factors that impede animal movement at slaughter plants. *Journal of the American Veterinary Medical Association*, **209**, 757–759.

Grandin, T. (1998). The feasibility of using vocalization scoring as an indicator of poor welfare during cattle slaughter. *Applied Animal Behaviour Science*, **56**, 121–128.

Grandin, T. (2000). Effect of animal welfare audits of slaughter plants by a major fast food company on cattle handling and stunning practices. *Journal of the American Veterinary Medical Association*, **216**, 848–851.

Grandin, T. (2001). Cattle vocalizations are associated with handling and equipment problems at beef slaughter plants. *Applied Animal Behaviour Science*, **71**, 191–201.

Grandin, T., Odde, K.G., Schutz, D.N. & Behrns, L.M. (1994). The reluctance of cattle to change a learned choice may confound preference tests. *Applied Animal Behaviour Science* **39**, 21–28.

Greene W.A., Gano A.M., Smith, K.L., Hogan, J.S. & Todhunter, D.A. (1991). Comparison of probiotic and antibiotic intramammary therapy of cattle with elevated somatic cell counts. *Journal of Dairy Science,* **74**, 2976–2981.

Greenough, P.R. (1991). A review of factors predisposing to lameness in cattle. In *Breeding for Disease Resistance* (eds J.B. Owen and R.F.E. Axford), pp. 371–393. CABI, Slough.

Gregory, N. (1998). *Animal Welfare and Meat Science*. CAB International, Wallingford.

Grondahl Nielsen, C. & Simonsen, H.B. (1999). Behavioural, endocrine and cardiac responses in young calves undergoing dehorning without and with use of sedation and analgesia. *The Veterinary Journal*, **158,** 14–20.

Gross, J.E., Shipley, L.A., Hobbs, N.T., Spalinger, D.E., & Wunder, B.A. (1993). Functional-response of herbivores in food-concentrated patches – tests of a mechanistic model. *Ecology*, **74**, 778–791.

Gupta, S.C., Gupta, N. & Nivsarkar, A.E. (1999). *Mithun – A Bovine of Indian Origin*. Indian Council of Agricultural Research, New Delhi.

Gustafson, G.M. & LundMagnussen, E. (1995). Effect of daily exercise on the getting up and lying down behaviour of tied dairy cows. *Preventive Veterinary Medicine*, **25**, 27–36.

Gwazdauskas, F.C., Lineweaver, J.A. & McGilliard, M.L. (1983). Environmental and management factors affecting oestrous activity in dairy cattle. *Journal of Dairy Science*, **66**, 1510–1514.

Hackett, A.J. & McAllister, A.J. (1984). Onset of oestrus in dairy cows maintained indoors year-round. *Journal of Dairy Science*, **67**, 1793–1797.

Hafez, E.S.E., Schwein, M.W. & Ewbank, R. (1969). The behaviour of cattle. In *The Behaviour of Domestic Animals* (ed. E.S.E. Hafez), pp. 235–295. Baillière Tindall and Cassell, London.

Hahn, M.V., McDaniel, B.T. & Wilk, J.C. (1977). Repeatability of measurements of variation in feet of dairy cattle. *Journal of Dairy Science*, **60** (Suppl. 1), 146 (Abstract).

Halachmi, I., Edan, Y., Maltz, E., Peiper, U.M., Moallem, U. & Brukental, I. (1998). A real-time control system for individual dairy cow food intake. *Computers and Electronics in Agriculture*, **20**, 131–144.

Haley, D.B., Rushen, J. & de Passillé, A.M. (2000). Behavioural indicators of cow comfort: activity and resting behaviour of dairy cows in two types of housing. *Canadian Journal of Animal Science*, **80**, 257–263.

Hall, S.J.G. & Moore, G.F. (1986). Feral cattle of Swona, Orkney Islands. *Mammal Review*, **16**, 89–96.

Hall, S.S., Vince, M.A., Walser, E.S. & Garson, P.J. (1988). Vocalisations of the Chillingham cattle. *Behaviour*, **104**, 78–104.

Halley, R.J. & Dougall, B.M. (1962). The feed intake and performance of dairy cows fed on cut grass. *Journal of Dairy Research*, **29**, 241–248.

Hammell, K.L., Metz, J.H.M. & Mekking, P. (1988). Sucking behaviour of dairy calves fed milk ad libitum by bucket or teat. *Applied Animal Behaviour Science*, **20**, 275–285.

Hammond, J.A. (1927). *The Physiology of Reproduction in the Cow*. Cambridge University Press, London.

Hancock, J. (1950). Studies in monozygotic cattle twins. IV. Uniformity trials: grazing behaviour. *New Zealand Journal of Science and Technology* A, **32**, 22–59.

Hancock, J. (1953). Grazing behaviour of cattle. *Animal Breeding Abstracts*, **21**, 1–13.

Hansen, S.W. & Damgaard, B.M. (1993). Behavioural and adrenocortical coping strategies and the effect on eosinophil leucocyte level and heterophil/lymphocyte-ratio in beech marten (*Martes foina*). *Applied Animal Behaviour Science*, **35**, 369–388.

Hard, C.A.F., Segerstad, A.F. & Hellekant, G. (1989). The sweet taste in the calf. *Physiology and Behaviour*, **45**, 633–638, 1043–1047.

Hart, R.H., Hepworth, K.W., Smith, M.A. & Waggoner, J.W. (1991). Cattle grazing behavior on a foothill elk winter range in southeastern Wyoming. *Journal of Range Management*, **44**, 262–266.

Hasegawa, N., Nishiwaki, A., Sugawara, K. & Ito, I. (1997). The effects of social exchange between groups of lactating primiparous heifers on milk production, dominance order, behavior and adrenocortical response. *Applied Animal Behavioural Science*, **51**, 15–27.

Hayakawa, H., Takahashi, H. & Kikuchi, T. (1984). Influence of the attack of tabanid flies on the daily behaviour pattern of grazing cattle. *Annual Report of the Society of Plant Protection of North Japan*, **35**, 162–164.

Haynes, R.J. & Williams, P.H. (1999). Influence of stock camping behaviour on the soil microbiological and biochemical properties of grazed pastoral soils. *Biology and Fertility of Soils*, **28**, 253–258.

Hearnshaw, H. & Morris, C.A. (1984). Genetic and environmental effects on a temperament score in beef cattle. *Australian Journal of Agricultural Research*, **35**, 723–773.

Heffner, R.S. & Heffner, H.E. (1983). Hearing in large mammals: horses (*Equus Caballus*) and cattle (*Bos taurus*). *Behavioural Neuroscience*, **97**, 299–309.

Heffner, R.S. & Masterton, R.B. (1990). Sound localisation in mammals: brain-stem mechanisms. In *Comparative Perception, Vol. 1. Basic Mechanism* (eds M.A. Berkley and W.C. Stebbins). John Wiley and Sons, Chichester.

Helmer, S.D. & Britt, J.H. (1985). Mounting behaviour as affected by stage of oestrous cycle in Holstein heifers. *Journal of Dairy Science*, **68**, 1290–1296.

Hemsworth, P.H., Breuer, K. Barnett, J.L., Coleman, G.J. & Matthews, L.R. (1995). Behavioural responses to humans and the productivity of commercial dairy cows. In *Proceedings of the 29th International Congress of the International Society for Applied Ethology*, pp. 175–176.

Henke Drenkard, D.V., Gorewit, R.C., Scott, N.R. & Sagi, R. (1985). Milk production, health, behavior, and endocrine responses of cows exposed to electrical current during milking. *Journal of Dairy Science*, **68**, 2694–2702.

Henney, S.R., Killian, C.J. & Denver, D.R. (1990). Libido, hormone concentrations in blood plasma and semen characteristics in Holstein bulls. *Journal of Animal Science*, **68**, 2784–2792.

Henning, P.A. (1993). Transportation of animals by road for slaughter in South Africa. *Proceedings of the 4th International Symposium on Livestock Environment*, 6–9 July, pp. 536–541. American Society of Agricultural Engineers, St. Joseph, MI.

Hinch, G.N. & Lynch, J.J. (1987). A note on the effect of castration on the ease of movement and handling of young cattle in yards. *Animal Production*, **45**, 317–320.

Hinch, G.N., Thwaites, C.J., Lynch, J.J. & Pearson, A.J. (1982a). Spatial relationships within a herd of young sterile bulls and steers. *Applied Animal Behaviour Science*, **8**, 27–44.

Hinch, G.N., Lynch, J.J. & Thwaites, C.J. (1982b). Patterns and frequency of social interactions in young grazing bulls and steers. *Applied Animal Behaviour Science*, **9**, 15–30.

Hinde, R.A. (1970). *Animal Behaviour, A Synthesis of Ethology and Comparative Psychology*. McGraw-Hill, New York.

Hoffman, D.E., Spire, M.F., Scwenke, J.R. & Unrah, J.A. (1998). Effect of source of cattle and distance transported to a commercial slaughter facility on carcass bruises in mature beef cows. *Journal of Animal Science*, **212**, 668–672.

Homewood, K., Rodgers, W.A. & Arheni, K. (1987). Ecology of pastoralism in Ngorongoro Conservation Area, Tanzania. *Journal of Agricultural Science, Cambridge*, **108**, 47–72.

Hoogeveen, H. & Meijering, A. (eds) (2000). *Robotic Milking*. Wageningen Pers, The Hague.

Hopster, H., O'Connell, J.M. & Blokhuis, H.J. (1995). Acute effects of cow–calf separation on heart-rate, plasma-cortisol and behavior in multiparous dairy-cows. *Applied Animal Behaviour Science*, **44,** 1–8.

Hopster, H., van der Werf, J.T.N. & Blokhuis, H.J. (1998). Side preference of dairy cows in the milking parlour and its effects on behaviour and heart rate during milking. *Applied Animal Behaviour Science*, **55**, 213–229.

Horning, B. & Tost, J. (2001). Factors influencing the lying behaviour of dairy cows in cubicle houses. In *Proceedings of the 35th International Congress of the International Society for Applied Ethology*, Davis, California, 4–9 August 2001. Centre for Animal Welfare, Davis.

Hornsby, M. (1990). Abattoir killing causes pain from faulty stunning. *The Times*, 23 February.

Horrell, R.I., Kilgour, R., MacMillan, K.L. & Bremner, K. (1984). Evaluation of fluctuations in milk yield and parlour behaviour as indicators of oestrus in dairy cows. *Veterinary Record*, **114**, 36–39.

Houpt, K.A. & Wollney, C. (1989). Frequency of masturbation and time budgets of dairy bulls used for semen production. *Applied Animal Behaviour Science*, **24**, 217–225.

Houpt, K.A., Rivera, W. & Glickstein, L. (1989). The flehman response of bulls and cows. *Theriogenology*, **32**, 343–350.

Houseal, G.A. & Olson, B.E. (1995). Cattle use of microclimates on a northern latitude winter range. *Canadian Journal of Animal Science*, **75,** 501–507.

Hurnik, J.F., King, C.J. & Robertson, H.A. (1975). Oestrus and related behaviour in post partum Holstein cows. *Applied Animal Ethology*, **2**, 55.

Iggo, A. (1984). Pain in animals. Hume Memorial lecture, 15 November 1984. University Federation for Animal Welfare, London.

Illius, A.W. & Gordon, I.J. (1990). Diet selection and foraging behaviour in mammalian herbivores. In *Behavioural Mechanisms of Food Selection* (ed. R.N. Hughes), pp. 370–392. NATO, ASJ Series Vol. 20. NATO, Brussels.

Immonen, K., Ruusunen, M., Hissa, K. & Puolanne, E. (2000). Bovine muscle glycogen concentration in relation to finishing diet, slaughter and ultimate pH. *Meat Science*, **55**, 25–31.

Ingrand, S. (2000). Feeding behaviour, intake and performance in beef cattle managed in groups. *Productions Animales*, **13**, 151–163.

Irps, H. (1983). Results of research projects into the flooring preference of cattle. In *Farm Animal Housing and Welfare*, pp. 200–215. Martinus Nijhoff, The Hague.

Jackson, P.G.G. (1995). *Handbook of Veterinary Obstetrics*. W.B. Saunders, London.

Jan, L.B. & Nichelmann, M. (1993). Differences in behavior of free-ranging cattle in the tropical climate. *Applied Animal Behaviour Science*, **37,** 197–209.

Jaramillo, V.J. (1990). Small-scale heterogeneity in a semiarid grassland: the role of urine deposition by herbicides. *Dissertation Abstracts International B, Sciences and Engineering*, **50** (8), 3283 B.

Jensen, M.B. (1995). The effect of age at tethering on behavior of heifer calves. *Applied Animal Behaviour Science*, **43**, 227–238.

Jensen, M.B. (2001). A note on the effect of isolation during testing and length of previous confinement on locomotor behaviour during open-field test in dairy calves. *Applied Animal Behaviour Science*, **70**, 309–315.

Jensen, M.B. & Kyhn, R. (2000). Play behaviour in group-housed dairy calves, the effect of space allowance. *Applied Animal Behaviour Science*, **67**, 35–46.

Jensen, M.B., Vestergaard, K.S., Krohn, C.C. & Munksgaard, L. (1997). Effect of single versus group housing and space allowance on responses of calves during open-field tests. *Applied Animal Behaviour Science*, **54**, 109–121.

Jensen, M.B., Vestergaard, K.S. & Krohn, C.C. (1998). Play behaviour in dairy calves kept in pens: the effect of social contact and space allowance. *Applied Animal Behaviour Science*, **56**, 97–108.

Jensen, M.B., Munksgaard, L., Mogensen, L. & Krohn, C.C. (1999). Effects of housing in different social environments on open-field and social responses of female dairy calves. *Acta Agriculturae Scandinavica Section A – Animal Science*, **49**, 113–120.

Jezierski, T.A. & Podluzny, M. (1984). A quantitative analysis of social behaviour of different crossbreeds of dairy cattle in loose housing and its relationship to productivity. *Applied Animal Behaviour Science*, **13**, 31–40.

Jezierski, T.A., Koziorowski, M., Goszczynski, J. & Sieradzka, I. (1989). Homosexual and social behaviours of young bulls of different geno- and phenotypes and plasma concentrations of some hormones. *Applied Animal Behaviour Science*, **24**, 101–113.

Johannesson, T. & Ladewig, J. (2000). The effect of irregular feeding times on the behavior and growth of dairy calves. *Applied Animal Behaviour Science*, **69**, 103–111.

Johnston, A.M. & Edwards, D.S. (1996). Welfare implications of identification of cattle by ear tags. *Veterinary Record*, **138**, 612–614.

Jordan, T.C., Coe, C.L., Patterson, J. & Levine, S. (1984). Predictability and coping with separation in infant squirrel monkeys. *Behavioral Neuroscience*, **98**, 556–560.

Kabuga, J.D. (1993). The standing behavior of ndama cattle during idling in a night paddock. *Applied Animal Behaviour Science*, **37**, 17–29.

Kaneene, J.B. & Hurd, H.S. (1990). The National Animal Health Monitoring Sustem in Michigan. I. Design, data and frequencies of selected dairy cattle diseases. *Preventive Veterinary Medicine*, **8**, 103–114.

Karatzias, H., Roubies, N., Polizopoulou, Z. & Papasteriades, A. (1995). (Tongue play and magnesium deficiency in dairy cattle). Zungenspielen und Manganmangel bei Milchkuhen. *Deutsch Tierarztliche Wochenschreib*, **102**, 352–353.

Keil, N.M., Audige, L. & Langhans, W. (2001). Is intersucking in dairy cows the continuation of a habit developed in early life? *Journal of Dairy Science*, **84,** 140–146.

Kelley, K.W., Oxbourne, C.A., Evermann, J.F., Parish, S.M. & Hinricks, D.G. (1981). Whole blood leukocytes vs separated mononuclear cell blastogenesis in calves. Time-dependent changes after shipping. *Canadian Journal of Comparative Medicine*, **45**, 249–258.

Kendler, K.S., Neale, M.C., Kessler, R.C., Heath, A.C. & Eaves, L.J. (1992). The genetic epidemiology of phobias in women. The interrelationship of agoraphobia, social phobia, situational phobia, and simple phobia. *Archives of General Psychiatry*, **49**, 273–281.

Kenny, F.J. & Tarrant, P.V. (1987a). The reaction of young bulls to short-haul road transport. *Applied Animal Behaviour Science*, **17**, 209–227.

Kenny, F.J. & Tarrant, P.V. (1987b). The behaviour of young Friesian bulls during social re-grouping at an abattoir: influence of an overhead electrified wire grid. *Applied Animal Behaviour Science*, **18**, 233–246.

Kiernm, W.R., Sherry, C.J., Schoke, L.M. & Sis, R.F. (1983). Homosexual behaviour in feedlot steers, an aggression hypothesis. *Applied Animal Ethology*, **11**, 187–195.

Kiley, M. (1972). The vocalisations of ungulates, their causation and function. *Zeitschrift fur Tierpsychologie*, **31**, 171–222.

Kiley-Worthington, M. (1976). The tail movements of ungulates, canids and felids with particular reference to their causation and function as displays. *Behaviour*, **56**, 69–115.

Kilgour, R. (1981). Use of the Hebb-Williams closed field test to study the learning ability of Jersey cows. *Animal Behaviour*, **29**, 850–860.

Kilgour, R. (1985). Libido – the sexual responsiveness of male farm animals. In *Ethology of Farm Animals* (ed. A.F. Fraser), pp. 313–322. World Animal Science Series AS, Elsevier Science Publishers, Amsterdam.

Kilgour, R. & Carnpin, D.N. (1973). The behaviour of entire bulls of different ages at pasture. *Proceedings of the New Zealand Society of Animal Production*, **33**, 125–133.

Kilgour, R., Spartholt, B.H., Smith, J.F., Bremner, K.J. & Morrison, M.C.L. (1977). Observations on the behaviour and factors influencing the sexually active group in cattle. *Proceedings of the New Zealand Society of Animal Production*, **37**, 128–135.

Kirchner, M. & Boxberger, J. (1987). Loading of the claws and the consequences of the design of slatted floors. In *Cattle Housing Systems, Lameness and Behaviour*, pp. 37–44. Martinus Nijhoff, The Hague.

Kirkden, R.D., Broom, D.M. & Phillips, C.J.C. (2001). Report on links between animal health, in the terms of the world trade organisation, and animal welfare. Cambridge University Animal Welfare Information Centre, Cambridge.

Klemm, W.R., Sherry, C.J., Schake, L.M. & Sis, R.F. (1983). Homosexual behaviour in steers – an aggression hypothesis. *Applied Animal Ethology*, **11**, 187–195.

Knierem, U. & Warran, N.K. (1993). The influence of the human-animal interaction in the milking parlour on the behaviour, heart-rate and milk yield of dairy cows. In *Proceedings of the 27th International Congress on Applied Ethology*, pp. 169–173. Humboldt University, Berlin.

Kondo, S. & Hurnick, J.F. (1987). Progress of social stabilisation in dairy cows after grouping. *Canadian Journal of Animal Science*, **67**, 1167 (Abstract).

Kondo, S., Sekeine, J., Okubo, M. & Asahida, Y. (1989). The effect of group size and space allowance on the agonistic and spacing behaviour of cattle. *Applied Animal Behaviour Science*, **24**, 127–135.

Konggaard, S.P., Krohn, C.C. & Agergaad, E. (1982). Investigations concerning feed intake and social behaviour among group fed cows under loose housing conditions. VI. Effects of different grouping criteria in dairy. *Beretning Jra Statens Husdyrbrugsforsog*, No. 553.

Kossaibati, M.A. & Esslemont, R.J. (2000). The incidence of lameness in 60 dairy herds in England. In *Proceedings of the XIIIth International Symposium on Disorders of the*

Ruminant Digit (eds C.M. Mortelaro, L. de Vecchis and A. Brizzi), p. 160:3. Fondazione Initiative Xooprofilattiche Zootechniche, Brescia, Italy.

Kovalcik, K. & Kovalcikova, M. (1974). Vplyv skupinoveho presumu prvostok cernos-trakateho plemena na priebeh ich laktacnej krivky. *Zivocisna Vyroba*, **19**, 945–952.

Kovalcik, K., Kovalcikova, M. & Brestensky, V. (1980). Comparison of the viour of newborn calves housed with the dam and in the calf-house. *Applied Animal Ethology*, **6**, 377–380.

Kovalcikova, M. & Kovalcik, K. (1984). Learning ability and memory in cattle of different age. In *Proceedings of the International Congress on Applied Ethology in Farm Animals* (eds J. Unshelm, G. Van Patten and C. Zeeb), pp. 65–69. KTBL, Darmstadt.

Krohn, C.C. (1978). The effect of group change on behaviour and production performance in large dairy herds. *Proceedings of the First World Congress on Ethology Applied to Zootechnology*, Madrid, Spain, 23–27 October 1978, E-1–26, 40.

Krohn, C.C. & Munksgaard, L. (1993). Behavior of dairy-cows kept in extensive (loose housing pasture) or intensive (tie stall) environments. 2. Lying and lying-down behavior. *Applied Animal Behaviour Science*, **37**, 1–16.

Krohn, C.C. & Rasmussen, M.D. (1992). (Dairy cows under extreme conditions: production, reproduction, health and stayability.) Malkekoer under ekstremt forskellige productionsbetingelser: ydelse, tilvaekst, reproduktion, sundhed og holdbarhed. *Landbrugsministeriet Statens Husdyrbrugsforsog (Danish Institute of Animal Science) Report No 70*. DIAS, Foulum.

Ladewig, J. & Smidt, D. (1989). Behavior, episodic secretion of cortisol, and adreno-cortical reactivity in bulls subjected to tethering. *Hormones and Behaviour*, **23**, 344–360.

Lang, H., Preisinger, R. & Kalm E. (1988). (Analysis of data on semen quality in Angeln cattle obtained from a breeding programme.) *Zuchthygiene*, **23**, 10–18.

Langbein, J. & Raasch, M.L. (2000). Investigations on the hiding behaviour of calves at pasture. *Archiv Fur Tierzucht – Archives of Animal Breeding*, **43**, 203–210.

Lanier, J.L., Grandin, T., Green, R.D., Avery, D. & McGee, K. (2000). The relationship between reaction to sudden, intermittent movements and sounds and temperament. *Journal of Animal Science*, **78**, 1467–1474.

Lawrence, P.R. & Stibbard, R.J. (1990). The energy costs of walking, carrying and pulling loads on flat surfaces by Brahman cattle and swamp buffalo. *Animal Production*, **50**, 29–39.

Lay, D.C., Randel, R.D., Friend, T.H., Jenkins, O.C., Neuendorff, D.A., Bushong, D.M., Lanier, E.K. & Bjorge, M.K. (1997). Effects of prenatal stress on suckling calves. *Journal of Animal Science*, **75**, 3143–3151.

Lazo, A. (1992). Facteurs déterminants du comportement grégaire de bovins retournés à l état sauvage. (The determinants of grouping behaviour in feral cattle.) *Revue d'Écologie – la Terre et al., Vie*, **41**, 51–66.

Lazo, A. (1994). Social segregation and the maintenance of social stability in a feral cattle population. *Animal Behaviour*, **48**, 1133–1141.

Le Du, Y.L.P., Baker, R.D. & Newberry, R.D. (1981). Herbage intake and milk production by grazing dairy cows. The effect of grazing severity under continuous stocking. *Grass and Forage Science*, **36**, 307–318.

Lee, D.H.K. (1953). Manual of field studies on the heat tolerance of domestic animals. Food and Agriculture Organisation Paper No. 38. FAO, Rome.

Le Neindre, P. (1993). Evaluating housing systems for veal calves. *Journal of Animal Science*, **71**, 1345–1354.

Le Neindre, P. (1989a). Influence of cattle rearing conditions and breed I relationships of mother and young. *Applied Animal Behaviour Science*, **23**, 117–127.

Le Neindre, P. (1989b). Influence of rearing conditions and breed on social and activity of cattle in novel environments. *Applied Animal Behaviour Science*, **23**, 129–140.

Le Neindre, P. & D'Hour, P. (1989). Effects of a postpartum separation on maternal responses in primiparous and multiparous cows. *Animal Behaviour*, **37**, 166–168.

Le Neindre, P. & Sourd, C. (1984). Influence of rearing conditions on subsequent social behaviour of Friesian and Salers heifers from birth to six months of age. *Applied Animal Behaviour Science*, **12**, 43–52.

Le Neindre, P., Veissier, I., Boissy, A. & Boivin, X. (1992). Effects of early environment on behaviour. In *Farm Animals and the Environment* (eds C.J.C. Phillips and D. Piggins), pp. 307–322. CAB International, Wallingford.

Le Neindre, P., Boivin, X. & Boissy, A. (1996). Handling of extensively kept animals. *Applied Animal Behaviour Science*, **49**, 73–81.

Lensink, B.J., Boivin, X., Pradel, P., Le Neindre, P. & Veissier, I. (2000a). Reducing veal calves' reactivity to people by providing additional human contact. *Journal of Animal Science*, **78**, 1213–1218.

Lensink, B.J., Fernandez, X., Boivin, X., Pradel, P., Le Neindre, P. & Veissier, I. (2000b). The impact of gentle contacts on ease of handling, welfare, and growth of calves and on quality of veal meat. *Journal of Animal Science*, **78**, 1219–1226.

Lensink, B.J., Raussi, S., Boivin, X., Pyykkoenen, M. & Veissier, I. (2001a). Reactions of calves to handling depend on housing condition and previous experience with humans. *Applied Animal Behaviour Science*, **70**, 187–199.

Lensink, B.J., Fernandez, X., Cozzi, G., Florand, L. & Veissier, I. (2001b). The influence of farmers' behavior on calves' reactions to transport and quality of veal meat. *Journal of Animal Science*, **79**, 642–652.

Leonard, F.C., O'Connell, J. & O'Farrell, K. (1994). Effect of different housing conditions on behaviour and foot lesions in Friesian heifers. *Veterinary Record*, **134**, 490–494.

Leonard, F.C., O'Connell, J.M. & O'Farrell, K.J. (1996). Effect of overcrowding on claw health in first-calved Friesian heifers. *British Veterinary Journal*, **152**, 459–472.

Leveteau, J. & Daval, G. (1981). Bases physiologiques de la localisation d'une source odorante. *Journal de Psychologie Normale et Pathologique*, **78**, 107–128.

Lewis, J.G. (1978). Game domestication for animal production in Kenya, behaviour and factors affecting the herding of eland, oryx, buffalo and zebu cattle. *Journal of Agricultural Science, Cambridge*, **90**, 587–595.

Lidfors, L. (1989). The use of getting up and lying down movements in the evaluation of cattle environments. *Veterinary Research Communications*, **13**, 307–324.

Lidfors, L.M. (1993). Cross-sucking in group-housed dairy calves before and after weaning off milk. *Applied Animal Behaviour Science*, **38**, 15–24.

Lidfors, L.M. (1996). Behavioural effects of separating the dairy calf immediately or 4 days post-partum. *Applied Animal Behaviour Science*, **49**, 269–283.

Little, W., Collis, K.A., Gleed, P.T., Sansom, B.F., Allen, W.M. & Quick, A.J. (1980). Effect of reduced water intake by lactating dairy cows on behaviour, milk yield and blood composition. *Veterinary Record*, **106**, 547–551.

Livesey, C.T., Johnston, A.M., Marsh, C., May, S.A. & Metcalf, J.A. (1998). The occurrence of hock injuries in primiparous Holstein cows in straw yards and cubicles with either butyl rubber mats or mattresses. In *Proceedings of the 10th International Symposium on Lameness in Ruminants*, pp. 42–43. Lucerne, Switzerland.

Livestock Auctioneers Association. (1996). *Code of Practice for the Guidance of Livestock Auctioneers in Livestock Auction Markets in England and Wales*. LAA, Coventry.

Livestock Auctioneers Association. (1998). *Conditions of Sale for Cattle, Calves, Sheep and Pigs, Recommended for Use by the Livestock Auctioneers Association*. LAA, Coventry.

Livingstone, A., Ley, S. & Waterman, A. (1992). Tactile and pain perception. In *Farm Animals and the Environment* (ed. C.J.C. Phillips), pp. 201–208. CAB International, Wallingford.

Llamas, L.F. (2001). An insight into the bullfighting industry in Spain. HND dissertation, Moulton College of Agriculture, University College Northampton.

Loberg, J. & Lidfors, L. (2001). Effect of milkflow rate and presence of a floating nipple on abnormal sucking between dairy calves. *Applied Animal Behaviour Science*, **72**, 189–199.

Loerch, S.C. & Fluharty, F.L. (2000). Use of trainer animals to improve performance and health of newly arrived feedlot calves. *Journal of Animal Science*, **78**, 539–545.

Loizos, C. (1966). Play in mammals. *Proceedings of the Symposium of the Zoological Society of London*, **18**, 1–9.

Longenbach, J.I., Heinrichs, A.J. & Graves, R.E. (1999). Feed bunk length requirements for Holstein dairy heifers. *Journal of Dairy Science*, **82**, 99–109.

Lopez, H., Orihuela, A. & Silva, E. (1999). Effect of the presence of a dominant bull on performance of two age group bulls in libido tests. *Applied Animal Behaviour Science*, **65**, 13–20.

LopezGatius, F., Rutllant, J., Labernia, J., Ibarz, A., LopezBejar, M. & Santolaria, P. (1996). Rheological behavior of the vaginal fluid of dairy cows at estrus. *Theriogenology*, **46**, 57–63.

Lorenz, K. (1966). *On Aggression*. Methuen, London.

Lorenz, K. (1996). *On Aggression*. Routledge, London.

Loscher, W. & Kas, G.(1998). Behavioural abnormalities in a dairy cow herd near a TV and radio transmitting antenna. *Praktische Tierarzt*, **79**, 437.

Lott, D. & Hart, B.L. (1977). Aggressive domination of cattle by Fulani herdsman and its relation to aggression in Fulani culture and personality. *Ethos*, **5**, 174–186.

Lovari, S. & Rosto, G. (1985). Feeding rate and social stress of female chamois foraging in groups. In *The Biology and Management of Mountain Ungulates* (ed. S. Lovari), pp. 102–105. Croom Helm, London.

Lowe, D.E., Steen, R.W.J., Beattie, V.E. & Moss, B.W. (2001). The effects of floor type systems on the performance, cleanliness, carcass composition and meat quality of housed finishing beef cattle. *Livestock Production Science*, **69**, 33–42.

Loynes, I.F. (1985). Dairy buildings – where now? *Farm Buildings Association Journal*, **34**, 39–41.

Lunstra, D.D., Boyd, G.W. & Corah, L.R. (1989). The effects of natural mating stimuli on serum luteinising hormones testosterone and oestradiol-17 beta in yearling beef bulls. *Journal of Animal Science*, **67**, 3277–3288.

Macaulay, A.S., Hahn, G.L., Clark, D.H. & Sisson, D.V. (1995). Comparison of calf housing types and tympanic temperature rhythms in Holstein calves. *Journal of Dairy Science*, **78**, 856–862.

MacFarlane, J.S. (1974). The effect of two post-weaning management systems on the social and sexual behaviour of zebu bulls. *Applied Animal Ethology*, **1**, 31–34.

Macha, J., & Olsarova, J. (1986). (Variability and heritabilities of grazing intensity in cattle). *Acta Universitatis Agriculturae Brno*, **34**, 313–320.

Machado, L.C.P., Hurnik, J.F. & Burton, J.H. (1997). The effect of amniotic fluid ingestion on the nociception of cows. *Physiology and Behavior*, **62**, 1339–1344.

Machado, L.C.P., Hurnik, J.F. & Ewing, K.K. (1998). A thermal threshold assay to measure the nociceptive response to morphine sulphate in cattle. *Canadian Journal of Veterinary Research – Revue Canadienne De Recherche Veterinaire*, **62**, 218–223.

Makarechian, M. & Berg, R.T. (1988). *Natural Service Fertility of Bulls in Pasture*. Agriculture and Forestry Bulletin, University of Alberta, Special Issue, pp. 10–12.

MacPhail, E. (1982). *Brain and Intelligence in Vertebrates*. Oxford University Press, Oxford.

Madsen, E.B. & Nielsen, K. (1985). A study of tail tip necrosis in young fattening bulls on slatted floors. *Nordic Veterinary Medicine*, **37**, 349–357.

Manson, F.J. & Appleby, M.C. (1990). Spacing of cows at a food trough. *Applied Animal Behaviour Science*, **26**, 69–81.

Manson, F.J. & Leaver, J.D. (1988). The influence of concentrate amount on locomotion and clinical lameness in dairy cattle. *Animal Production*, **47**, 185–190.

Marian, G.B., Smith, V.R., Wiley, J.E. & Barrett, G.R. (1950). The effect of sterile copulation on time of ovulation in dairy heifers. *Journal of Dairy Science*, **33**, 885–889.

Mattiello, S., Pozzi, A., Leggeri, P., Trabalza-Marinucci, M., Redaelli, W. & Carenzi, C. (1997). Social and spatial interactions between red deer and cattle in the Italian Alps. *Zeitschrift Fur Saugetierkunde–International Journal of Mammalian Biology*, **62**, 134–138.

Mattoni, M., Mukasa-Mugerwa, E., Cecchini, C. & Sovani, S. (1988). The reproductive performance of East African (*Bos indicus*) zebu cattle in Ethiopia.I. Estrous cycle length, duration, behaviour and ovulation time. *Theriogenology*, **30**, 961–971.

McDaniel, B.T., Verbeek, B., Hahn, M.V., Wilk, J.C. & Keown, J.F. (1984). Genetics of hoof measurements: repeatabilities, heritabilities and correlations with yields by lactation. *Journal of Dairy Science*, **67** (Suppl.), 199 (Abstract).

McDonald, C.L., Beilharz, R.G. & McCutchan, J.C. (1981). Training cattle to control by electric fences. *Applied Animal Ethology*, **7**, 113–121.

McMeekan, C.M., Mellor, D.J., Stafford, K.J., Bruce, R.A., Ward, R.N. & Gregory, N.G. (1998). Effects of local anaesthesia of 4 to 8 hours' duration on the acute cortisol response to scoop dehorning in calves. *Australian Veterinary Journal*, **76**, 281–285.

McNaughton, S.J. (1984). Grazing lawns, animals in herds, plant form and evolution. *American Naturalist*, **124**, 863–886.

Meddis, R. (1975). On the function of sleep. *Animal Behaviour*, **23**, 676–691.

Meddis, R. (1987). Sleep. In *The Oxford Companion to Animal Behaviour* (ed. D. McFarland), pp. 512–517. Oxford University Press, Oxford.

Melizi, M. (1985). Effect of different amounts of forced exercise on patella morphology in young beef bulls. II Morphology of the menisci in cattle in relation to age and exercise. *Veterinary Bulletin*, Abstract 055, 05334.

Mendoza-Ordones, G., Wilke, A. & Secland, G. (1988). The importance of certain feeding traits of dairy calves as an aid to selection. *Berichte, Humboldt Universitat zu Berlin*, **8**, 62–67.

Metz, J.H.M. (1984). The reaction of cows to short term deprivation of lying. *Applied Animal Behaviour Science*, **13**, 301–307.

Metz, J. & Metz, J.H.M. (1987). Behavioural phenomena related to normal and difficult deliveries in dairy cows. *Netherlands Journal of Agricultural Science*, **35**, 87–101.

Mialon, M.M., Renand, G., Krauss, D. & Menissier, F. (1999). Puberty of Charolais heifers in relation to growth rate. 1. Phenotypic variability. *Annales De Zootechnie*, **48**, 413–426.

Mialon, M.M., Renand, G., Krauss, D. & Menissier, F. (2000). Genetic variability of the length of postpartum anoestrus in Charolais cows and its relationship with age at puberty. *Genetics Selection Evolution*, **32**, 403–414.

Michalkiewicsz, M., Brzozowski, P. & Korwin-Kossakowski, J. (1984). Estrus manifestation in relation to milk yield, post-partum period, age and milk progesterone levels in dairy cows. In *Proceedings of the 10th International Congress on Animal Reproduction and Artificial Insemination*, Illinois, USA.

Milinski, M. & Parker, G.A. (1991). Competition for resources. In *Behavioural Ecology, an Evolutionary Approach* (eds J.R. Krebs and N.B. Davies), pp. 137–168. Blackwell Scientific Publications, Oxford.

Milk Marketing Board (MMB). (1991). *Dairy Facts and Figures*. The Dairy Federation of UK, MMB, Surrey.

Mill, J.M. & Ward, W.R. (1994). Lameness in dairy cows and farmers' knowledge, training and awareness. *Veterinary Record*, **134**, 162–164.

Miller, C. (2001). Childhood animal cruelty and interpersonal violence. *Clinical Psychology Review*, **21**, 735–749.

Ministry of Agriculture, Fisheries and Food. (1997). *The Welfare of Animals Transport Order*. MAFF, London.

Ministry of Agriculture, Fisheries and Food. (1998). *Guidance on the Transport of Casualty Animals*. MAFF, London.

Ministry of Agriculture, Fisheries and Food. (2000). Enforcement of animal welfare. http://www.maff.gov.ac.uk/animalh/welfare/on-farm/on-farm-oindex.htm

Minon, D.P., Cauhepe, M.A., Lorenzo, M.S., Colombo, I., Brizuela, M.A. & Miguel, M.C. (1984). Comparative analysis of diets of two breeds of cattle on pasture in the Salado basin (Buenos Aires). Botanical composition of the diet. *Reysista Argentina de Produccio Animal*, **4**, 789–801.

Mishra, R.R., Chauhan, R.S. & Gupta, S.C. (1975). Studies of dairy temperament of Karan Swiss cows. *Indian Journal of Dairy Science*, **28**, 83–88.

Mistleberger, R.E. (1994). Circadian food-anticipatory activity: formal models and physiological mechanisms. *Neuroscience and Biobehavior Reviews*, **18**, 171–195.

Mitchell, C.D. (1974). Are the passageways in your cubicle building too slippery? *Farm Building Progress*, **37**, 17–20.

Mogensen, L., Krohn, C.C., Sorensen, J.T., Hindhede, J. & Nielsen, L.H. (1997a). Association between resting behaviour and live weight gain in dairy heifers housed in pens with different space allowance and floor type. *Applied Animal Behaviour Science*, **55**, 11–19.

Mogensen, L., Nielsen, L.H., Hindhede, J., Sorensen, J.T. & Krohn, C.C. (1997b). Effect of space allowance in deep bedding systems on resting behaviour, production and health of dairy heifers. *Acta Agriculturae Scandinavica Section A – Animal Science*, **47**, 178–186.

Mohamed, M.O. & Phillips, C.J.C. (2001). The effect of sodium supplementation of pregnant cows on the preference of their calves for concentrate with added sodium. *Proceedings of the British Society of Animal Science*, 135.

Mokhov, B.P. (1983). (Breeding of cattle for stereotyped behaviour.) *Doklady Vsesoyuznoi Akademi Sel skokkozyoistvennykh Nauk,* **9**, 32–35.

Monin, G. (1981). Double-muscling and sensitivity to stress. In *The Problem of Dark-cutting in Beef. Current Topics in Veterinary Medicine and Animal Science*, Vol. 10 (eds D.E. Hood and P.V. Tarrant), pp. 3–35. Martinus Nijhoff, The Hague.

Morrison, D.G., Williamson, W.D. & Humes, P.E. (1986). Estimates of heritabilities and correlations of traits associated with pelvic area in beef cattle. *Journal of Animal Science*, **63**, 432–437.

Mueller, C., Ladewig, J., Thielscher, H.H. & Smidt, D. (1989). Behavior and heart rate of heifers housed in tether stanchions without straw. *Physiology and Behavior*, **46**, 751–754.

Mulkens, F. & Geers, R. (1995). The influence of human–animal interactions in farm animal production and reproduction – a review. *Vlaams Diergeneeskundig Tijdschrift*, **64**, 157–162.

Muller, C.J.C., Botha, J.A. & Smith, W.A. (1996). Effect of confinement area on production, physiological parameters and behaviour of Friesian cows during winter in a temperate climate. *South African Journal of Animal Science – Suid-Afrikaanse Tydskrif Vir Veekunde*, **26**, 1–5.

Muller, M. & Brem, G. (1996). Intracellular, genetic or congenital immunisation – transgenic approaches to increase disease resistance of farm animals. *Journal of Biotechnology,* **44**, 233–242.

Munksgaard, L. & Herskin, M.S. (2001). Does milking frequency and energy concentration of the diet affect time budgets of high yielding cows. *Proceedings of the 35th International Congress of the International Society for Applied Ethology*, Davis, 4–9 August, 2001, p. 190. Center for Animal Welfare, Davis, CA.

Munksgaard, L. & Simonsen, H.B. (1995). Behavioral and pituitary–adrenal axis responses of tethered cows or cows kept in pens with slatted floors. *Acta Agriculturae Scandinavica Section A – Animal Science*, **45**, 132–138.

Munksgaard, L. & Simonsen, H.B. (1996). Behavioral and pituitary adrenal-axis responses of dairy cows to social isolation and deprivation of lying down. *Journal of Animal Science*, **74**, 769–778.

Munksgaard, L., Ingvartsen, K.L., Pedersen, L.J. & Nielsen, V.K.M. (1999). Deprivation of lying down affects behaviour and pituitary–adrenal axis responses in young bulls. *Acta Agriculturae Scandinavica Section A – Animal Science*, **49**, 172–178.

Murphey, R.M. & Moura-Duarte, F.A. (1983). Calf control by voice in a Brazilian dairy. *Applied Animal Ethology*, **11**, 7–18.

Murphey, R.M., Moura-Duarte, F.A., Coelho-Novoes, W. & Torres, M.C. (1981). Age group differences in bovine investigatory behaviour. *Developmental Psychobiology*, **14**, 117–125.

Murphey, R.M., Ruiz Miranda, C.R. & Duarte F.A. (1990). Maternal recognition in Gyr (*Bos indicus*) calves. *Applied Animal Behaviour Science*, **27**, 183–191.

Murphey, R.M., Paranhos da Costa, M.J.R., Gomes da Silva, R. & de Souza, R.C. (1995). Allonursing in river buffalo, *Bubalus bubalis*: neoptism, incompetence, or thievery? *Animal Behaviour*, **49**, 1611–1616.

Murray, M., Stear, M.J., Trail, J.C.M., Ieteren, G.D.M., Agyemang, K. & Dwinger, R.H. (1991). Trypanomiasis in cattle: prospects for control. In *Breeding for Disease Resistance* (eds J.B. Owen and R.F.E. Axford), pp. 203–223. CABI, Slough.

Murray, R.D., Downham, D.Y., Merritt, J.R., Russel, W.B. & Manson, F.J. (1994). Observer variation in field data describing foot shape in dairy cattle. *Research in Veterinary Science*, **56**, 265–269.

Murray, R.D., Cartwright, T.A., Downham, D.Y. & Murray, M.A. (1999). Some maternal factors associated with dystocia in Belgian Blue cattle. *Animal Science*, **69**, 105–113.

Nanging, C. (1989). Feeding dairy cattle in tropical regions of China. In *Feeding Dairy Cows in the Tropics* (eds A. Speedy and P.R. Sansoucy). Book No. 86. FAO Proceedings, Bangkok.

Nash, R. (1990). Adam's place in nature: respect or domination? *Journal of Agricultural Ethics*, **3**, 102–113.

National Research Council (1978). Nutrient Requirements of Dairy Cattle. In *Nutrient Requirements of Domestic Animals*, No. 3. National Academy of Science, Washington, DC.

Nayak, S. & Mishra, M. (1984). Dairy temperament of Red Sindhi, crossbred cows and Murrah buffaloes in relation to their milking ability and composition. *Indian Journal of Dairy Science*, **37**, 20–23.

New Zealand Dairy Board. (1961). 37th Farm Production Report, 1960–61. Farm Production Division, NZ Dairy Board, Wellington.

Nicholson, M.J. (1989). Depression of dry matter and water intake in Boran cattle, owing to physiological, volumetric and temporal limitations. *Animal Production*, **49**, 29–34.

Nickel, R., Schummer, A., Seiferle, E. & Frewein, J. (1986). *The Locomotor System of the Domestic Mammals*. Verlag Paul Parey, Berlin.

Nocek, J.E. & Braund, D.G. (1985). Effect of feeding frequency on diurnal dry matter and water consumption, liquid dilution rate, and milk yield in first lactation. *Journal of Dairy Science*, **68**, 2238–2247.

Nogge, G. & Staack, W. (1969). Flying behavior of the warble-fly and the panicking of cattle. *Behaviour*, **35**, 200–211.

O'Bleness, G.V., Van Vleck, L.E. & Henderson, C.R. (1960). Heritabilities of some type appraisal tests and their genetic and phenotypic correlations with production. *Journal of Dairy Science*, **43**, 1490–1498.

O'Connell, J., Giller, P.J. & Meaney, W. (1989). A comparison of dairy cattle behavioural patterns at pasture and during confinement. *Irish Journal of Agricultural Research*, **28**, 65–72.

Odagiri-Shimizu H. & Shimizu, K. (1999). Experimental analysis of the human perception threshold of a DC electric field. *Medicine and Biology in Engineering and Computing*, **37**, 727–732.

Odyuo, L.T., Jana, D.N. & Das, N. (1995). Maintenance behavior of Murrah buffalo under an intensive management system. *Applied Animal Behaviour Science*, **45**, 293–299.

O'Farrell, R.J. (1978). Heat detection – an observation problem. *Food and Farm Research*, **9**, 95–97.

Olofsson, J. & Wiktorsson, H. (2001). Competition for total mixed diets fed restrictively using one or four cows per feeding station. *Acta Agriculturae Scandinavica Section A – Animal Science*, **51**, 59–70.

Olson, K.C. & Malechek, J.C. (1988). Heifer nutrition and growth of short duration grazed crested wheatgrass. *Journal of Range Management*, **41**, 259–263.

Orihuela, A. (2000). Some factors affecting the behavioural manifestation of oestrus in cattle, a review. *Applied Animal Behaviour Science*, **70**, 1–16.

Orr, R.J., Penning, P.D., Harvey, A. & Champion, R.A. (1997). Diurnal patterns of intake rate by sheep grazing monocultures of ryegrass or white clover. *Applied Animal Behaviour Science*, **52**, 65–77.

Osterman, S. & Redbo, I. (2001). Effects of milking frequency on lying down and getting up behaviour in dairy cows. *Applied Animal Behaviour Science*, **70**, 167–176.

Owen, J.B. (1989). Welfare problems in animal breeding. In *Proceedings of the Farm Animal Behaviour and Welfare Course*, 12–13 September, 1989, University of Wales, Bangor, pp. 56–62.

Owen, J.B. (1990). Weight control and appetite: nature over nurture. *Animal Breeding Abstracts*, **58**, 583–591.

Paranhos da Costa, M.J.R. & Broom, D.M. (2000). Suckling and allosuckling in river buffalo calves and its relation with weight gain. *Applied Animal Behaviour Science*, **66**, 1–10.

Paranhos da Costa, M.J.R. & Broom, D.M. (2001). Consistency of side choice in the milking parlour by Holstein-Friesian cows and its relationship with their reactivity and milk yield. *Applied Animal Behaviour Science*, **70**, 177–181.

Paul, M.L., Currie, R.W. & Robertson, H.A. (1995). Priming of a D1 dopamine receptor behavioural response is dissociated from striatal immediate-early gene activity. *Neuroscience*, **66**, 347–359.

Pearson, R.A. (1989). A comparison of draft cattle (*Bos indicus*) and buffalos (*Bubalis bubalis*) carting loads in hot conditions. *Animal Production*, **49**, 355–363.

Pearson, R.A., Zerbini, E., & Lawrence, P.R. (1999). Recent advances in research on draught animals. *Animal Science*, **68**, 1–17.

Penning, P.D., Parsons, A.J., Newman, J.A., Orr, R.J. & Harvey, A. (1993). The effects of group size on grazing time in sheep. *Applied Animal Behaviour Science*, **37**, 101–109.

Pennington, I.A., Albright, J.L., Diekman, M.A. & Callahan, C. (1985). Sexual activity of Holstein cows: seasonal effects. *Journal of Dairy Science*, **68**, 3023–3030.

Persson, E. (1978). (Analysis of test milking data.) *Husdjur*, **11**, 16.

Petrie, N.J., Mellor, D.J., Stafford, K.J., Bruce, R.A. & Ward, R.N. (1996). Cortisol responses of calves to two methods of disbudding used with or without local anaesthetic. *New Zealand Veterinary Journal*, **44**, 9–14.

Pfister, J.A., Panter, K.E. & Gardner, D.R. (1998). Pine needle consumption by cattle during winter in South Dakota. *Journal of Range Management*, **51**, 551–556.

Phillips, C.J.C. (1983). Conserved forage as a buffer feed for dairy cows. PhD thesis, University of Glasgow.

Phillips, C.J.C. (1988). Review article: The use of conserved forage as a buffer feed for grazing dairy cows. *Grass and Forage Science*, **43**, 215–230.

Phillips, C.J.C. (1989). New techniques in the nutrition of grazing cattle. In *New Techniques in Cattle Production* (ed. C.J.C. Phillips), pp. 106–120. Butterworths, London.

Phillips, C.J.C. (1990a). Pedometric analysis of cattle locomotion. In *Update in Cattle Lameness* (ed. R.O. Murray), Proceedings of the VIth International Symposium on Diseases of the Ruminant Digit, pp. 163–176. British Cattle Veterinary Association, Liverpool.

Phillips, C.J.C. (1990b). Adverse effects on reproductive performance and lameness of feeding grazing dairy cows partially on silage indoors. *Journal of Agricultural Science, Cambridge*, **115**, 253–258.

Phillips, C.J.C. (1991). Restriccion de la ingestion de pasto en la vaca lechera [in Spanish]. *Archivos Medicina Veterinaria*, **23**, 5–20.

Phillips, C.J.C. (1993). *Cattle Behaviour*. Farming Press, Ipswich.

Phillips, C.J.C. (1997). Review article: Animal welfare considerations in future breeding programmes for farm livestock. *Animal Breeding Abstracts*, **65**, 645–654.

Phillips, C.J.C. (2001). *Principles of Cattle Production*. CAB International, Wallingford.

Phillips, C.J.C. & Arab, T.M. (1998). The preference of individually-penned cattle to conduct certain behaviours in the light or the dark. *Applied Animal Behaviour Science*, **58**, 183–187.

Phillips, C.J.C. & Denne, S.K.P.J. (1988). Variation in the grazing behaviour of dairy cows measured by a Vibrarecorder and bite count monitor. *Applied Animal Behaviour Science*, **21**, 329–339.

Phillips, C.J.C. & Hecheimi, K. (1989). The effect of forage supplementation, herbage height and season on the ingestive behaviour of dairy cows. *Applied Animal Behaviour Science*, **24**, 203–216.

Phillips, C.J.C. & James, N.L. (1998). The effects of including white clover in perennial ryegrass swards and the height of mixed swards on the milk production, sward selection and ingestive behaviour of dairy cows. *Animal Science*, **67**, 195–202.

Phillips, C.J.C. & Leaver, J.D. (1985a). Effect of restriction of silage intake and the provision of an alternative forage on the performance of dairy cows. *Grass and Forage Science*, **40**, 419–427.

Phillips, C.J.C. & Leaver, J.D. (1985b). Supplementary feeding of forage to grazing dairy cows. 1. Offering hay to dairy cows at a high and low stocking rate. *Grass and Forage Science*, **40**, 183–192.

Phillips, C.J.C. & Leaver, J.D. (1985c). Seasonal and diurnal variation in the grazing behaviour of dairy cows. In *Grazing*, BGS Occasional Symposium, No. 19, pp. 98–104. British Grassland Society, Reading.

Phillips, C.J.C. & Leaver, J.D. (1986). The effect of forage supplementation on the behaviour of grazing dairy cows. *Applied Animal Behaviour Science*, **16**, 233–247.

Phillips, C.J.C. & Lomas, C.A. (2001). The perception of color by cattle and its influence on behavior. *Journal of Dairy Science*, **84**, 801–813.

Phillips, C.J.C. & Morris, I.D. (2000). The locomotion of dairy cows on concrete floors that are dry, wet or covered with a slurry of excreta. *Journal of Dairy Science*, **83**, 1767–1772.

Phillips, C.J.C. & Morris, I.D. (2001). The locomotion of dairy cows on floor surfaces with different frictional properties. *Journal of Dairy Science*, **84**, 623–628.

Phillips, C.J.C. & Morris, I.D. (2002). The ability of cattle to distinguish between, and their preference for, floors with different levels of friction, and their avoidance of floors contaminated with excreta. *Animal Welfare*, **11**, 21–29.

Phillips, C.J.C. & Rind, I. (2002a). The effects of social dominance on the production and behaviour of grazing dairy cows offered forage supplements. *Journal of Dairy Science*, **85**, 51–59.

Phillips, C.J.C. & Rind, I. (2002b). The effects on production and behaviour of mixing uniparous and multiparous cows. *Journal of Dairy Science*, **84**, 2424–2429.

Phillips, C.J.C. & Rind, M.I. (2002c). The effects of frequency of feeding a total mixed ration on the production and behavior of dairy cows. *Journal of Dairy Science*, **84**, 1979–1987.

Phillips, C.J.C. & Schofield, S.A. (1989). The effect of supplementary light on the production and behaviour of dairy cows. *Animal Production*, **48**, 293–303.

Phillips, C.J.C. & Schofield, S.A. (1990). The effect of environment and stage of the oestrous cycle on the behaviour of dairy cows. *Applied Animal Behaviour Science*, **27**, 21–31.

Phillips, C.J.C. & Schofield, S.A. (1994). The effect of cubicle and straw yard housing on the behaviour, production and hoof health of dairy cows. *Animal Welfare*, **3**, 37–44.

Phillips, C.J.C. & Weiguo, L. (1991). Brightness discrimination abilities of calves relative to that of humans. *Applied Animal Behaviour Science*, **31**, 25–33.

Phillips, C.J.C., Margerison, J.K., Azazi, S., Chamberlain, A.G. & Omed, H. (1991). The effect of adding surface water to herbage on its digestion by ruminants. *Grass and Forage Science*, **46**, 333–338.

Phillips, C.J.C., Patterson, S.J., Ap Dewi, I. & Whittaker, C.J. (1996). Volume assessment of the bovine hoof. *Research in Veterinary Science*, **61**, 125–128.

Phillips, C.J.C., Lomas, C.A. & Arab, T.M. (1997). Differential response of dairy cows to supplementary light during increasing or decreasing daylength. *Animal Science* **66**, 55–64.

Phillips, C.J.C., Youssef, M.Y.I., Chiy, P.C. & Arney, D.R. (1999). Sodium chloride supplements increase the salt appetite and reduce sterotypies in confined cattle. *Animal Science*, **68**, 741–748.

Phillips, C.J.C., Morris, I.D. & Lomas, C.A. (2000). The locomotion of cattle in passageways with different light intensities. *Animal Welfare*, **9**, 421–431.

Phillips, C.J.C., Morris, I.D. & Lomas, C.A. (2001). A novel operant conditioning test to determine whether dairy cows dislike passageways that are dark or covered with slurry. *Animal Welfare*, **10**, 65–72.

Pierscionek, B.K. (1994). Refractive Index of decapsulated bovine lens surfaces measured with a reflectometric sensor. *Vision Research*, **34**, 1927–1933.

Plath, U., Knierim, U., Schmidt, T., Buchenauer, D. & Hartung, J. (1998). Group housing of veal calves older than two to eight weeks of age. *Deutsche Tierarztliche Wochenschrift*, **105**, 100–104.

Plusquellec, P. & Bouissou, M.F. (2001). Behavioural characteristics of two dairy breeds of cows selected (*Herens*) or not (*Brune des Alpes*) for fighting and dominance ability. *Applied Animal Behaviour Science*, **72**, 1–21.

Politiek, R.D. (1981). (Does selection for characteristics of the udder, teats, ease of milking and udder health offer any prospects of improvement of resistance to mastitis?) Biedt selectie op kenmerken van uier, spenen, melkbaarheid en uiergezondheidskenmerken een perspectief voor de verbetering van de weerstand tegen mastitis? *Tijdschrift Diergeneeskd*, **106**, 546–553.

Pordomingo, A.J. & Rucci, T. (2000). Red deer and cattle diet composition in La Pampa, Argentina. *Journal of Range Management*, **53**, 649–654.

Porzig, E. & Laube, R. B. (1977). Investigations into the long-term visual memory of cattle (*Bos taurus* L.) with reference to the recognition of colours and shapes. *Studia Psychologica*, **19**, 218–220.

Potter, M.J. & Broom, D.M. (1987). The behaviour and welfare of cows in relation to cubicle house design. In *Cattle Housing Systems, Lameness and Behaviour* (eds H.K. Wierenga and D.J. Peterse), pp. 129–147. Current Topics in Veterinary Medicine and Animal Science, No. 40. Martinus Nijhoff, Dordrecht.

Potter, M.J. & Broom, D.M. (1990). Behaviour and welfare aspects of cattle lameness in relation to building design. In *Proceedings of the VI International Symposium on Diseases of the Ruminant Digit*, pp. 80–84. British Cattle Veterinary Association, University of Liverpool.

Prescott, M.L., Havstad, K.M., Olsonrutz, K.M., Ayers, E.L. & Petersen, M.K. (1994). Grazing behavior of free-ranging beef-cows to initial and prolonged exposure to fluctuating thermal environments. *Applied Animal Behaviour Science*, **39**, 103–113.

Presicce, G.A., Brockett, C.C., Cheng, T. & Foote, R.H. (1993). Behavioral responses of bulls kept under artificial breeding conditions to compounds presented for olfaction, taste or with topical nasal application. *Applied Animal Behaviour Science*, **37**, 273–284.

Price, E. O. & Wallach, S.J.R. (1990). Rearing bulls with females fails to enhance sexual performance. *Applied Animal Behaviour Science*, **26**, 339–347.

Price, E.O., Martinez, C.L. & Coe, B.L. (1985). The effects of twinning on mother–offspring behaviour in range beef cattle. *Applied Animal Behaviour Science*, **13**, 309–320.

Price, E.O., Smith, V.M., Thos, J. & Anderson, G.B. (1986). The effects of twinning and maternal experience on maternal–filial social relationships in confined beef cattle. *Applied Animal Behaviour Science*, **15**, 137–146.

Price, E.O., Harris, J.E., Borgward, R.E. & Sween, M.L. (2001). Fenceline contact reduces the negative effects on weaning on the behavior and growth of beef calves. In *Proceedings of the 35th International Congress of the ISAE*, Davis, 4–9 August (eds J. Garner, J. Mench and S. Heekin), p. 41. International Society for Applied Ethology, Davis, California.

Provenza, F.D. & Balph, D.F. (1987). Diet learning by domestic ruminants, theory, evidence and practical implications. *Applied Animal Behaviour Science*, **18**, 211–232.

Provenza, F.D. & Balph, D.F. (1990). Applicability of five diet-selection models to various foraging challenges ruminants encounter. In *Behavioural Mechanisms of Food Selection* (ed. R.N. Hughes), pp. 423–459. NATO, ASI Series Vol. 20. NATO, Brussels.

Pruett, J.H., Guillot, F.S. & Fisher, W.F. (1986). Humoral and cellular immunoresponsiveness of stanchioned cattle infested with *Psoroptes ovis*. *Veterinary Parasitology*, **22**, 121–133.

Purcell, D., Arave, C.W. & Walters, J.L. *et al.* (1998). Relationship of three measures of behavior to milk production. *Applied Animal Behaviour Science*, **21**, 307–313.

Ralley, W.E., Galloway, T.D. & Crow, G.H. (1993). Individual and group behaviour of pastured cattle in response to attack by biting flies. *Canadian Journal of Zoology*, **71**, 725–734.

Ralphs, M.H. (1999). Lithium residue in milk from doses used to condition taste aversions and effects on nursing calves. *Applied Animal Behaviour Science*, **61**, 285–293.

Rathore, A.K. (1982). Order of cows entry at milking and its relationships with milk yield, and consistency of the order. *Applied Animal Ethology*, **8**, 45–52.

Redbo, I. (1990). Changes in duration and frequency of sterotypies and their adjoining behaviours in heifers, before, during and after the grazing period. *Applied Animal Behaviour Science*, **26**, 57–67.

Redbo, I. (1992). The influence of restraint on the occurrence of oral stereotypies in dairy-cows. *Applied Animal Behaviour Science*, **35**, 115–123.

Redbo, I. (1998). Relations between oral stereotypies, open-field behavior, and pituitary–adrenal system in growing dairy cattle. *Physiology and Behavior*, **64**, 273–278.

Redbo, I. & Nordblad, A. (1997). Stereotypies in heifers are affected by feeding regime. *Applied Animal Behaviour Science*, **53**, 193–202.

Redbo, I., Jacobsson, K.G, van Doorn, C. & Petterson, G. (1992). A note on relations between oral sterotypies in dairy cows and milk production, health and age. *Animal Production*, **54**, 166–168.

Redbo, I., Emanuelson, M., Lundberg, K. & Oredsson, N. (1996a). Feeding level and oral sterotypies in dairy cows. *Animal Science*, **62**, 199–206.

Redbo, I., Mossberg, I., Ehrlemark, A. & Stahl Hogberg, M. (1996b). Keeping growing cattle outside during winter: behaviour, production and climatic demand. *Animal Science*, **62**, 35–41.

Rehkamper, G. & Gorlach, A. (1998). Visual identification of small sizes by adult dairy bulls. *Journal of Dairy Science*, **81**, 1574–1580.

Rehkamper, G., Perrey, A., Werner, C.W., Opfermann Rungeler, C. & Gorlach, A. (2000). Visual perception and stimulus orientation in cattle. *Vision Research*, **40**, 2489–2497.

Reinhardt, V. (1973). Social rank order and milking order in cows. *Zuchstungskunde Tierpsychologie*, **32**, 281–292.

Reinhardt, V. (1983a) Movement orders and leadership in a semi-wild cattle herd. *Behaviour*, **83**, 251–264.

Reinhardt, V. (1983b). Flehman, mounting and copulation among members of a semi-wild cattle herd. *Animal Behaviour*, **31**, 641–650.

Reinhardt, V. & Reinhardt, A. (1981). Cohesive relationships in a cattle herd (*Bos indicus*). *Behaviour*, **77**, 121–151.

Reinhardt, V., Reinhardt, A. & Reinhardt, C. (1987). Evaluating sex differences in aggressiveness in cattle, bison and rhesus monkeys. *Behaviour*, **102**, 58–66.

Ribeiro, J.M. de C.R., Brockway, J.M. & Webster, A.J.F. (1977). A note on the energy cost of walking. *Animal Production*, **25**, 107–110.

Rind, M.I. & Phillips, C.J.C. (1999). The effects of group size on the ingestive and social behaviour of grazing dairy cows. *Animal Science*, **68**, 589–596.

Riol, J.A., Sanchez, J.M., Egwen, U.G. & Gaudioso, U.R. (1989). Colour perception in fighting cattle. *Applied Animal Behaviour Science*, **23**, 199–208.

Robinson, P.H. & Sniffen, C.J. (1985). Forestomach and whole tract digestibility for lactating dairy cows as influenced by feeding frequency. *Journal of Dairy Science*, **68**, 857–867.

Roche, J.A.F. (1989). New techniques in hormonal manipulation of cattle production. In *New Techniques in Cattle Production* (ed. C.J.C. Phillips), pp. 48–60. Butterworths, London.

Rogers, G.W., Hargrove, G.L., Lawlor, T.J. Jr & Ebersole, J.L. (1991). Correlations among linear type traits and somatic cell counts. *Journal of Dairy Science,* **74**, 1087–1091.

Rohler, R. (1962). Die Abbildungseigenschaften der Augenmedien. *Vision Research*, **2**, 391–429.

Rottensten, K. & Touchberry, R.W. (1957). Observations on the degree of expression of oestrus in cattle. *Journal of Dairy Science,* **40**, 1457–1465.

Roy, P.K. & Nagpaul, P.K. (1986). The influence of genetic and non-genetic factors on temperament and milking parameters in dairy animals. *Indian Journal of Animal Production and Management*, **2**, 11–15.

Ruckebush, Y. (1972). The relevance of drowsiness in the circadian cycle of farm animals. *Animal Behaviour*, **20**, 637–643.

Ruh, H. (1989) (Animal rights – new questions about animal ethics.) Tierrechte – neue Fragen zur Tierethik. *Schweiz Archiv fur Tierheilkund,* **131**, 5–11.

Rushen, J., Boissy, A., Terlouw, E.M.C. & de Passillé, A.M.B. (1999a). Opioid peptides and behavioral and physiological responses of dairy cows to social isolation in unfamiliar surroundings. *Journal of Animal Science*, **77**, 2918–2924.

Rushen, J., de Passillé, A.M.B. & Munksgaard, L. (1999b). Fear of people by cows and effects on milk yield, behavior, and heart rate at milking. *Journal of Dairy Science*, **82**, 720–727.

Rushen, J., Taylor, A.A. & de Passillé, A.M. (1999c). Domestic animals' fear of humans and its effect on their welfare. *Applied Animal Behaviour Science*, **65**, 285–303.

Rutter, S.M., Jackson, D.A., Johnson, C.L. & Forbes, J.M. (1987). Automatically recorded competitive feeding behaviour as a measure of social dominance in dairy cows. *Applied Animal Behaviour Science*, **17**, 41–50.

Rybarzyk, P., Koba, Y. Rushen, J., Tanida, H. & de Passillé, A.M. (2001). Can cows discriminate people by their faces? *Applied Animal Behaviour Science*, **74**, 175–189.

Salcido, C.P. & Eugenio, L. (1979). (Estimation of heritability indices for body weight at weaning, one year and 550 days, pigmentation and temperature in a herd of Brahman cattle in Playa Vicente, Veracruz.) *Veteriiiaria*, **10**, 194 (Abstract).

Sambraus, H.H. (1979). Rank related factors in cattle. *Animal Behaviour Abstracts*, **8**, 17.

Sambraus, H.H. (1999). The behaviour of yaks (*Bos grunniens*). *Tierarztliche Praxis Ausgabe Grobtiere Nutztiere*, **27**, 239–244.

Sambraus, H.H. & Gotthardt, A. (1985). Prepuce sucking and tongue rolling in intensively fattened bulls. *Deutsche Tierarztliche Wockenschrift,* **92**, 465–468.

Sambraus, H.H., Fries, B. & Osterhorn, K. (1979). Social relationships in a herd of dehorned dairy cattle. *Animal Behaviour Abstracts*, **7**, 228.

Sanchez, R. & Febles, I. (1999). Behaviour of grazing Holstein cows in natural shade. *Cuban Journal of Agricultural Science*, **33**, 241–246.

Sandøe, P., Crisp, R. & Holtug, N. (1997). Animal ethics. In *Animal Welfare* (eds M. Appleby and B. Hughes). CABI, Wallingford.

Santha, T., Prieger, K., Keszthelyi, T. & Czako, J. (1988). (Genetic analysis of feeding behaviour of cows.) *Allaltenyesztes-es-Takarmanyozas*, **37**, 501–514.

Sato, S. (1981). Factors associated with temperament of beef cattle. *Japanese Journal of Zootechnical Science,* **52**, 595–605.

Sato, S. (1984). Social licking pattern and its relationships to social dominance and liveweight gain in weaned calves. *Applied Animal Behaviour Science*, **12**, 25–32.

Sato, S., Sassa, H. & Sonoda, T. (1990). Effect of dominance rank of partner cows on social behaviour of newly introduced heifers. *Japanese Journal of Livestock Management*, **26**, 64–69.

Sato, S., Tarumizu, K. & Hatae, K. (1993). The influence of social factors on allogrooming in cows. *Applied Animal Behaviour Science*, **38**, 235–244.

Sato, S., Nagamine, R. & Kubo, T. (1994). Tongue-playing in tethered Japanese Black cattle: diurnal patterns, analysis of variance and behaviour sequences. *Applied Animal Behaviour Science*, **39**, 39–47.

Sauter, C.M. & Morris, R.S. (1995). Dominance hierarchies in cattle and red deer (*Cervus elaphus*), their possible relationship to the transmission of bovine tuberculosis. *New Zealand Veterinary Journal*, **43**, 301–305.

Schein, M.W. & Fohrman, M.H. (1955). Social dominance relationships in a herd of dairy cattle. *British Journal of Animal Behaviour*, **3**, 45–55.

Schilling, E. & Hartwig, H.H. (1984). Behaviour in cows before and during parturition. In *Proceedings of International Conference on Applied Ethology in Farm Animals* (eds J. Unshelm, C. Van Putten and K. Zeeb), pp. 391–394. Kiel. KTBL, Darmstadt.

Schloeth, R. (1961). Das Sozialleben des Camargue-Rindes. Qualitatif und quantitatif Untersuchungen uber die socialen Beziehungen – insbesondere die soxaile Rangordnung – des halbwinlden franzosisschen Kampfirndes. *Zuchtungskunde Tierpsychologie*, **18**, 574–627.

Schofield, D. & Hall, D.M. (1986). A recording penetrometer to measure the strength of soil in relation to the stresses exerted by a walking cow. *Journal of Soil Science*, **37**, 165–176.

Schofield, S.A. (1988). Oestrus in dairy cows. Technical Report No. 3. Dairy Research Unit, University of Wales, Bangor.

Schofield, S.A., Phillips, C.J.C. & Owens, A.R. (1991). Variation in the milk production, activity rate and electrical impedance of cervical mucus over the oestrous period of dairy cows. *Animal Reproduction Science*, **24**, 231–248.

Schrama, J.W., Roefs, J.P.A., Gorssen, J., Heetkamp, M.J.W. & Verstegen, M.W.A. (1995). Alteration of heat-production in young calves in relation to posture. *Journal of Animal Science*, **73**, 2254–2262.

Schukken, Y.H., Kremer, W.D. & Lohuis, J.A. (1989). (*Escherichia coli* mastitis in cattle. I. Clinical diagnosis and epidemiological aspects.) *Escherichia coli*-mastitis bij het rund. I. Klinische diagnostiek en epidemiologische aspecten. *Tijdschrift und Diergeneeskd*, **114**, 829–838.

Schwartzkopf Genswein, K.S., Stookey, J.M. & Welford, R. (1997). Behavior of cattle during hot-iron and freeze branding and the effects on subsequent handling ease. *Journal of Animal Science*, **75**, 2064–2072.

Scott, G.B. (1989). Change in limb loading with lameness for a number of Friesian cattle. *British Veterinary Journal*, **145**, 28–38.

Seabrook, M.F. (1984). The psychological interaction between the stockman and his animals and its influence on performance of pigs and dairy cows. *Veterinary Record*, **115**, 84–87.

Seabrook, M.F. & Bartle, N.C. (1992). Human factors influencing the production and welfare of farm animals. In *Farm Animals and the Environment*. (eds C.J.C. Phillips and D. Piggins), pp. 111–130. Commonwealth Agricultural Bureaux, Slough.

Seo, T., Sato, S., Kosaka, K., Sakamoto, N, Tokumoto, K. & Katoh, K. (1998a). Development of tongue-playing in artificially reared calves: effects of offering a dummy-teat, feeding of short cut hay and housing system. *Applied Animal Behaviour Science*, **56**, 1–12.

Seo, T., Sato, S. Kosako, H., Sukamoto, K., Tokumoto, K. & Kakah, K. (1998b). Tongue-playing and heart rate in calves. *Applied Animal Behaviour Science*, **58**, 179–182.

Seufert, H. (1997). Stall barn forms for daily cows under regard of animal physiology and profitability. *Zuchtungskunde*, **69**, 421–434.

Seykora, A.J. & McDaniel, B.T. (1985) Udder and teat morphology related to mastitis resistance: a review. *Journal of Dairy Science*, **68**, 2087–2093.

Sharman, D.F. & Stephens, D.B. (1974). The effect of apomorphine on the behaviour of farm animals. *Journal of Physiology*, **242**, 25P.

Shingler, A.B., Harvard, A., Jones, M.G.S. & Morgan, D.E. (1979). Nutritional aspects of complete diets for dairy cows – a survey on commercial farms, winter 1977–78. Ministry of Agriculture, Fisheries and Food, London.

Shrode, R.R. & Hammock, S.P. (1971). Chute behaviour of yearling beef cattle. *Journal of Animal Science*, **33**, 193 (Abstract).

Silver, G.V. & Price, E.O. (1986). Effects of individual vs. group rearing on the sexual behaviour of prepubertal beef bulls, mount orientation and sexual responsiveness. *Applied Animal Behaviour Science*, **15**, 287–294.

Singh, S.S., Ward, W.R., Lautenbach, K. & Murray, R.D. (1993). Behaviour of lame and normal dairy cows in cubicles and in a straw yard. *Veterinary Record*, **133**, 204–208.

Smit, J., Verbeek, B., Peterse, D.J., Jansen, J., McDaniel, B.T. & Politiek, R.D. (1986). Genetic aspects of claw disorders, claw measurements and 'type' scores for feet in Friesian cattle. *Livestock Production Science*, **15**, 205–217.

Smith, C.A. (1955). Studies on the Northern Rhodesia Hyporrhemia veld. *Journal of Agricultural Science, Cambridge*, **52**, 369–375.

Smith, M.E., Linnell, J.D.C., Odden, J. & Swenson, J.E. (2000). Review of methods to reduce livestock depradation.). Guardian animals. *Acta Agricultural Scandinavica Section A – Animal Science*, **50**, 279–290.

Soffie, M. & Zayan, R. (1977). Responsiveness to social releasers in cattle, 1. A study of the differential and additive effects of visual and sound stimatic, with special reference to the law of heterogenous summation. *Behavioural Processes*, **2**, 75–97.

Soffie, M., Thines, G. & de Marneffe, G. (1976). Relation between milking order and dominance value in a group of dairy cows. *Applied Animal Ethology*, **2**, 271–276.

Sommer, T. (1985). Untersuchungen zur Tiergerchtreit praxisublicher Gestaltung von Laufflachen fur Milchvieh im Boxenlaufstal. Report of the Ethologische Station Hasli, Zoological Institute, Berne.

Sowerby, M.E. & Polan, C.E. (1977). Milk production responses of shifting cows between intraherd groups. *Journal of Dairy Science*, **61**, 455–460.

Spinka, M. (1992). Intersucking in dairy heifers during the 1st 2 years of life. *Behavioural Processes*, **28,** 41–50.

Stefanowska, J., Plavsic, M., Ipema, A.H. & Hendriks, M.M. (2000). The effect of omitted milking on the behaviour of cows in the context of cluster attachment failure during automatic milking. *Applied Animal Behaviour Science*, **67**, 277–291.

Stephens, D.B. (1974). Studies on the effect of social environment on the behavioural growth of artificially-reared British Friesian male calves. *Animal Production*, **18**, 23–34.

Stephens, D.B. & Jones, J.N. (1975). Husbandry influences on some physiological parameters of emotional responses in calves. *Applied Animal Ethology*, **1**, 233–243.

Stricklin, W.R. (1983). Matrilinear social dominance and spatial relationships among Angus and Hereford cows. *Journal of Animal Science*, **57**, 1397–1405.

Stricklin, W.R.T., Graves, H.B., Wilson, L.L. & Singh, R.K. (1980). Social organisation among young beef cattle in confinement. *Applied Animal Ethology,* **6**, 211–219.

Syme, G.J. & Syme, L.A. (1979). *Social Structure in Farm Animals*. Elsevier Scientific Publishing Co., Amsterdam.

Tarlton, J.F., Holah, D.E., Evans, K.M., Jones, S., Pearson, G.R. & Webster, A.J.F. (2001). Biomechanical and histopathological changes in the support tissues of bovine hooves around the time of first calving. *The Veterinary Journal* (in press).

Tarrant, P.V. (1981). The occurrence, causes and economic consequences of dark-cutting in beef – a survey of current information. In *The Problem of Dark-cutting in Beef. Current Topics in Veterinary Medicine and Animal Science*, Vol. 10 (eds D.E. Hood and P.V. Tarrant), pp. 3–35. Martinus Nijhoff, The Hague.

Tarrant, V. & Grandin, T. (2000). Cattle transport. In *Livestock and Transport* (ed. T. Grandin), pp. 151–174. CAB International, Wallingford.

Taschke, A.C. & Folsch, D.W. (1997). Ethological, physiological and histological aspects of pain and stress in cattle when being dehorned. *Tierarztliche Praxis*, **25**, 19–27.

Terlouw, E.M.C., Boissy, A. & Blinet, P. (1998). Behavioral responses of cattle to the odours of blood and urine conspecifics and to the odour of faeces from carnivores. *Applied Animal Behaviour Science*, **57**, 9–21.

Thorpe, W.H. (1963). *Learning and Instinct in Animals*, 2nd edn. Methuen, London.

Thoules, C.R. (1990). Feeding competition between grazing red deer hinds. *Animal Behaviour*, **40**, 105–111.

Thysen, I. (1987). Foot and leg disorders in dairy cattle in different housing systems. In *Cattle Housing Systems, Lameness and Behavior*, pp. 166–178. Martinus Nijhoff, Dordrecht.

Tizol, C., Martinez, C., Nunez, E.A. & Garcia, H. (eds Wierenga, H.K. and Peterse, D.J.) (1987). Effect of different levels of exercise on semen quality in Holstein-Friesian bulls. *Revista de Salud Animal*, **9**, 129–137.

Tom, E., Rushen, J., Duncan, I.J.H. & de Passille, A.M.B. (2001). Acute method of tail docking on young calves. In *Proceedings of the 35th International Congress of the International Society for Applied Ethology*, Davis, California, p. 51. 4–9 August 2001, Centre for Animal Welfare, Davis.

Tyrrell, H.F., Moe, P.W., Collis, K. A. & Stark, A.J. (1970). In *Energy Metabolism of Farm Animals. Proceedings of the 5th Symposium* (eds A. Schurch and C. Wenk), pp. 68–72. Juris Verlag, Zurich.

Uetake, K. & Kudo, Y. (1994). Visual dominance over hearing in feed acquisition procedure of cattle. *Applied Animal Behaviour Science*, **42**, 1–9.

Uetake, K., Hurnik, J.F. & Johnson, L. (1997). Effect of music on voluntary approach of dairy cows to an automatic milking system. *Applied Animal Behaviour Science*, **53**, 175–182.

Ungar, E.D., Ravid, N. & Bruckental, I. (2001). Bite dimensions for cattle grazing herbage at low levels of depletion. *Grass and Forage Science*, **56**, 35–45.

Vailes, L.D. & Britt, J.H. (1990). The influence of footing surface on mounting and other sexual behaviours of oestral Holstein cows. *Journal of Animal Science*, **68**, 2333–2338.

Vajner, L. (1978). K vlivu stability socialni struktury skupine dojnic na dojivost. *Veterinarstvi*, **28**, 468–470.

Vanderlee, J., Udo, H.M.J. & Brouwer, B.O. (1993). Design and validation of an animal traction module for a smallholder livestock systems simulation model. *Agricultural Systems*, **43**, 1997–227.

Veissier, I., le Neindre, P. & Trillat, G. (1989). The use of circadian behaviour to measure adaptation of calves to changes in their environment. *Applied Animal Behaviour Science*, **22**, 1–12.

Veissier, I., Gesmier, V., Leneindre, P., Gautier, J.Y. & Bertrand, G. (1994). The effects of rearing in individual crates on subsequent social-behavior of veal calves. *Applied Animal Behaviour Science*, **41**, 199–210.

Veissier, I., de la Fe, A.R.R. & Pradel, P. (1998). Nonnutritive oral activities and stress responses of veal calves in relation to feeding and housing conditions. *Applied Animal Behaviour Science*, **57**, 35–49.

Veissier, I., Rushen, R., Colwell, D. & de Passillé, A.M. (2000). A laser-based method for measuring thermal nociception of cattle. *Applied Animal Behaviour Science*, **66**, 289–304.

Venis, J., Bajnar, Z. & Navratil, I. (1980). Daily behaviour of dairy cows in groups of different size and at different stages of lactation under conditions of free housing in a large cowshed with cubicles. *Dairy Science Abstracts*, 1984, 046–00258.

Vetoshkina, C.A. (1985). Effect of exercise on heart in morphometry in cattle II. Effect of age on dimensions of the heart in bulls, in relation to the amount of exercise. *Veterinary Bulletin*, Abstract 055, 05319.

Vitale, A.F., Tenucci, M., Papiri, M. & Lovari, S. (1986). Social behaviour of the calves of semi-wild Maremma cattle, *Bos primigenius taurus*. *Applied Animal Behaviour Science*, **126**, 217–231.

Voisinet, B.D., Grandin, T., O'Connor, T.F., Tatum, J.D. & Deesing, J.M.J. (1997a). *Bos indicus* cross feedlot cattle with excitable temperaments have tougher meat and a higher incidence of borderline dark cutters. *Meat Science*, **46**, 367–377.

Voisinet, B.D., Grandin, T., Tatum, J.D., O'Connor, S.F. & Struthers, J.J. (1997b). Feedlot cattle with calm temperaments have higher average daily gains than cattle with excitable temperaments. *Journal of Animal Science*, **75**, 892–896.

Vokey, F.J., Guard, C.L., Erb, H.N. & Garlton, D.M. (2001). Effects of alley and stall surfaces on indices of claw and leg health in dairy cattle housed in a freestall barn. *Journal of Dairy Science*. **84**, 2686–2699.

Von Borell, E. & Ladewig, J. (1992). Relationship between behaviour and adrenocortical response pattern in domestic pigs. *Applied Animal Behaviour Science*, **34**, 195–206.

Wakelin, D. (1991). Model systems on the genetic basis of disease resistance. In *Breeding for Disease Resistance* (eds J.B. Owen and R.F.E. Axford), pp. 54–70. CABI, Slough.

Wallis DeVries, M.F. (1996). Effects of resource distribution patterns on ungulate foraging behaviour, a modelling approach. *Forest Ecology and Management*, **88**, 167–177.

Warriss, P.D. (1990). The handling of cattle pre-slaughter and its effects on carcass and meat quality. *Applied Animal Behaviour Science*, **28**, 171–186.

Warwick, V.D., Arave, C.W. & Mickelsen, C.M. (1977). Effects of group, individual and isolated rearing of calves on weight gain and behaviour. *Journal of Dairy Science*, **50**, 947–953.

Wassmuth, R. & Alps, H. (2000). Recording of reed intake in stationary testing of potential AI bulls. *Archiv Fur Tierzucht – Archives of Animal Breeding*, **43**, 561–571.

Watt, D.C. & Seller, A. (1993). A clinico-genetic study of psychiatric disorder in Huntington's chorea. *Psychological Medicine,* **23**, 1–46.

Watts, J.M. & Stookey, J.M. (1999). Effects of restraint and branding on rates and acoustic parameters of vocalization in beef cattle. *Applied Animal Behaviour Science*, **62**, 125–135.

Watts, J.M. & Stookey, J.M. (2000). Vocal behaviour in cattle, the animal s commentary on its biological processes and welfare. *Applied Animal Behaviour Science*, **67**, 15–33.

Waynert, D.F., Stookey, J.M., Schwartzkopf Genswein, K.S., Watts, J.M. & Waltz, C.S. (1999). The response of beef cattle to noise during handling. *Applied Animal Behaviour Science*, **62**, 27–42.

Webb, N.C. & Nilsson, C. (1983). Flooring and injury – an overview. In *Farm Animal Housing and Welfare*, pp. 226–259. Martinus Nijhoff, The Hague.

Webb, W.B. (1979). Theories of sleep functions and some clinical functions. In *The Functions of Sleep* (eds C.R. Drucker, M. Shkurovich and M.B. Sterman), pp. 19–35. Academic Press, New York.

Weber, R. & Wechsler, B. (2001). Reduction in cross-sucking in calves by the use of a modified automatic teat feeder. *Applied Animal Behaviour Science*, **72**, 215–223.

Webster, A.J.F. (1984). *Calf Husbandry, Health and Welfare*. Granada Publishing, London.

Webster, A.J.F. (1987). *Understanding the Dairy Cow,* pp. 330–332. BSP Professional Books, Oxford.

Webster, A.J.F., Saville, C. & Welchman, D. (1986). *Improved Husbandry Systems for Veal Calves.* Farm Animal Care Trust, London.

Webster, J. (1995). *Animal Welfare, A Cool Eye Towards Eden*. Blackwell Scientific Publications, London.

Weigand, E., Meyer, U. & Guth, N. (1993). Intake, chewing activity and carbohydrate digestibility by lactating dairy-cows fed maize silage with a different physical structure. *Journal of Animal Physiology and Animal Nutrition – Zeitschrift für Tierphysiologie Tierernahrung und Futtermittelkunde*, **69**, 120–132.

Weiguo, L. & Phillips, C.J.C. (1991). The effects of supplementary light on the behaviour and performance of calves. *Applied Animal Behaviour Science*, **30**, 27–34.

Wickham, D.W. (1979). Genetic parameters and economic values of traits other than production for dairy cattle. *Proceedings of the New Zealand Society of Animal Production*, **39**, 180–193.

Wiepkema, P.R. (1983). On the significance of ethological criteria for the assessment of animal welfare. *Current Topics in Veterinary Medicine*, **23**, 71–79.

Wiepkema, P.R., Broom, D.M., Duncan, L.J.H. & van Putten, C. (1983). Abnormal behaviours in farm animals. Report of the CEC, Brussels.

Wiepkema, P.R., Van Hellemond, K.K., Roessing, P. & Romberg, H. (1987). Behaviour and abomasal damage in individual veal calves. *Applied Animal Behaviour Science*, **18**, 257–268.

Wierenga, H.K. (1990). Social dominance in dairy cattle and the influences of housing and management. *Applied Animal Behaviour Science*, **27**, 201–229.

Wiese, M. (1996). Searching for the biological roots of self-care and care behaviour. 1. The evolutional importance of self-care and care. *Pflege*, **9**, 105–112.

Wijeratne, W.V. & Curnow, R.N. (1990). A study of the inheritance of susceptibility to bovine spongiform encephalopathy, (comment). *Veterinary Record*, **126**, 92.

Wilesmith, J.W., Wells, G.A., Cranwell, M.P. & Ryan, J.B. (1988). Bovine spongiform encephalopathy: epidemiological studies. *Veterinary Record*, **123**, 638–644.

Wilkinson, J.M. (1999). Silage and animal health. *Natural Toxins*, **7**, 221–232.

Williamson, N.B., Morris, R.S., Blood, D.C. & Cannon, C.M. (1972). A study of oestrus detection methods in a large commercial herd. *Veterinary Record*, **91**, 50–62.

Wilson, L.L., Terosky, T.L., Stull, C.L. & Stricklin, W.R. (1999). Effects of individual housing design and size on behavior and stress indicators of special-fed Holstein veal calves. *Journal of Animal Science*, **77**, 1341–1347.

Winder, J.A., Walker, D.A. & Bailey, C.C. (1995). Genetic aspects of diet selection in the Chihuahuan desert. *Journal of Range Management*. **48**, 549–553.

Womack, J.E. (1996). The bovine gene map. In *Progress in Dairy Science* (ed. C.J.C. Phillips), pp. 89–104. CAB International, Wallingford.

Wood, M.T. (1977). Social grooming patterns in two herds of monozygotic twin dairy cows. *Animal Behaviour*, **25**, 635–642.

Yadav, A.S., Dhaka, S.S. & Kumar, B. (2001). Effect of working on physiological, biochemical and haematological parameters in Hariana bullocks. *Asian-Australian Journal of Animal Sciences*, **14**, 1067–1072.

Yarney, T.A., Rahnefield, C.W. & Konefal, C. (1979). Time of day of parturition in beef cows. *Canadian Journal of Animal Science*, **59**, 836.

Yeruham, I. & Markusfeld, O. (1996). Self destructive behaviour in dairy cattle (comment). *Veterinary Record*, **138**, 308.

Zaitser, E.A. (1985). Preventing hock arthrosis in breeding bulls. *Veterinary Bulletin*, Abstract 055, 05168.

Zeeb, K. (1983). Locomotion and space structure in six cattle units. In *Farm Animal Housing and Welfare*, pp. 129–136. Martinus Nijhoff, The Hague.

Zeeb, K. & Bammert, J. (1984). Locomotion and number of cubicles for dairy cows. In *Proceedings of the 15th International Conference on Angewandite Ethologie bei Nutztierea*, Freiburg, 16 November 1983.

Zeeb, K., Bock, C. & Heinzler, B. (1983). Control of social stress by consideration of suitable space. In *Social Stress in Domestic Animals* (eds R. Zayan and R. Dantzer), pp. 275–281. Kluwer Academic, Dordrecht.

Zimmerman, P.H. & Koene, P. (1998). The effect of frustrative nonreward on vocalisations and behaviour in the laying hen, *Gallus gallus domesticus*. *Behavioural Processes*, **44**, 73–79.

Zinn, S.A., Chapin, L.T., Lookingland, K.J., Moore, K.E. & Tucker, H.A. (1989). Effects of photoperiod on tuberoinfundibular dopaminergic (TIDA) nerone aid on lactotropes in Holstein bull calves. *Journal of Dairy Science*, **72** (Suppl. 1), 338–339.

Index